American Bodies

AMERICAN BODIES

Cultural Histories of the Physique

Edited by

Tim Armstrong

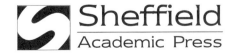

Sheffield
Academic Press

Copyright © 1996 Sheffield Academic Press

Published by Sheffield Academic Press Ltd
Mansion House
19 Kingfield Road
Sheffield S11 9AS
England

Printed on acid-free paper in Great Britain
by The Cromwell Press
Melksham, Wiltshire

British Library Cataloguing in Publication Data

A catalogue record for this book is available
from the British Library

ISBN 1-85075-753-4
ISBN 1-85075-790-9 pbk

CONTENTS

Science Fiction

Gender

Acknowledgments

Most of the essays collected here are based on papers given at the 1994 British Association for American Studies annual conference at Halifax Hall, Sheffield. Thanks are due to members of the University of Sheffield's Departments of English Literature and History who assisted at the conference, particularly Beverley Eaton.

Contributors

Tim Armstrong is Lecturer in English at Royal Holloway, University of London. He has has published in *Textual Practice* and other journals, edited *Thomas Hardy: Selected Poems* for Longmans Annotated Texts, and co-edited *Beyond the Pleasure Dome: Writing and Addiction from the Romantics*. A study of the body in Modernism will appear in 1997.

James Annesley recently completed a PhD at the University of Sussex. His study of 'Blank Fiction' will appear in 1997.

Kasia Boddy is Lecturer in English at University College London. She is working on a book on boxing fiction and film, and on a collection of criticism on Raymond Carver.

Amanda Boulter is completing a PhD on women science fiction writers at the University of Southampton. She co-founded the journal *diatribe* and has published in *OverHere*, *New Formations* and elsewhere.

Richard Canning is Lecturer in English at the University of Sheffield. He is currently writing a book on AIDS narratives.

Brian Caldwell teaches American Studies at Nene College of Higher Education, specializing in literature and film. His current research interests include the concept of excess as a cinematic function.

Lee Grieveson is completing a PhD on early American Film in relation to the discourses of social reform at the University of Kent. He has published in *Screen*.

Margaret Jones is a Lecturer at the University of the West of England, Bristol. She is author of *Heretics and Hellraisers: Woman Contributors to 'The Masses'* and editor of Elsie Clews Parsons' previously unpublished *The Journal of a Feminist*. She is working on *Mapping the Margins*, a study of post-colonial texts.

Louis J. Kern is Professor of History at Hofstra University, New York. His publications include *An Ordered Love: Sex Roles and Sexuality in Victorian Utopias: the Shakers, the Mormons, and the Oneida Community*, and (co-edited with Wendy Chmielewski and Marilyn Klee-Hartzell) *Women in Spiritual and Communitarian Societies in the United States*. He is working on a book on masculine role construction among nineteenth-century American free-lovers.

John Moore is Lecturer in American Literary Studies at the University of Luton. He is author of *Anarchy and Ecstasy, Lovebite: Mythography and the Semiotics of Culture*, and is currently preparing a critical edition of Thomas Morton's *New English Canaan*. His research interests include American science fiction and alternative America.

Simon P. Newman teaches in the Department of History at Northern Illinois University. He is the author of *Parades, Festivals and the Politics of the Street: Popular Political Culture in the Early American Republic* (forthcoming), and co-author of *Vue d'Amérique: La révolution française jugée par les américains.*

Peter Thompson is Sydney L. Mayer Lecturer in American History and a Fellow of St. Cross College, Oxford. He is currently completing a book on tavern-going in colonial Philadelphia and researching the cultural politics of maritime famine.

Sue Vice is Lecturer in English Literature at the University of Sheffield. She has edited *Malcolm Lowry Eighty Years On* and *Psychoanalytic Criticism: A Reader*, co-edited *Beyond the Pleasure Dome: Writing and Addiction from the Romantics*, and is currently completing *Introducing Bakhtin: From Formalism to Feminism.*

Barbara Will is Assistant Professor of English at Dartmouth College, New Hampshire. She is completing a book on Gertrude Stein, gender and the modernist concept of 'genius'.

INTRODUCTION

The essays in this collection deal with issues relating to the body in American culture in the period from 1900 to the present. In approach they range from cultural and intellectual history to film and literary studies, a number of them crossing disciplinary boundaries in order to explore the meanings of the body, its social locations, and the mechanisms which reproduce its images. Throughout, two interrelated topics are explored—topics which are constantly impinging on each other. In some cases the actual body is at issue—its shape, markings, reproductive status, even its use as food; in others the body serves as a metaphor for social formations and cultural processes, while also being the object of those relations, as in the discourses of birth-control or social diseases.

If such an embodiment of social relations is intrinsic to capitalism, as a variety of writers from Marx and Veblen to Foucault and Bourdieu have observed, then the essays collected here exemplify the intensification of historical knowledge and discourse about the body which has taken place since the eighteenth century. The different areas addressed in relation to the body—from tattoos to diet, from reproduction to filmic representation—are also illustrative of the extent to which work on the body has broadened from the focus on regulative positions in Foucault's earlier work. For the later Foucault, the body is the site of a 'bio-politics' which operated both at the level of the individual and the population, constructing the body—and the subject—as a set of interlinked discursive practices, with their attendant institutional sites of intervention.[1] Foucault's investigations into the penal system, mental health, and sexology have been elaborated and contested by a huge range of scholars who have provided a more detailed sense of shifts in the understanding of such issues as the gendered body, sex, techniques of medical intervention, and the representation of the body, from classical texts to the postmodern.[2] In the period considered in this collection, Foucault's attack on the 'repressive hypothesis' (the idea that the Victorians suppressed reference to bodily and sexual functions) has provided a framework for an impressive body of work on the nineteenth century fascination with sexual knowledge, even if others (most recently Peter Gay and Michael Mason) have found his work inattentive to historical detail, to areas of contestation, and to the recorded experience of historical subjects.[3] A number of essays in this volume attempt to contribute to that ongoing debate, describing the way in which the nature of bodies is a political question in which other discourses—for example those of eugenics, economics, and social hygiene—are part of the description of the body; or even looking at the way in which systems of representation like cinema constitute themselves as a mode of bodily extension. Recent theorists, notably Donna Haraway, have attempted to posit a body with a utopian technology and bio-politics, moving beyond those gendered constructions of the modern body which tend, in Foucault, to be monolithic (though as the essays by Brian Caldwell and Amanda Boulter suggest here, such utopianism is always compromised by its interaction with existing categories).[4]

If Foucault's work concerns itself with the interaction of 'sexuality and textuality' (to borrow the title of a recent collection), we can turn to a number of other writers for an elaboration of relations between text and body which provides a context for a collection which includes a number of discussions of literary texts.[5] For Barthes and Derrida the production of writing is itself a bodily function, with terms such as 'jouissance' and 'dissemination' implying the impossibility of a dualism which separates text and body, writing and experience. Writing cannot simply be said to be about the body; it is embodied in a way which constantly engages with and traverses accepted codes of gender, taste, decorum (as the essays here by Sue Vice and Tim Armstrong argue).

The textuality of the body implies that any account of bodily experience is mediated; it cannot serve, as many modernists suggest, as the source of a primitive 'reality'. Moreover, a sense of the body's presence informed by psychoanalysis suggests that there is no stable relation set of meanings attached to bodily symptoms; as Barbara Will argues here, the body (particularly the neurasthenic or hysterical body) is an open text which is constantly re-interpreted and re-written; which can achieve no stable relation to that core of the self which we call the unconscious, even if we must inevitably ground the unconscious in our embodiment. If Freud could argue that the ego is a projection of the surface of the body, then that surface is always a site of inscription, over-inscription and conflict, a fact nicely suggested by the essays in this collection dealing with tattoos and plastic surgery.

Thus, as Bryan Turner has argued, the body as an object of investigation conflates any ready distinction between a philosophy of experience and a philosophy of knowledge.[6] Writers on language like George Lakoff and Elaine Scarry have suggested the way in which bodily categories permeate thinking about the organization of social relations and the world of objects or technology; and, in reciprocal fashion, representations of the body are never 'natural', they enter a charged social and conceptual field (as Richard Canning's essay below shows).[7] The body is at once the point at which a nexus of structures—political, cultural, medical, technological, and linguistic—intersect, and the experiential ground on which resistance to or engagement with those structures begins. We act, as we write, with the body. The best recent work on the body and culture has thus stressed the way in which bodily and textual relations constantly interpenetrate.[8]

A historical trajectory underlies the variety of the essays collected here. In the later nineteenth century and early part of the twentieth century the dominant bodily paradigm is, Anson Rabinbach argues, the 'Human Motor': the body conceived in terms of energy, work, and the conversion of energy, with an accompanying stress on quantifying the body's throughput, efficiency and productivity in electro-chemical terms.[9] A variety of techniques aim to categorize, discipline and regulate bodies, both at the level of populations and individual bodies: Eugenics, Sexology, birth-control, Taylorism and Fordism, fashion, exercise-movements and eating regimes. Medical techniques (from the stethoscope and speculum at one end of the century to the X-ray at the other) increasingly open up the body, and tend to render it as a series of dispersed systems and parts, culminating in the early twentieth century technocratic reforms of Flexnerian medicine.

At the turn of the century, Hillel Schwartz suggests, a more dynamic conception of the body and of movement also begins to develop: the 'modern' body becomes streamlined, lighter and more mobile, and is defined in terms of torque—in dance, handwriting, weight-reduction; in posture-release regimes like the Alexander technique.[10] We might also note that in the twentieth century the lightest form of body of all begins to dominate its representation: the film image, which increasingly renders the body as pure spectacle. As a number of essays here suggest, the body as commodity and image must be conceived in terms which lie outside the nineteenth century calculus of work and production. Advertising, from the patent medicines of the late nineteenth century to the body-care products of the 1920s and 1930s, links bodies and consumption; while in a reverse cycle bodies sell products as images of erotic attainment.[11] Fetishized and abstracted, the body takes on the burden of modernity itself, of the circulation of image, desire, and ultimately of capital. In gender terms, this body is of course most readily stereotyped as 'feminine', though that characterization itself returns to the social sphere as a fear of commodified feminine sexuality which reaches its culmination in the 1930s.

In the postmodern world, the body has again been re-positioned: in terms of the discourses of control generated by cybernetics and genetics, which focus on biological, chemical and psychological or electronic programmability; and in terms of a more fluid understanding of gender-relations and sexuality.[12] Nonetheless, the postmodern body inherits many of the problems associated with the body in modernity: its perfectability, commodification and status as image are all at issue, as well as the status of work. Beyond that, the redundancy of the body has been posited by cyber-theory, a development which can be read as an expression of utopian possibilities; or on the other hand as a further and more attenuated stage in the reification of the human, reflected, perhaps, in the violence directed at the body in recent film and fiction, its status as image or waste generated by a society of informatics.[13] Our present fascination with the body as image and topic—and here the *Zone* series is exemplary, for its emphasis on spectacle and even for a certain sensationalism, as much as for its content—suggests the way in which bodily experience, visual pleasure, and social discourse have become interconnected.

The paired essays collected here address a number of the issues summarized above. The earliest bodies examined, historically, are those of merchant seamen in the early years of the nineteenth century. Marcus Redikker has argued that seamen constitute the first industrial proletariat, selling their labour to joint-stock owners. They were also among the first groups of workers whose bodies are constituted as the subjects of a capitalist economy, with its sense of the commodification of the self and its calculus of use.[14] Defoe had already, in 1697, drawn up tables of compensation which

placed a cash value on their legs, arms, and lives.[15] That sense of subordination—
though also a countervailing sense of collective identity—is examined here by Simon
Newman, via the records of American seamen's tattoos. These markings had a status
which relates to ownership and self-ownership, since the records involved were
compiled for documents which helped them to escape impressment onto British
ships. They marked the body for a possible death at sea, attesting to religion, identity,
and loved ones; but they also reflect the way in which professional sailors constituted
a potentially politicized group of outsiders, with their own markings and lore reflected
in the tattoos. The tattoo is thus a contradictory sign, signalling both subordination
and identity. One might compare Melville's use of tattoo: Qweeqweg's Polynesian
tattoos involve a potential commoditization of the body (the shrunken heads he sells),
as well as the identity-in-death which he copies onto his coffin.

Peter Thompson's paper looks at the issue of maritime cannibalism: a recurrent
topos familiar to readers of Byron and Poe, present in the subtexts of Gericault's
painting *The Raft of the Medusa*, and the subject of famous trials.[16] In these texts and
in the pamphlet accounts of the wreck of the *Peggy* which Thompson discusses (an
episode used in Poe's *Narrative of Arthur Gordon Pym*), the status of the human is
central, as well as the question raised by Newman: who owns a body? How does the
the body relate to the hierarchy which places animals at the bottom and humans,
segregated by rank, at the top? The narratives of mercantile enterprise and cannibalism which Thompson examines display a separation of civilization and its 'others'
rendered problematic by the pragmatics of survival.

If the first two essays deal with the significances of historically existing bodies,
the second pair of essays examine the way in which discourse about the body takes
on a social significance in the debates on women's rights in the late nineteenth and
early twentieth century. Louis J. Kern's essay on 'Sex Radicals' nicely captures the
ambivalence of an avant-gardism which constantly needed to defend its morality. On
the one hand, Ezra Heywood, Moses Harman and other radicals wished to enhance
the sexual freedom of both women and men; on the other hand fears of racial purity
and of feminine desire meant a sense of the dangers of that freedom. One outcome
was a stress on self-regulation; on a personal discipline which would fill the vacuum
left by a weakening of external constraints on sexuality. Margaret Jones illustrates the
parallel position of feminist reformers like Elsie Clews Parson, Margaret Sanger and
Emma Goldman, for whom justification for women's management of their own
sexuality and reproduction could most readily be found in eugenics, which subsumed
individual desire to a calculus of populations. Jones also considers utopian fiction like
Inez Irwin's *Angel Island* (1914) and Charlotte Perkins Gilman's *Herland* (1915), in
which feminine self-fashioning is expressed as social reformation. In both these papers
we see sexology operating at a political level, regulating the reproduction of desire as
a social and economic force.[17]

In two other papers these concerns are broadened towards what we could call a
bodily economics, in which the social and personal constantly act as interlocking metaphors. Barbara Will examines the widespread diagnosis of neurasthenia, the disease
of nervous exhaustion popularized by psychologist George Beard. In Will's account,
neurasthenia is central to the experience of modernity, providing a mobile set of

symptoms through which the individual's relations with rapidly changing social and historical circumstances could be expressed. Beard attributed neurasthenia to the pace of modern life. It was an ailment which fell most heavily on those who were most subject to the debilitating burdens of modern civilization, and whose energy levels were, in theory, readily depleted: women and intellectual men. Beard treated neurasthenia with top-ups of electricity and even advocated the use of chemical stimulants to replenish nervous systems (he wrote a book on recreational drugs[18]). Dr Silas Weir Mitchell's 'cure', on the other hand, was more pessimistic in its sense of bodily energies: he advocated complete rest and the cessation of brain-work, a treatment mocked by Charlotte Perkins Gilman in *The Yellow Wallpaper* (1892). As Will points out, Mitchell's treatment was also used on men: the Western-writer Owen Wister's cure was matched by his emphasis on healthy masculinity and the outdoors. Since Beard's work influenced Freud's early work, we can see the beginnings of a debate on gender and neurosis.[19]

Tim Armstrong's essay also attempts to bridge actual and metaphorical practices, relating Henry James's unlikely adherence to the dietary prescriptions of Horace Fletcher, the advocate of complete mastication, to his sense of his literary corpus. Fletcher was part of that eccentric world of Progressive-Era dietary reform described in T. Coraghessan Boyle's novel *The Road to Wellville* (1993); his work can also be linked to Taylorism (the body as a well-managed factory) and Pragmatism. Beginning with the timing of James's Fletcherism, which overlaps with his massive self-revisions for the New York Edition, Armstrong argues that Fletcherism provides a metaphor for a re-engineering of the corpus. Fletcher's insistence on taste as the regulatory mechanism which polices consumption is also useful in mediating James's sense of unease at engagement with a market.

Film is considered in a number of papers in this volume; two focus exclusively on the subject, and provide a useful sense of a continuous link between the making of the body and the cinematic apparatus. Lee Grieveson examines cinema as a disciplinary mechanism, placing the body within an emerging structure of narrative which aims at the simultaneous production of pleasure and control. Using Griffith's *The Drive for a Life* (1909), he notes that the early cinema attempted to legitimize its cultural position by its use of the discourse of social hygiene. Grieveson relates the protagonist's mistress, who in revenge poisons her lover, to the impact of venereal disease on the body politic. Like the contemporary 'topic' film (*Fatal Attraction*, for example), *The Drive for a Life* encodes social messages within a narrative in which suspense and identification are carefully modulated in order to suggest penalties for the failure of social hygiene.

Brian Caldwell's paper on the muscle-obsessed contemporary films of Stallone, Schwarzenegger and others explores the relationship between the (male) gaze and a body which has, like that of the female star, been rendered an object of pleasure. Using the notion of cinematic 'excess' (the obsessive gaze directed at musculature isolated from the body of which it forms a part), Caldwell argues that these films express pressure on the concept of the masculine through a representational hyperbole. If Stallone is always a male-impersonator, his body may ultimately bear no organic relation to the work it does—as in his unlikely appearance as a rock-climber in *Cliffhanger*.

We could thus speculate that the male body in cinema is caught in the crisis engendered by modern modes of production: 'work' in the sense which is so important in the nineteenth century has been replaced by the commoditization and marketing of the self, with particular emphasis on beauty and on the body as image (as in the elaborate and non-productive musculature which Caldwell discusses. The body as commodity is also discussed by James Annesley, who examines the penetration of the body as evidence of the violence of its commodification in late capitalism, using two 'blank generation' novels, Brian D'Amato's *Beauty* (1993) and Dennis Cooper's *Frisk* (1993). The former's focus is plastic surgery as self-fashioning, dependent only on the ability to pay. In the latter, murder and dismemberment serve as metaphors for that reduction of the body to the status of object and waste which Annesley sees as endemic to the postmodern. *Frisk* becomes postmodern satire, challenging the reader with the blankness of its response to pornographic violence; while *Beauty* literalizes the equivalence of money and beauty.

Richard Canning's discussion of the discourse of sexuality in Armistead Maupin's *Tales from the City* trilogy (1978-82) focuses on the absence of the body rather than its presence. He argues that for all that the novel parodies patriarchal structures like the family, the gay body represents a limit point for the early Maupin, before AIDS: his texts see an elision of the sexual body, prompted by his need, in the context of original publication in a mass-market newspaper, to address an audience outside the gay community. Writing on an author from a milieu similar to Maupin's, John Moore considers Samuel R. Delany's cult science-fiction novel *Dhalgren* (1974), and attempts to explain its success—a success maintained despite its formal experimentation. Linking *Dhalgren* to Delany's candid bisexual autobiographies, Moore concludes that the novel's popularity must be attributed in part to its focus on sexuality. Where Maupin's satirical engagement with a popular audience tempers his treatment of the body, Delany's more experimental work finds an audience through privileging the body.

The paired essay on science fiction by Amanda Boulter examines the Afro-American writer Octavia Butler's *Xenogenesis* trilogy, which uses alien colonization of Earth and genetic manipulation to explore race and gender in a context conditioned by 1980s debates on sociobiology and the human genome. Butler's benign aliens, the Oankali with their multiple genders and their hybridization with the people of Earth, create a situation which both sharpens and problematizes the category of the 'human'. Butler's characters wish to assert their biological difference from the aliens, but find that their unity is challenged by differences of gender, race, and power. Boulter also shows how involuntary hybridization in Butler's work recalls the histories of slavery and colonialism in America, founded as they were on rape and bodily appropriation. Nonetheless, she detects a utopian, 'curative' trust in Butler's trilogy which points towards a 'polymorphous future' in which essentialism has melted away.

A final pair of essays continue the recurrent interest in this volume in relationships between gender and the body. Sue Vice contests Mark Anderson's contention that the modernist text operates by a refusal of meaning which might be thought of as 'anorexic' (an anorexia embodied in such texts as Melville's 'Bartelby the Scrivener' and Kafka's 'The Hunger Artist'). In Vice's account, recent texts by women writers explore more productive relationships between eating, body and writing than those present in the minimalist texts of male modernists. Finally, Kasia Boddy explores the issues of performance and the reified body in an essay that shares some of the pre-occupations of the essays by Annesley and Moore. The naturalist text's fascination with boxing finds its focus, in Jack London's boxing stories, on the figure of the woman spectator. The woman is supposed to see the performance as masculine virility; instead, she often sees it as an æsthetic performance closer in its coding to the 'feminine'. In Joyce Carol Oates's *On Boxing* (1987) and in her fiction Boddy sees an existential approach to the fight which places Oates close to male writers like Norman Mailer and Ishmael Reed. But Oates also—in a step beyond this paradigm—compares boxing to childbirth, a simile which reaffirms sexual difference.

Taken together, these essays suggest that the current preoccupation with the body remains productive of a dialogue between modernism and postmodernism; between a body which retains a privileged status as the carrier of meanings and physical or metaphorical work, with a potential for creativity and threat, and, on the other hand, a body which has become enmeshed in less tangible forms of repro-duction. Terry Eagleton's recent call for a moratorium on work on the body and sexuality reflects an irritation with the latter possibility (and with a politics which, it seems to him, effaces class in favour of representational categories). That seems pre-mature, enmeshed as we are in a historical dialectic in which the postmodern and modern conceptions of the body co-exist; in which the body is both the site of dis-course and of political intervention. More prosaically, one could argue that the body has been for so long the site of repression, and (in the period treated here) of suc-cessive efforts to police the body politic, that the current enthusiasm for exploring its meanings reflects an emancipatory pressure which has not yet been dissipated. As recent developments in American cultural politics suggests—the disbanding of the NEA and NEH was being debated as this publication went to press, two institutions attacked for reasons at least related to the representation of the body—bodies are still subject to cultural fears which impinge on political structures.

Tim Armstrong

Notes

1.   Michel Foucault, *The Birth of the Clinic, An Archæology of Medical Perception* (London: Tavistock, 1973); *The History of Sexuality* (3 vols; trans. Robert Hurley; Harmondsworth: Penguin, 1981-88).

2.   The range of work on the body is such that the most recent articles are already dated; see, for example, A. Frank, 'Bringing Bodies Back in: a Decade Review', *Theory, Culture and Society* 7 (1990), pp. 131-62. A selection of relevant texts in the field of gender alone would include Gena Corea, *The Mother Machine: Reproductive Technologies from Artificial Insemination to Artificial Wombs* (New York: (Harper & Row, 1985); Emily Martin, *The Woman in the Body: A Cultural Analysis of Reproduction* (Milton Keynes: Open University, 1987); Frank Mort, *Dangerous Sexualities: Medical-Moral Politics in England* (London: Routledge, 1987); Cynthia Eagle Russett, *Sexual Science: The Victorian Construction of Womanhood* (Cambridge,

MA: Harvard University Press, 1989); Thomas Laqueur, *Making Sex: Body and Gender from the Greeks to Freud* (Cambridge, MA: Harvard University Press, 1990); Roy Porter and Mikulas Teich, eds; *Sexual Knowledge, Sexual Science: The History of Attitudes to Sexuality* (Cambridge: Cambridge University Press, 1994) among many other texts.

3.   M. Mason, *The Making of Victorian Sexuality* (Oxford: Oxford University Press, 1994); P. Gay, *The Bourgeois Experience: Victoria to Freud* (2 vols; New York: Oxford University Press, 1984-86).

4.   Donna Haraway, *Primate Visions: Gender, Race and Nature in the World of Modern Science* (New York: Routledge, 1989).

5.   Judith Still and Michæl Worton, eds, *Textuality and Sexuality* (Manchester: Manchester University Press, 1993).

6.   Bryan S. Turner, *Regulating Bodies: Essays in Medical Sociology* (London: Routledge, 1992), p. 8.

7.   George Lakoff, *Women, Fire and Dangerous Things: What Categories Reveal About the Mind* (Chicago: University of Chicago Press, 1987); Elaine Scarry, *The Body in Pain: The Making and Unmaking of the World* (New York: Oxford University Press, 1985).

8.   See, for example, Friedrich Kittler, *Discourse Networks 1800/1900* (trans. Michæl Metteer; Stanford: Stanford University Press, 1990); Mark Seltzer, *Bodies and Machines* (New York: Routledge, 1992).

9.   Anson Rabinbach, *The Human Motor: Energy, Fatigue and the Origins of Modernity* (New York: Basic Books, 1990).

10.   Hillel Schwartz, 'Torque: The New Kinæsthetic of the Twentieth Century', in *Incorporations* (ed. Jonathan Crary and Sanford Kwinter; New York: Urzone, 1992).

11.   On patent medicines, advertising and the body in the nineteenth century, see Thomas Richards, *The Commodity Culture of Victorian England: Advertising and Spectacle 1851–1914* (London: Verso, 1990), ch. 4.; on twentieth-century extension of the tendency, Stuart and Elizabeth Ewen, *Channels of Desire: Mass Images and the Shaping of American Consciousness* (New York: McGraw-Hill, 1982).

12.   See for example N. Katherine Hayles, 'Designs on the Body: Norbert Weiner, Cybernetics, and the Play of Metaphor', *History of the Human Sciences* 3 (1990), pp. 211-28.

13.   See, for example, Arthur and Marylouise Kroker, 'Theses on the Disappearing Body in the Hyper-Modern Condition', in *Body Invaders: Panic Sex in America* (ed. Arthur and Marylouise Kroker; Montreal: New World Perspectives, 1987), pp. 20-34.

14.   Marcus Rediker, *Between the Devil and the Deep Blue Sea: Merchant Seamen, Pirates, and the Anglo-American Maritime World, 1700–1750* (Cambridge: Cambridge University Press, 1987).

15.   Daniel Defoe, *An Essay Upon Projects* (London, 1697), pp. 129-30.

16.   A.W.B. Simpson, *Cannibalism and the Common Law* (Chicago: University of Chicago Press, 1984).

17.   Compare Lawrence Birkin, *Consuming Desire: Sexual Science and the Emergence on a Culture of Abundance, 1871–1914* (Ithaca: Cornell University Press, 1988).

18.   George M. Beard, *Stimulants and Narcotics; Medically, Philosophically and Morally Considered* (New York: G.P. Putnam, 1971).

19.   M.B. Macmillan, 'Beard's Concept of Neurasthenia and Freud's Concept of the Actual Neuroses', *Journal of the History of the Behavioral Sciences* 12 (1976), pp. 376-90.

Seafarers and the Body
in the Age of Revolution

Simon P. Newman

WEARING THEIR HEARTS ON THEIR SLEEVES:
READING THE TATTOOS OF EARLY AMERICAN SEAFARERS

Three-quarters of a century ago in his *Maritime History of Massachusetts Bay* Samuel Eliot Morison spun a romantic tale of adventuresome young boys running away from home in order to spend an exciting few years at sea. They returned as men, he believed, ready for solid and productive lives as model American citizens.[1] Historians have dismissed much of this as fanciful nonsense, but Admiral Morison's description of short-term seafaring has held firm. Daniel Vickers, for example, has recently argued that 'every piece of evidence' supports the conclusion that 'seafaring was a stage in life' for young men, with the exception of the very few who 'rose into officers' ranks'.[2]

In truth we know very little about the hundreds of thousands of sailors who dominated the early national urban landscape. And dominate they most surely did: all of the young republic's major towns and cities were ports, and more of their male residents worked as sailors than as anything else. But when they were not at sea or in far distant ports these sailors inhabited the wretched dockland sections of port towns, living with their families in the direst of poverty. Consequently their names rarely appear in the tax lists, the militia rolls, the city directories and the probate records that historians have employed to reconstruct the lives of working people in early America.[3]

If we turn to literature, however, there is at least some evidence to suggest that a good many of these men spent the great majority of their adult years at sea, living and working as members of a highly skilled seafaring fraternity. In a subtle and sympathetic sketch of the declining years of the old sailor Daniel Orme, Herman Melville told us much about one old tar compelled by old age to retire from the sea. This was a lonely end, for on land Orme was regarded with profound suspicion by his fellow countrymen and women. Melville describes how Orme's words, his actions and his very body all distinguished him as an outsider, a man with an alternative identity constructed in the liminal world of seafarers. His 'moody ways' and 'tanned' complexion, his job-related scars, the crucifix tattooed upon his chest and his 'darned Guernsey frock' all marked him as a professional seafarer, forever alien to those who were not members of the seafaring fraternity.[4]

If we are to establish the existence of these long-term professional seafarers and learn more about their world, we must approach their history in unconventional ways. They rarely figure in many of our more traditional sources, but there are ways in which their very bodies can still talk to us, telling us about them and the events, the people and the beliefs that were important in their lives. For like Daniel Orme, many of these professional seafarers wore tattoos, and with these bodily markings these men self-consciously constructed and displayed identities that were simultaneously personal and public, marking themselves not just as professional sailors but as individuals within that fraternity.

Records of tattoos exist, quite by chance, because of 'An Act for the relief and protection of American Seamen', passed by Congress in 1796, that was intended to respond to the impressment of American sailors into the British Royal Navy.[5] It ordered the collectors of customs in American ports to issue 'certificates of citizenship' to those mariners who could prove their American citizenship and pay a fee of twenty-five cents.[6]

In the quarter-century following the passage of this act tens and probably hundreds of thousands of American sailors applied for Seamen's Protection Certificates in every major American seaport. Between 1796 and 1819 some twenty-six thousand seamen received 'protections' in Philadelphia alone, and almost ten thousand of their applications still exist.[7] These documents yield a wealth of information about these seafarers, for they recorded the applicant's date and place of birth, his race, height, and complexion, and detailed descriptions of the scars and marks on his body. Over ten percent of all of these men were tattooed, and I believe that they were usually members of the long-term professional seafaring fraternity. This essay is based upon a survey of 500 of the applications that contain descriptions of tattoos, all filed between 1798 and 1816.[8]

There are a number of reasons for concluding that tattoos marked professional sailors. In early national America sailors were probably the only white and black men to wear tattoos, and consequently tattoos functioned as emblems of membership in their seafaring community.[9] Almost all of these tattoos would have been inscribed by the mariners or their friends during long ocean voyages. Using several needles tied together, dipped in a mixture of urine and Indian, Chinese, or gunpowder-based ink, the tattooists stretched the skin as tightly as possible, and then pricked the needles into the skin deep enough to deposit the ink into the dermis, below the epidermis.[10] This was a painful process that could easily result in infection, the transmission of disease, and even death.[11] These five hundred seafarers shared some 1,329 tattoos between them, and each wore an average of 2.65 tattoos. Given the pain and danger involved in acquiring just one tattoo, a sailor was unlikely to acquire all of these tattoos during one voyage: these were the marks of men who had spent a good deal of time plying the oceans. It seems extremely unlikely that short-term seafarers would have marked themselves in this manner.

Some mariners had actual dates tattooed upon their bodies. Lawrence Rugans of Philadelphia, for example, had the date 'Nov. 8. 1793' tattooed upon his left arm.[12] There is evidence to suggest that it was common for seafarers to record the dates of momentous events in their professional lives, thereby affirming and commemorating their membership in the long-term seafaring community.[13] For sailors like William Story and Jacob McKinsey, over twenty years had elapsed between the date tattooed on their bodies and the date on which they applied for a protection. On average, close to nine years had elapsed between a tattooed date and an application date, providing further evidence that these men were far more than casual sailors, and that they were spending much or even all of their working lives at sea.

Like Daniel Orme these men were outsiders in the non-seafaring world, and they self-consciously modified their bodies in such a way as to symbolically demonstrate their disregard for the prevailing behavioral norms of a larger society. Their tattoos show that seafarers were acutely aware of their own role in creating their individual and group identities, and that they actively constructed their appearance, displaying their status, their lifestyle, their belief systems, their masculinity, and a variety of other identity features on their very bodies.[14] Thus the descriptions of their bodily adornments provide us with some fascinating insights into the identities of these lowly seafarers, as they chose to express and record them.

Why did so many professional seafarers choose to undergo this painful and dangerous ritual? Individual motives may have varied widely, from drunkenness, to the overwhelming boredom of a long voyage, to the desire to record a significant event, experience or person.[15] It is clear, however, that for many eighteenth-century seafarers the construction of their identity was central to their decision to acquire tattoos. These were men who lived in poverty, worked in what was perhaps their age's most dangerous occupation, and often owned little more than their own bodies. Tattoos allowed them to celebrate, commemorate and record all manner of things on their own canvas, reminding themselves and telling others about their individual lives and identities, and their beliefs and accomplishments.[16]

When one of these men acquired a tattoo, he symbolically and irrevocably identified himself as a member of the professional seafaring community, while simultaneously providing symbolic information about his own interests, experience and values. They clearly functioned as professional badges, showing landsmen and women that the bearers were seafarers, and showing other seafarers that the bearer was a member of their community. Almost 92% of the tattoos in this sample were inscribed on the hands or the arms, and as such they were highly visible public marks of identity.

To a degree, seafarer and landsman alike could see and interpret these tattoos, but they were part of a language available—and perhaps fully understandable—only to the initiated. In a literal sense these tattoos were symbols of deviance, appropriated by lowly seafarers in order to retain some control over the definition of themselves, their profession and their very bodies.[17] The wearing of these tattoos was, of course, gendered. Only available to the all-male community of seafarers they constituted public displays of masculinity, and could function as badges of strength, courage and manhood, and it seems likely that they played important roles in these sailors' constructions of distinct masculine identities.[18]

Many of the seafarers who passed through the port cities of the early republic wore tattoos that identified their profession: close to 22% were of maritime images such as ships, the North Star, mermaids or foul anchors.[19] Twenty-two-year-old James Powers of Philadelphia was 'marked with India Ink on the left Arm with an Anchor and Mermaid'.[20] A foul anchor could be seen on the back of each of the hands of Benjamin Miles,[21] and John Campbell of Baltimore displayed a star on his right arm.[22]

While images of mermaids, the North Star and anchors were traditional symbols of good fortune amongst the maritime community, these and other images suggest that the men who wore them on their bodies took pride in their profession. From the gentry's powdered wigs, to the continental army veteran's black cockade, to the artisan's leather apron, many eighteenth-century Americans wore emblems of their class and trade. Tattoos of seafaring images showed mariners advertising their class and profession, and celebrating their membership in a lowly paid yet highly skilled proletariat.[23]

And perhaps the 20% of these tattoos that featured the initials or name of the mariner served a somewhat similar purpose. In defiance of his poverty and power-lessness in the larger society, a seafarer asserted and celebrated his own identity by tattooing his name or initials upon his body. When Joseph Shourds of Tuckertown, New Jersey applied for a 'protection' in 1807, Justice Richard Palmer recorded that Shourd's initials were inscribed on his left hand and right arm, along with 'his name in full length...done with Indian Ink'. In addition to using this lettering to assert his own individuality and to prove that he was the American named on the 'protection' he carried, Shourds may well have wanted to record his identity in case he died at sea or in a distant land. As late as 1823 Jeremy Bentham took note of this 'common usage among English sailors', explaining that seafarers had their names or initials tattooed upon their bodies in order 'that they may be recognized in case of ship-wreck'. The initials R.R. appeared next to Joseph Shourds' initials on his right arm, while the initials R.S. were inscribed on his left hand, perhaps the initials of his companion before and after she married him. Should the twenty-five-year-old sea-man have died away from her, his tattoo might have helped to save him from an entirely anonymous fate, and word of his demise may have reached loved ones.[24]

A further 16% of the tattoos recorded the initials or names of people other than the mariner applying for a 'protection'. William Newark of Salem County, New Jersey had the initials MNS on his right hand, and TNA on his left leg, perhaps the initials of a spouse or companion, or even of parents, siblings or friends. In twentieth-century America it is not unusual for gay men to affirm their relationships by having the initials of their companions tattooed on their bodies: this raises the interesting possibility that some of these late eighteenth-century mariners were either gay or bisexual, but used only the initials of their companions in order to avoid homophobic reactions. Within the seafaring world homosexuality may well have been common, but it was far from condoned.[25] It is also possible that some of these mariners were not who they claimed to be: perhaps William Newark was a Briton who had changed his identity since having his initials recorded on his body.[26]

Seven percent of the tattoos of these five hundred seafarers addressed love and loved ones. John Peters of Philadelphia had the name Rachel Peters tattooed on his right arm. For men like Peters and John Hancurne of Charleston, on whose left arm the name Ann Jackson appeared over two interlocked hearts, the name or initials of loved ones indelibly inscribed on their skin served as a comforting reminder of a distant companion.[27] Thirty-five-year-old Peter Mende of Charleston carried the representation of 'a Woman' on his left arm, next to the dual sets of initials PM and SM, each circumscribed by interlocking hearts. Such a design was common, as was

the representation of a heart with 'darts' or arrows piercing it: on each of Philadelphia-born William Lane's shoulders could be found the letters ES tattooed above
a heart transfixed by crossed arrows.[28]

Later in the nineteenth century, as Margaret Creighton has shown, American
sailors came to reject affection for women as an inappropriate emotion, but many of
these early national sailors appear to have been quite comfortable advertising their
relationships with loved ones through their tattoos.[29] And although these tattoos may
have helped sailors to affirm their masculinity and their power over a woman, love
and affection appear to have been the dominant tone. Virtue was as yet as much a
male as a female quality, and these seafarers appear to have regarded love and affection
as legitimate male emotions.[30]

Religious symbols comprised some 9% of the tattoos in this sample. For many
seafarers who wore tattooed anchors on their bodies, images of their lives at sea and
their religious beliefs were combined in one symbol. In early Christian art the anchor
had served as a disguised form of the cross, and from that time forward the anchor
had been a symbol of hope based on the cross of Christ, representing safety, security
and good luck.[31] Twenty-two-year-old James Head had 'the mark of hope' on his
breast, just as thirty-six-year-old Bartlett Wrangham had 'the Figure of hope' on his
right arm.[32] Twenty-seven-year-old William Cox of Philadelphia County bore two
of the most common religious tattoos on his breast, a crucifix, and the figures of
Adam and Eve and 'the Tree of Life'. On his right arm, Nicholas Welsh of Philadelphia bore the less common letters IHS below a cross.[33]

The popularity of religious designs and symbols is less surprising than is the large
number of crucifixes. More common to Catholicism than Protestantism, it is no wonder
that crucifixes were tattooed on a dozen of the thirty mariners from New Orleans.
In English America, the most evangelical Protestant nation on earth, crucifixes were
more readily associated with Papist idolatry. Yet it is extremely unlikely that men like
John Brown of Norfolk, Virginia, New York City-born James Hutton, and John
Dixon from Boston were all Catholics, even though they and some 75 of their fellow
mariners had 'the mark of Christ on the Cross' on their bodies.[34] The burgeoning Episcopalian church and the growing influx of Scottish and Irish Catholics may have con-
tributed to this popularity of crucifixes.[35] It is also possible that a tradition of tattooed
crucifixes that dated back to the Crusades was flourishing amongst seafarers. Given
the diverse peoples and traditions encountered by sailors, and their familiarity with
the Mediterranean world, one might speculate that they had appropriated this tradition, originally adopted by European Crusaders to ensure that they would be marked
for a Christian burial should they die in battle.[36] Herman Melville recorded that
Catholic sailors commonly had tattooed crucifixes to ensure 'a decent burial in consecrated ground' should they 'die in a Catholic land'.[37] The pathetic plea of one Philadelphia mariner in the spring of 1809 suggests that Protestant sailors had similar ideas.
Dying in abject poverty in the Pennsylvania hospital, he pleaded with the Reverend
Nicholas Collin for a burial in consecrated ground, for otherwise 'I shall be thrown
into a pit like another beast without christian ceremonies'.[38]

It also seems probable that many seafarers had considerable faith in the
redeeming power of representations of the crucified Christ. In his short sketch of the

sailor Daniel Orme, Melville made a tattoo of the crucified Christ on Orme's chest the defining characteristic of the old mariner. A long scar, 'such as might ensue from the slash of a cutlass', ran across the tattoo, and Melville implies that the image served a talismanic purpose for Orme and for other sailors. In *White Jacket* Melville relates that seafarers believed a tattooed crucifix would protect them from harm should they fall overboard, even in shark infested waters.[39]

Marcus Rediker has suggested that most early American seamen had 'few religious beliefs central to their identities', and that religion was 'a distinctly secondary matter'.[40] Although the nature of life and work in the seafaring world minimized the impact of organized religion, these tattoos show that religious beliefs were neither absent nor unimportant. The image of Christ on the Cross, Adam and Eve, and other religious symbols served as reminders of religious beliefs, and may have been as much of a comfort to an illiterate mariner as a Bible was to a more literate landsman.[41]

Thirty-year-old James Henry of Philadelphia had 'a Compass & Square, a Ladder, an hour Glass, and five points of fellow Ship, [and] the all seeing Eye' tattooed on his left arm, while thirty-one-year-old John Berry of Baltimore had 'a Free Masons Coat of Arms' on his right breast.[42] Although these tattoos suggest that their bearers were freemasons, historians have commonly assumed that such lowly members of society were excluded from these fairly elite organizations. Most urban freemasons were artisans, merchants, retailers, lawyers and manufacturers, and by 1786 the initiation fees for membership in Philadelphia lodges were between $24 and $30, over a month's wages for a laborer and even more for a mariner.[43]

But perhaps these seafarers were amongst the first of a new class of masons. In the years following the American Revolution the elitist character of 'Modern' lodges had been undermined by the rise of 'Ancient' lodges, drawing their members from a broad social coalition of those who had supported the Patriot cause.[44] Throughout the 1790s, as the Democratic Republican party coalesced around Painite and Jeffersonian democratic ideology, its supporters assumed control of American freemasonry.[45] In 1810, 1813 and again in 1816, unauthorized masonic meetings were held in various taverns throughout Philadelphia, which may have been accessible to and even aimed at members of the lower sort. The few seamen with masonic tattoos may well have been amongst the first of the lower orders to be initiated into masonic lodges.[46]

Professional seafarers were, then, a good deal more involved in religion and even freemasonry than most historians have realized. Much the same was true of politics. Their burning hatred of impressment and the cruel treatment many suffered at the hands of the British informed these sailors' self-constructed identities, giving them a distinctly Anglophobic patriotism that was often expressed in fiercely political patriotic tattoos.[47] Their Anglophobia grew stronger during the 1790s and early 1800s as the British, intent on blockading and destroying revolutionary France, seized more and more American ships and impressed growing numbers of American seamen. However, the patriotism of American seafarers transcended a simple self-interested hatred of England, and in a variety of civic festivals and crowd actions during the 1790s sailors manifested their support for revolutionary French republicanism. For many of them, the liberty, equality and fraternity of the French Revolution represented a powerful extension of the as yet unfulfilled radical promise of the American Revolution.[48]

Consequently Federalists who desired good relations with Britain and who distrusted the French constantly found themselves at odds with the mariners who suffered at the hands of the British. The Federalists' Jay Treaty of 1795 did virtually nothing to protect American ships and their sailors, and enormous crowds protested the treaty in every major port, their ranks swelled by thousands of seamen.[49] A year later on the eve of the presidential election of 1796, a large crowd of seamen marched through the streets of Philadelphia 'with a drum and colors', wearing French republican tri-colored cockades in their hats, while some of their number prepared a banner bearing the motto 'Jefferson the Man of the People'.[50]

The point here is that tattoos of eagles, liberty trees and American flags were more than simple emblems of patriotism. We should not regard seafarers and other lowly Americans as nothing more than pawns in the political battle between elite Founding Fathers, but should instead acknowledge their limited yet significant role as actors in this political contest. The role of the seafaring community in articulating a stridently Anglophobic republicanism was a significant one, and from the mid-1790s on, the Democratic Republican leadership was under constant pressure to articulate and represent the concerns of hundreds of thousands of American sailors.[51]

Despite the fact that these professional seafarers were disenfranchised outsiders in the political world of terra firma, many chose to identify with America as a republican enemy of Britain, and as a bastion of popular freedom and liberty. In the early republic, this kind of patriotism had deeply partisan implications: a seafarer walking through the streets of Philadelphia with an American flag or liberty tree tattooed on his arm was no friend to the Federalist gentleman wearing a black cockade who walked past him.

The most common of the patriotic tattoos were representations of an American Eagle. With a classical republican heritage, the eagle had grown in popularity in the years after it first appeared on the Great Seal of the United States, and 40 seamen had eagles emblazoned on their bodies. Boston-born John Curtis had 'an Eagle on the Right Arm', as did John Clay of Delaware, and John Brown of Norfolk, Virginia.[52] Often the eagle appeared in conjunction with other patriotic symbols. Twenty-one-year-old William Sweeny of Baltimore, for example, had 'a Spread Eagle & 15 Stars' on his right arm, representing the fifteen states of the union in the mid-1790s.[53] Twenty-six-year-old Samuel Anderson who also hailed from Maryland, displayed his patriotism with a Spread Eagle and 13 stars on his left arm, and the date '1776' on his right arm.[54] Anderson had not been born in the year America declared its independence, but his decision to have the date tattooed on his arm a quarter-century later invested his patriotism with strongly Democratic Republican overtones. By the end of the eighteenth century, few Federalists countenanced the radical democratic ideology espoused by Paine and Jefferson in the heady year of independence. But this ideology was at the heart of the Democratic Republican movement, and when Jefferson was elected in 1800 his supporters regularly drank celebratory toasts to '1776', and 'The Spirit of '76'.[55]

Other seamen such as the Bostonian William Carson were marked 'with the Flag of the United States' and 'the word Liberty'. Philadelphia-born John Thompson, his face 'very much pitted with the Small pox', had 'the figure of a Spread Eagle,

Stars and flag', his initials and the date 1801 all tattooed on his left arm. These patriotic symbols, probably inscribed in the year of Jefferson's inauguration, illustrated Thompson's patriotism and the partisan sympathies that informed it.[56]

The rather less common tattoos of Liberty Trees and Liberty Caps confirm the partisan character of seafaring patriotism. These symbols of republicanism and liberty had become popular during the American Revolution, and in the early 1790s the Democratic Republican David Rittenhouse had placed them upon the coins of the young republic, against the wishes of Federalists who would have preferred Washington's stately head. Infused with a new radicalism by the French Revolution, they had become badges of Democratic Republican affiliation, and from the days of the Whiskey Rebellion on, Democratic Republicans erected Liberty Poles and often placed Liberty Caps atop them.[57]

Thus the patriotic symbols favored by these American seamen had an unmistakably partisan significance, advertising the political identities of sailors who wore them, and suggesting that common seamen played a heretofore unseen role in both the construction of and support for the Democratic Republican party. But these seafarers were far more than simple plebeian supporters of Jefferson's Democratic Republicans, for they had constructed their own strongly patriotic identity, informed by an enduring hatred of the British and their policies, and an identification with the cause of radical democratic republicanism. Although they might choose to affiliate themselves with the Democratic Republicans, their support was conditional: when Jefferson's Embargo misfired and brought seafaring communities to the brink of starvation, seamen mounted major protests in the nation's port cities.[58]

These, then, were long-term seafarers who had been or who expected to be at sea for many years. With their tattoos they identified themselves as significantly different from short-term sailors, and as wholly dissimilar from the men and women who lived and worked ashore. Desperately poor, they enjoyed little control over their relative illiteracy, their occupational scars, dark complexions, short stature and the marks of disease that could all help identify them as some of the lowest members of society. With the words and the images inscribed upon their bodies, however, these men exerted some control over the construction of their individual and social identities, displaying pride in their beliefs, their values, their achievements, and their membership in the seafaring fraternity.

And yet for all of the assertions of individuality and power expressed in these tattoos, many of these images betrayed seafarers' awareness of their vulnerable position in an extremely dangerous profession. When they inscribed their own names, those of loved ones, and symbols of religious belief on their hands and arms, seafarers were marking their bodies for the death that was never far away, acknowledging their subordinate role in the world of maritime commerce. On both levels, as badges of pride and as symbols of subservience, the tattoos of these professional seafarers furnish us with a few fascinating glimpses of the values and beliefs they cherished, the people they loved, and their pride in their craft.

Notes

1.   Samuel Eliot Morison, *The Maritime History of Massachusetts, 1783–1860* (Boston: Houghton Mifflin, 1921), p. 16.
2.   Daniel Vickers, 'Beyond Jack Tar', *The William and Mary Quarterly*, III, 50 (1993), p. 422.
3.   Marcus Rediker, *Between the Devil and the Deep Blue Sea: Merchant Seamen, Pirates, and the Anglo-American Maritime World, 1700-1750* (New York, 1987), pp. 77-78, 288-89; Billy G. Smith, *The 'Lower Sort': Philadelphia's Laboring People, 1750–1800*, (Ithaca: Cornell University Press, 1990), pp. 64, 112-113; Gary B. Nash, *The Urban Crucible: Social Change, Political Consciousness, and the Origins of the American Revolution* (Cambridge, MA: Harvard University Press, 1979), p. 16.
   Despite the lack of sources, several historians have attempted to find out more about the lives and experiences of American merchant seamen. See Rediker, *Between the Devil and the Deep Blue Sea*; Jesse Lemisch, 'Jack Tar in the Streets: Merchant Seamen in the Politics of Revolutionary America', *William and Mary Quarterly* III, 25 (1968), pp. 371-407, and 'Listening to the "Inarticulate": William Widger's Dream and the Loyalties of American Revolutionary Seamen', *Journal of Social History* 3 (1969), pp. 1-29. However, were we to rely on the works of social and labor historians such as Bruce Laurie, *Working People of Philadelphia, 1800–1850* (Philadelphia: Temple University Press, 1980), we would find virtually no references to the mariners who comprised the largest single occupational group in the towns and cities of early national America.
4.   Herman Melville, 'Daniel Orme', in *Billy Budd, Sailor & Other Stories* (New York: Penguin Books, 1970), pp. 414-15, 417.
5.   Under the principle of Indefeasible Nationality, British authorities argued that any man born a British subject remained one until the day he died, which to their minds justified the impressment of Americans whenever the Royal Navy was short-handed: see Christopher Lloyd, *The British Seaman, 1200–1860: A Social Survey* (Rutherford: Fairleigh Dickinson University Press, 1970 [1968]), pp. 115, 117-18, 215, 265-66. During the first decade of the Wars of the French Revolution, over twenty-four hundred Americans secured their release from His Majesty's service, but many more were less fortunate. By the turn of the century at least three thousand native-born citizens of the republic were fighting and dying for a foreign monarch, to say nothing of the thousands of British-born impressed mariners who had become legal residents and citizens of the United States. For some first hand accounts of impressment see Joshua Davis, *A Narrative of Joshua Davis, An American Citizen, Who Was Pressed and Served on Board Six Ships of the British Navy* (Boston: B. True, 1811), and Samuel Leech, *Thirty Years from Home, or, A Voice From the Main Deck: Being the Experiences of Samuel Leech, Who Was for Six Years in the British and American Navies* (Boston: Tappan & Dennet, 1843).
6.   The Debates and Proceedings in the Congress of the United States, Fourth Congress—First Session (Washington: G.P.O., 1849), V, p. 802; Richard Peters (ed.), *The Public Statutes at Large of the United States of America, From the Organization of the Government in 1789, to March 3, 1845* (Boston: G.P.O., 1845), I, p. 477.
7.   Ira Dye, 'The Philadelphia Seamen's Protection Certificate Applications', *Prologue: Sources at the National Archives for Genealogical and Local History Research* 18 (1986), p. 51. The Seamen's Protection Certificate Applications (SPCA's) are in the National Archives, Record Group 36, Records of the Bureau of Customs. Few applications filed in any other American ports have survived, and almost all of the protection certificates themselves have long since

disappeared. Ira Dye, a retired navy captain and research professor of civil engineering, is one of the few people to have researched these fascinating records, spending countless hours in the National Archives, and willingly sharing the fruits of his work with other scholars. See Dye, 'Early American Merchant Seafarers', *Proceedings of the American Philosophical Society* 120 (1976), pp. 340-44; Dye, 'Physical and Social Profiles of Early American Seafarers, 1812-1815', in *Jack Tar in History: Essays in the History of Maritime Life and Labour* (ed. Colin Howell and Richard J. Twomey; Fredricton, New Brunswick: Acadiensis Press, 1991), pp. 220-35; Dye, 'The Tattoos of Early American Seafarers, 1796-1818', *Proceedings of the American Philosophical Society* 133 (1989), pp. 520-54. While the latter essay provides a splendid overview of the designs and physical location and frequency of seafarers' tattoos, Dye made little reference to either their cultural significance or to their utility for a 'reading' of the bodies of early national sailors.

8.   Most of the applications were prepared on printed forms, and they usually documented the seaman's name, age, race, height, complexion, eye and hair color, descriptions of scars, marks and tattoos, his birthplace (or the date and place of his naturalization), his signature or mark, and the name and signature of a witness. The 500 applications were filed between 1798 and 1816, and were selected from the larger group for the completeness of information contained therein.

British impressment was justified by the fact that a large number of British sailors and deserters from the Royal Navy were working in the American merchant marine, and many of these may well have fraudulently applied for American protection certificates. Consequently Royal Navy officers frequently impressed seamen who they suspected were British 'without respect to their protections, which were often taken from them and destroyed' (Leech, *A Voice From the Main Deck*, p 80). Thus, some of the 500 applicants for protection certificates who are the subjects of this essay in all probability lied about their place of birth. This does not detract from my interpretation, however. All of the men in this sample were members of the American seafaring community, a heterogeneous mix of ethnicities and races: whether or not they lied about their birthplace, they were sailors on American ships, and sometime members of the American seaport communities. Their tattoos, the central focus of this essay, were certainly real enough.

9.   An ancient art form, tattooing may have been introduced into the seafaring community in the wake of Captain Cook's South Pacific voyages of the 1770s. However, the heavy incidence of tattooing amongst late-eighteenth-century mariners throughout the Atlantic world suggests that exposure to the ornate tattooing of the South Sea Islanders simply increased interest in a practice already well established amongst seamen. See, for example, Robert Brain, *The Decorated Body* (New York: Harper & Row, 1979); R.W.B. Scutt and Christopher Gotch, *Art, Sex and Symbol: The Mystery of Tattooing* (London: P. Davies, 1974); W.D. Hambly, *The History of Tattooing and its Significance* (London: H.F. & G. Witherby, 1925); Samuel M. Steward, *Bad Boys and Tough Tattoos: A Social History of the Tattoo with Gangs, Sailors and Street-Corner Punks* (New York: Haworth, 1990).

10.   Dye, 'The Tattoos of Early American Seafarers', pp. 529-31.

11.   Gangrene, tetanus and lymphadenitis are often the result for men and women tattooed in a similar fashion in the twentieth century. Arkady G. Bronnikov, 'Telltale Tattoos in Russian Prisons', *Natural History* 102 (November 1993), p. 50.

12.   Lawrence Rugans, SPCA, 24 December 1803.

13.   Other sources suggest a possible meaning for this use of dates. Thomas Ellison, one of the mutinous crew of H.M.S. *Bounty*, was recorded by Captain William Bligh as having the date 25 October 1788 tattooed on his right arm, the date on which the *Bounty*'s crew first saw Tahiti. Greg Dening, *Mr. Bligh's Bad Language: Passion, Power and Theatre on the Bounty*

(New York: Cambridge University Press, 1992), p. 36.

14.   Lyn H. Lofland, *A World of Strangers: Order and Action in Urban Public Space* (New York: Basic Books, 1973), p. 79-80; Clinton R. Sanders, *Customizing the Body: The Art and Culture of Tattooing* (Philadelphia: Temple University Press, 1989), pp. 1-2; Erving Goffman, *Behavior in Public Places: Notes on the Social Organization of Gatherings* (New York: Free Press of Glencoe, 1963); Alison Lurie, *The Language of Clothes* (New York: Random House, 1981). The detailed British prisoner-of-war records for the 1990 American soldiers held at Quebec during the War of 1812 provide further evidence of the fact that only sailors were tattooed. These prisoners were drawn from urban and rural areas throughout the United States, but only 11 were tattooed, and at least four of these were sailors. See Dye, 'The Tattoos of Early American Seafarers', pp. 548-49.

15.   According to Herman Melville it was 'the long, tedious hours' of shipboard life that led many seafarers on a mid-nineteenth century American warship to visit the 'prickers' who could tattoo them. Melville, *White Jacket: Or The World in a Man-of-War* (New York: G. Putnam's Sons, 1892 [1850]), p. 160.

16.   The arguments I am making in this paragraph mirror those of Bronnikov, who has established that tattoos fulfilled similar functions within the criminal community inhabiting post-World War II Russian prisons. See Bronnikov, 'Telltale Tattoos', pp. 50-59.

17.   Robert K. Merton, *Social Theory and Social Structure* (New York: Free Press of Glencoe, 1968), pp. 217-18.

18.   For discussion of gender and masculinity within the seafaring community, see Margaret S. Creighton, 'Fraternity in the American Forecastle, 1830-1870', *New England Quarterly* 63 (1990), pp. 531-57, and 'American Mariners and the Rites of Manhood, 1830-1870', in *Jack Tar in History*, pp. 143-63.

        For sailors and other men tattooed in mid twentieth-century America, 'feelings of manliness' often accompanied the inscribing of tattoos, which were generally expressed in bouts of drinking, violence and sex. See Steward, *Bad Boys and Tough Tattoos*, p. 41.

19.   A foul or fouled anchor was an anchor with a chain wound around it. The distribution of these 1192 tattoos were as follows: 240 (20.13%) comprised the seaman's initials or name; 197 (16.52%) were the initials or names of others; 33 (2.76%) were of the date on which an accompanying tattoo was drawn; 262 (21.97%) were of seafaring and maritime images such as mermaids, fouled anchors, the North Star, or a ship; 89 (7.46%) were representations of loved ones or of hearts, which were often transfixed by arrows; 110 (9.22%) were of religious images; 13 (1.09%) were of masonic symbols; 66 (5.53%) were pictures of various people, animals and flowers, 71 (5.95%) portrayed political and patriotic images; and 111 (9.31%) were of miscellaneous objects such as patterns, groups of dots, or could not be identified.

20.   James Powers, SPCA, 23 November 1809.

21.   Benjamin Miles, SPCA, 29 October 1805.

22.   John Campbell, SPCA, 2 September 1805.

23.   It was Marcus Rediker who introduced the idea of seafarers as amongst the earliest free wage laborers, with a shared class consciousness, culture and mentalities. See *Beneath the Devil and the Deep Blue Sea*, *passim*.

24.   Joseph Shourds, SPCA, 14 February 1807; Jeremy Bentham, *The Theory of Legislation* (ed. C.K. Ogden; London: K. Paul, Trench, Trubner, 1931 [1823]), p. 416.

25.   Steward, *Bad Boys and Tough Tattoos*, pp. 52-56. In the contemporary Royal Navy a man accused of buggery was more likely to be convicted than one accused of murder or even mutiny, and in almost all cases the penalty was death: close to a third of all executions in the Royal Navy between 1700 and 1861 were for buggery. For more information see Arthur N. Gilbert, 'Buggery and the British Navy, 1700-1861', *Journal of Social History* 10 (1976), pp.

81-82, 87.

26.   William Newark, SPCA, 28 August 1809.

27.   John Peters, SPCA, 22 July 1806; John Hancurne, SPCA, 10 October 1805. The majority of these tattoos are of hearts, many of which featured names or initials beside or inside them, but sometimes the names or initials of wives appeared without this familiar image.

28.   Peter Mende, SPCA, 29 October 1803; William Lane, SPCA, 6 November 1807.

29.   By the middle of the nineteenth century, according to Margaret Creighton, American sailors 'in distancing themselves from female relatives and women's work, sought to protect and enhance distinct masculine identities'. Older sailors, according to Creighton, ridiculed greenhands for their sentimental attachments to women on shore, and acceptance 'in the forecastle was contingent upon the shift of allegiance from home to ship'. Creighton, 'American Mariners and the Rites of Manhood', pp. 155, 148.

30.   On virtue see Ruth H. Bloch, 'The Gendered Meanings of Virtue in Revolutionary America', *Signs: Journal of Women and Culture and Society* 13 (1987), pp. 37-58. For discussion of the ways in which emotions were 'sentimentalized' and 'feminized' as the nineteenth century progressed see Ann Douglas, *The Feminization of American Culture* (New York: Knopf, 1977), and Jane Tompkins, *Sentimental Designs: The Cultural Work of American Fiction, 1790-1860* (New York: Routledge, 1985).

31.   J.C. Cooper, *An Illustrated Encyclopedia of Traditional Symbols* (London: Thames & Hudson, 1978), p. 12.

32.   James Head, SPCA, 13 May 1804; Bartlett Wrangham, SPCA, 2 October 1807.

33.   William Cox, SPCA, 24 August 1804; Nicholas Welsh, SPCA, 25 October 1803. The letters IHS had two possible meanings: they were probably an abbreviation of 'In Hoc Signo Vinces', meaning 'By this sign [of the Cross] thou shalt conquer', but they may also have been a popular latinized contraction of the Greek word for Jesus. See F.L. Cross and E.A. Livingstone, *The Oxford Dictionary of the Christian Church* (2nd ed.; New York: Oxford University Press, 1974), p. 696.

34.   John Brown, SPCA, 12 December 1805; William Brown, SPCA, 13 June 1804; James Dixon, SPCA, 30 September 1805. This figure includes the dozen mariners from New Orleans who wore tattooed crucifixes on their bodies.

35.   Raymond W. Albright, *A History of the Protestant Episcopalian Church* (New York, 1964), pp. 101, 141-43; Frederick V. Mills, Sr, *Bishops By Ballot: An Eighteenth-Century Ecclesiastical Revolution* (New York: Oxford University Press, 1978), pp. 7-16.

36.   Having encountered the Coptic Christian tradition of tattooing, some of the European Crusaders had crucifixes tattooed upon their bodies to mark them for a Christian burial, and the practice soon became quite popular. Often acquired in the tattoo parlors of Jerusalem, religious tattoos became common souvenirs and badges of piety for the European Christians who made pilgrimages to the Holy Land. Alan Governar, 'Christian Tattoos', *Tattootime* 2 (1983), pp. 7-8; Sanders, *Customizing the Body*, pp. 13-14; Scutt and Gotch, *Art, Sex and Symbol*, pp. 65-66.

37.   Melville, *White Jacket*, p. 161.

38.   This sailor was Olaf Melin who, according to Collin, had 'sailed from this Port for several years'. Gloria Dei Burial Records, 20 April 1809, Pennsylvania Genealogical Society, Historical Society of Pennsylvania.

39.   Melville, 'Daniel Orme', p. 415; *White Jacket*, p. 161.

40.   Rediker, *Between the Devil and the Deep Blue Sea*, p. 173.

41.   It also seems likely that images of crosses and crucifixes had an æsthetic appeal to seafarers in the early republic. Stark and relatively simple, these designs had an immediate

impact. In post-World War II Russian prisons, tattooed crosses symbolized subordination, and this universal symbol of pain and suffering may have served a similar purpose for some seafarers. We can only guess what the image of the crucified Christ meant to these sailors, many of whose bodies had been broken by the rigors of life at sea. For some, perhaps, it was a lucky badge, emblematic of vaguely defined religion beliefs. But for others the cross and the crucifix may have said as much about the pain and suffering endured by their own bodies as it did about a belief in the divine. Bronnikov, 'Telltale Tattoos', p. 53.

42.   James Henry, SPCA, 26 December 1805; John Berry, SPCA, 14 June 1809. Masonic images appeared only on the bodies of seamen from the Southern or Middle Atlantic states: none of the New England-born mariners in this sample wore them.

43.   Wayne A. Huss, *The Master Builders: A History of the Grand Lodge of Free and Accepted Masons of Pennsylvania, Vol. 1: 1731-1873* (Philadelphia: The Grand Lodge, 1986), pp. 53, 82, 297-98. While the average age of the white seafarers in this sample was just under 26, Henry, Berry and the other sailors who wore Masonic tattoos were generally several years older: perhaps these men had experienced a decline in circumstances from a social position that had allowed them access and membership to the free masons.

44.   Steven C. Bullock, 'The Revolutionary Transformation of American Freemasonry, 1752-1792', *William and Mary Quarterly* III, 47 (1990), pp. 359, 363, 367.

45.   John L. Brooke, 'Ancient Lodges and Self-Created Societies: Voluntary Associations and the Public Sphere in the Early Republic', unpublished paper delivered at the United States Capitol Historical Society, March 1990, pp. 10, 64-65.

46.   Huss, *The Master Builders*, pp. 85-87. Few if any of their fellow lodge members would have worn masonic tattoos: these seamen may have worn them to identify themselves to fellow masons elsewhere. After all, one of the principle benefits of freemasonry was the guarantee of aid and friendship from masons the world over, a useful benefit to a sailor far from home and down on his luck.

47.   For a discussion of how Revolutionary ideology informed the ideas and actions of laboring people, see Alfred F. Young, 'George Robert Twelve Hewes (1742-1840): A Boston Shoemaker and the Memory of the American Revolution', *William and Mary Quarterly* III, 38 (1981), pp. 561-623. Hewes began as a lowly and deferential shoemaker, but revolutionary ideology transformed his attitudes towards himself and his supposed 'superiors', and by the end of the war he refused on principle to take his hat off to an officer of a privateer on which he had engaged to serve.

48.   One such event occurred in 1793: after the people of Boston had mounted a huge festival in celebration of the French victory at Valmy, 'a number of citizen seamen' affirmed their own support of revolutionary French republicanism by taking the horns of the oxen on which the townspeople had feasted, marching to the liberty pole, and then having the horns gilded and placed atop the pole. See *The New-York Journal* (6 February 1793). For a more detailed discussion of this festival, see Simon P. Newman, '"Tis the Worlds Jubilee and Mankind Must Be Free": Boston Celebrates the Victory at Valmy' (unpublished paper presented at the annual meeting of the American Historical Association, December 1991).

The Federalist party, with its economic program based on close cooperation with Britain, a growing fear of the social radicalism of the French Revolution, and a deep dislike of the radical democratic impulses of the American Revolution, regularly condemned the political participation of seamen and other members of the 'lower sorts'. One Boston Federalist ridiculed the ideology that had informed Boston's Valmy celebration as one that 'gave Tars and tailors a civic feast and taught the rabble that they were viceroys'. Joseph Dennie to Joseph Dennie, Sr and Mary Green Dennie, 25 April 1793, Joseph Dennie Papers, Houghton Library, Harvard University.

49. Simon P. Newman, 'American Popular Political Culture in the Age of the French Revolution', (PhD dissertation, Princeton University, 1991), pp. 248-97.

50. Political activity of this sort by disenfranchized mariners drew the wrath of Federalist authorities who forbade the display of the banner and forcibly broke up the procession: by the end of the day 'near 40 of these Rioters' were in custody, and '2 or 3 of them [were] much hurt'. Samuel Coates to William Moyer, Jr, 4 November 1796, Samuel Coates Letter Book, September 1795–May 1802, Coates Family Papers, Historical Society of Pennsylvania, pp. 142-43.

51. Further evidence of the impact of American seafarers on political discourse can be found in sources as diverse as a play about American sailors imprisoned in North Africa performed in Philadelphia in 1794, the Seamen's Protection Act of 1796, and a song celebrating American seafarers as 'independent, Brave & Free'. See Susanna Rowson, *Slaves in Algiers* (Philadelphia: The Author, 1795); The Debates and Proceedings in the Congress, V, p. 802; Rowson, 'Independent and Free', from her play *The American Tar*, quoted in Susan Branson, 'Politics and Gender: The Political Consciousness of Philadelphia Women in the 1790s' (PhD dissertation, Northern Illinois University, 1992), p. 82. For further discussion of the American sailors imprisoned in Algiers and Rowson's play, see Gary E. Wilson, 'American Hostages in Moslem Nations, 1784-1796: The Public Response', *Journal of the Early Republic* 2 (1982), pp. 123-41, and Branson, 'Politics and Gender', pp. 61-66.

52. John Curtis, SPCA, 7 January 1807; John M. Clay, SPCA, 14 August 1809; John Brown, SPCA, 12 December 1805.

53. William Sweeney, SPCA, 13 June 1804.

54. Samuel Anderson, SPCA, 4 September 1804.

55. *Aurora. General Advertiser* (Philadelphia), 15 April, 9 March 1801. By this time celebrations of the anniversary of independence had become Democratic-Republican festivals, and by the early nineteenth-century many Federalists refused to participate in July Fourth celebrations and even attacked as 'improper' the reading of the Declaration of Independence at these events: 'Oliver Oldschool's Portfolio', 12 April 1801, quoted in Edward G. Everett, 'Some Aspects of Pro-French Sentiment in Pennsylvania, 1790-1800', *The Western Pennsylvania Historical Magazine* 43 (1960), p. 26. See also Simon P. Newman, '"Principles or Men?" George Washington and the Political Culture of National Leadership, 1776-1801', *Journal of the Early Republic* 12 (1992), pp. 477-507, and 'American Popular Political Culture', pp. 163-65, 171-76, 338-41.

56. William Carson, SPCA, 6 January 1806; John Thompson, SPCA, 16 November 1805.

57. See Newman, 'Principles or Men', pp. 490-93; Arthur M. Schlesinger, 'The Liberty Tree: A Genealogy', *The New England Quarterly* 25 (1952), pp. 435-58; Jennifer Harris, 'The Red Cap of Liberty: A Study of Dress Worn by French Revolutionary Partisans, 1789-1794', *Eighteenth-Century Studies* 14 (1980-81), pp. 283-312.

Such was the symbolic power of these liberty poles that by the end of the decade Federalists condemned them as 'sedition poles', and used the Sedition Act of 1798 to imprison those responsible for erecting them. See, for example, *Aurora*, 20 September 1794; 'The Tree of Liberty', *Porcupine's Gazette and United States Daily Advertiser* (Philadelphia), 25 March 1797; 'Sedition Poles', *Porcupine's Gazette*, 2 February 1799.

58. In January of 1808 there were protests in Boston, New York City, Philadelphia and other ports. *L'Oracle and Daily Advertiser* (New York), 8 January 1808; *American Citizen*, (Philadelphia), 16 January 1808. See also Frank Folsom, 'Jobless Jack Tars, 1808', *Labor's Heritage: Quarterly of the George Meany Memorial Archives* 2 (1990), pp. 6, 8-10, 12-14.

Peter Thompson

No Chance in Nature:
Cannibalism as a Solution to Maritime Famine,
c.1750–1800

In November 1773, during his second visit to New Zealand, Captain James Cook invited a party of Maori on board the *Resolution*. 'Now tho' it was pretty certain that those people were Cannibals' Lt. John Elliott recalled, and

> Captain Cook had told them so in his former Voyage, yet he was doubted. He therefore thought this a very good opportunity to bring the Matter to a Proof. Having brought two of the principal Men with him, he told them we would not believe him that they eat Man's flesh. They said, Yes, they always eat their Enemies. He then asked them if they would eat part of the Man's head before them; they said Yes, only let it be broiled on the fire. For this purpose, two slices were cut from the lower part of the Cheeks (for the Lower Jaw had been taken out to decorate the inside of their War Canoes) and…broiled on a grid-iron. When ready, it was brought to the two Men, who instantly [ate] it with all the avidity of a Beef Steak, to the utmost horror of the whole Quarter deck …Many of the people…said a great deal…to induce [them] to relinquish so Horrid a custom, but to no purpose, we suppose, for they only laughed at…us.[1]

The human body had a crucial part to play in dramas such as this, wherein Europeans invented or reinvented a savage 'other' in the course of their voyages of exploration. Whether through the clothing and bodily adornments they did or did not wear, or the food they ate, or their sexual practices, or their attitudes toward the dead, the ways in which strangers related to the body encapsulated, for Europeans, an 'otherness' which was often construed as savage. Often but not always. What is striking about the encounter Cook staged on the *Resolution* to 'tell' the Maori they were cannibals is that, as a strategy for establishing the civility of the Europeans and the savagery of the Maori, it was a less than complete success. Despite nearly three hundred years of post-Columbian meditation on savage cannibalism, Cook's crew doubt that cannibalism—in the perjorative, 'savage' sense that Cook sought to establish—existed. On Elliott's testimony, the crew found the sight of human flesh-eating ghastly. Some, but not all, called on their visitors to desist. But it is by no means clear that the *Resolution*'s crew concluded that they had seen cannibalism. Elliott, who understood what Cook was trying to show, also carefully noted the

Maori's explanation of their actions—that they eat their *enemies*. He recorded the preparations they insisted on, and reported enough of their speech and action as to hint that they had their own reasons for participating in Cook's morality play. In other words some of Cook's officers and men harboured the suspicion that savage 'others', in this case Maori, might have their reasons for eating human flesh; and this suspicion or scepticism undermined the unequivocal association of cannibalism with pathology which the polarity between savage and civilized demanded.

Sailors were more likely to demonstrate such suspicion or scepticism than eighteenth-century landsmen. It had its roots and sustenance in the willingness of blue-water sailors to engage in all kinds of cultural exchange and appropriation with non-Europeans. Already suspect in light of a long western tradition equating nomadic migration with savagery, European sailors brought to their encounters with 'others' a willingness to exchange and experiment in matters of clothing, and bodily adorn-ment, food and drink, and, above all, sexual practice. Cook knew this, which is why he staged a morality play on the quarter deck of the *Resolution*. For Cook, and many of land based readers, the point of voyages of exploration was to demonstrate the reach and rectitude of civilization not barbaric savagery. Yet because civilization, embodied in the very acme of pre-industrial civilization, the ocean-going ship, was conveyed by sailors it was conveyed imperfectly.

This paper seeks to explore and develop the general imperfection or equivo-cality with which encounters with the 'other'—in which bodily practices and con-structions were key texts—conveyed the polarity civilized and savage, by reference to some of the specific problems raised for landbased 'civilization' by the pragmatism or, if you like, relativism of its sea-going agents. The discussion which follows is based on one of many narratives describing the eating of human flesh as a means of allevi-ating maritime famine. In keeping with the spirit of de Certeau's work on 'the other,' I shall be arguing that savage otherness, ostensibly a device upon which the authority of a text might be built, was frequently in practice a deeply subversive concept.[2]

In July 1765, New York newspapers reported the departure of the sloop *Peggy* for Fayal in the Azores.[3] The *Peggy* carried a cargo of pipe staves, bees wax, and fish. *Peggy*'s captain, David Harrison, took with him a slave, named Wiltshire, whom he hoped to sell in the Azores. The *Peggy* arrived in Fayal in early October and Harrison set about gathering a cargo for the return voyage to New York.[4] On 24 October 1765, the *Peggy* sailed for New York laden with 'wine, brandy, etc.' Captain Harrison had not found a buyer for Wiltshire, and the slave returned with the ship and its crew.

Almost immediately the *Peggy* ran into a series of storms. The ship's rigging was severely damaged, most of her sails were blown away, and the *Peggy* was essentially beyond control. Harrison put the crew on a strict allowance of two pounds of bread per person per week, one quart of water and one pint of wine per day. As the threat of starvation increased, Captain Harrison gradually 'contracted' the allowance 'granted' each man. Meanwhile the crew seized control of the ship's cargo and, according to Harrison, were in a state of near constant drunkenness.[5]

The crew of the *Peggy*, whose piety did not impress Captain Harrison, believed that salvation would come on Christmas Day. And indeed on 25 December, with the wind and sea temporarily calm, a ship appeared. Attracted by *Peggy*'s distress signal, this stranger bore down and her captain entered into negotiation with Harrison. The strange ship was itself, her captain explained, on short rations. The captain could spare no water and refused to take Harrison and his crew off the *Peggy*. However he did agree to hand over a small quantity of bread as soon as he had finished taking a navigational observation. Harrison described what happened next: 'I retired to rest myself in the cabbin, being much emaciated with fasting and fatigue; and labouring at the same time, not only under a dreadful flux, but a severe rheumatism in my right knee.'[6] A little while after he retired, Harrison was dragged on deck by his crew and watched with them as their rescue ship sailed away without having rendered any assistance. (Harrison subsequently refused to name this ship or identify her captain beyond the initial 'B.')[7] The men consoled themselves by sharing two 'pigeons' which had become entangled in the rigging. On Boxing Day, nine men, including Harrison, shared the meat gained by killing the ship's cat and dog. They divided these spoils by lot. The cat's head fell to Harrison. He recalled later that he had never feasted on anything which tasted so delicious to his appetite.

Thereafter the men on the *Peggy* fell into 'general distress.' Harrison lay confined in his bed. He refused wine, and subsisted on what he described as 'dirty water,' scorned by the crew, to which he added drops of a preparation called Turlington's Balsam. He ran out of space in his logbook and began to make notes in chalk on the deck. The men drank wine, chewed lead bullets, ate buttons, and attempted to scrape barnacles from the hull. Harrison's account admitted that he had now lost all control of the ship.

On 13 January, the crew, led by Archibald Nicholson Peggy's mate, entered Harrison's cabin and told him that:

> they could hold out no longer; that their tobacco was exhausted...that now they had no chance in nature but to cast lots, and to sacrifice one of themselves for the preservation of the rest.[8]

Although they were bent on going ahead with this scheme with, or without, Harrison's approval, the crew informed him that his name would be among the lots. Harrison would be obliged to take his chance because 'the general misfortune has levelled all distinctions of persons.'[9] Harrison recalled what happened, when, a few minutes later, they returned:

> [the crew said] they had taken a chance for their lives, and that the lot had fallen on a negro, who was part of my cargo—The little time taken to cast the lot, and their private manner of conducting the decision, gave me some strong suspicions that the poor Ethiopian was not altogether treated fairly; but, on recollection, I almost wondered that they had given him even the appearance of an equal chance with themselves.

Before he was shot by crewman James Doud, the 'miserable black' Wiltshire ran to Harrison for protection, which Harrison, possessed of a brace of pistols, was unwilling to give.[10] 'They suffered him to lye but a very little time before they ripped him open,' Harrison noted, 'intending to fry his entrails for supper.'[11]

Crewman James Campbell couldn't wait for this plan to be executed. He snatched and ate the slave's raw liver. (Campbell went 'raving mad' three days later, and quickly died. There were those of his crewmates who proposed preserving Campbell's body as a source of sustenance. However, a majority believed that to eat Campbell's flesh would be to be risk madness, and the body was thrown overboard.) Harrison lay in his bunk while above him on deck the remainder of the crew made a 'luxurious banquet' of the murdered slave. The next morning the crew, led by the mate Nicholson, asked Harrison's advice on how to preserve the 'carcass'. Harrison expressed outrage at this instance of 'shocking brutality' and threatened to shoot Nicholson. Nicholson relieved Harrison of command, taking his pistols. The crew retreated and held a 'council' where 'they unanimously agreed to cut the body into small pieces, and to pickle it, after chopping off the head and fingers, which they threw overboard by common consent.' They called the remaining small pieces, which they pickled in wine, 'stakes,' and Harrison had to admit that, 'notwithstanding the excesses into which my people ran, they nevertheless husbanded the negro's carcass with the severest economy, and stinted themselves to an allowance which made it last for many days.' On more than one occasion the crew tried to induce Harrison to eat a 'stake,' and he claimed that he consistently refused. 'Fearful,' he wrote, [that] 'if I closed my eyes they would surprize and murder me for their next supply, it is no wonder that I lost all relish for sustenance.'[12]

On the 29 January the crew told Harrison that it was once again necessary to draw lots, 'since it was better to die separately than all at once.' Harrison argued with them, advising prayer in place of further killing. The crew told him 'that they were now hungry and must have something to eat; and therefore it was no time to pray; and if I did not instantly consent to cast lots, they would instantly proceed without me.'[13] Harrison ordered the crew fetch pen and paper to his bedside, from where he supervized the drawing of the lots in 'the same manner as for a lottery at the Guild-hall.'[14] The victim chosen was David Flatt, a popular man, who Harrison described as the one remaining survivor 'on whom I could place any certain dependence.' 'The shock of the decision was great' and a profound silence fell.[15] However, Flatt appeared quite resigned. He asked that James Doud who despatched Wiltshire might also kill him, and that he be given the night to prepare himself. Flatt's bearing impressed all the men. Harrison was prevailed upon to lead prayers for the young man. He then retired to his cabin, leaving the crew to comfort Flatt, who during the night went 'deaf,' and was oblivious to the crew's assurances that 'something would mitigate the severity of his sentence.' There was some talk of sparing Flatt and killing Harrison.

At daybreak the delirious crew managed to attract the attention of a ship which had appeared on the horizon. They then proposed drinking a communal 'cann of joy,' a motion which Harrison refused on the grounds that the other ship might not take them on board if they were drunk. Nicholson, the mate, went below to initiate his own celebrations. The strange sail was the *Susannah*, Captain Evers, out of Virginia bound for London. Harrison recalled that, in the excitement of rescue, 'they almost forgot' to bring off Nicholson, who had been boozing down below. The *Susannah* reached Plymouth on 1 March 1766. David Flatt remained out of his senses. James Doud, Wiltshire's executioner, and the mate Archibald Nicholson had died *en route* to England. In all only three of the men who sailed on *Peggy* reached Plymouth alive and in their senses.

Although weak, Harrison was interviewed by the Governor of Plymouth, who treated him with 'remarkable civility.' Harrison travelled on to London with Captain Evers, stopping in Ramsgate, Evers' home town, where Harrison told his tale once more.[16] In London, Harrison was interviewed by the Lord Mayor, George Nelson, and he wrote and notarized a private account of the voyage, which he sent to New York to satisfy *Peggy*'s owners and insurers, before giving it out that he was to publish an account of his ordeal. *The Melancholy Narrative of the Distressful Voyage and Miraculous Deliverance of Captain David Harrison, of the Sloop Peggy* appeared in June 1766, and was heavily excerpted in British, and, in due course, American journals, newspapers, and anthologies.[17]

Against the unquantifiable authenticity of Harrison's *Melancholy Narrative* we can set one unimpeachable fact: very nearly every English-language newspaper in the North Atlantic basin offered its readers some account of Harrison's adventures.[18] On the other hand, while the case was widely reported, it attracted very little in the way of editorial comment. This broad but shallow coverage cannot be explained as a function of the sensational or unprecedented content of Harrison's story. Harrison's was not the first published account of the recourse to cannibalism to relieve famine and the casting of lots to choose 'a sacrifice for ravenous hunger to feed upon.'[19] Moreover, Harrison's narrative was not the only account of famine-induced cannibalism in circulation at the time it was published.[20] It was not uncommon for such cases to receive both wide attention and lengthy exegesis. Harrison's account does seem to have been the first published in English which admits to the murder of a living human as a means of creating 'food'. Hence the peculiarities of Harrison's narrative make the editorial silence which accompanied its dissemination all the more puzzling. The answer to this puzzle, which illuminates some of the difficulties attendant upon establishing, let alone utilizing, the polarity between savage and civilized in the case of actions undertaken by European sailors, lie in the manner in which Harrison's authorial intent, imperfectly realized, infuses the text.

Harrison wrote his narrative from a thoroughly 'civilized' perspective. 'It would look like a want of gratitude to the great disposer of all things,' he wrote, 'if I neglected to employ a few hours in the recital of some particulars where his Providence has been singularly manifested.'[21] The text attempts to depict Harrison as a victim of circumstance: one whose conduct met the dictates of piety, calling, and commerce. In Harrison's view, killing would have been unnecessary had not a wretch, who Harrison was too charitable to name, refused to aid the *Peggy*. Thereafter, Harrison had attempted first to prevent and then to control the commission of crime by abstaining from its fruits.

This self-portrait gained some degree of acceptance. For example, initial reports of the voyage in *Lloyd's Evening Post and British Chronicle* were buttressed by editorial interpolations reminding readers that Harrison had eaten no food of any kind for forty-two days and that the ghastly events aboard the *Peggy* were the fault of 'Captain B' who had withheld aid on 25 December.[22] Sympathy for Harrison's plight was a feature of very nearly all rehearsals of the voyages, even those which did not express the kind of confidence in Harrison's version of events shown in *Lloyd's Evening Post*. The one exception was the *Gentleman's Magazine*, which in June 1766 published a lengthy summary of the material contained in Harrison's *Melancholy Narrative* into which it interpolated sceptical editorial comment.

The *Gentleman's Magazine* was disturbed by a number of problems within the narrative. For example, the magazine faulted Harrison for not saying how he survived from 25 December to 17 January: 'we must suppose the dirty water and drops kept him alive.'[23] The precise periodization adopted by this editorial comment obliquely disputed Harrison's claim that he had eaten no part of the slave's 'meat.' The editors pointedly did not wonder how Harrison survived after the slave had been killed, that is after 17 January. Although it was prepared to admit that Harrison would have found it difficult to spare the life of the slave Wiltshire, (an admission which carried implications concerning Harrison's competency), the *Gentleman's Magazine* found fault with Harrison's refusal to advise on pickling the body. It noted with 'regret':

> that [Harrison] did not make the same effort to save the poor fellow's life, that he did to prevent the pickling of the body. The best thing he could have done when he was dead, was, to give such orders as might make the food, that was so dearly obtained, go as far as possible, that it might be longer before they were again urged by the same horrid necessity to commit another murder…[24]

Harrison, who had eaten the head of the ship's cat with 'indescribable relish' found Nicholson request for advice on pickling disgusting. Harrison's claim was that he respected the human body, indeed life itself. He invited his readers to compare his attitudes to those of the crew, particularly Archibald Nicholson's. Taking up this invitation, the *Gentleman's Magazine*, by arguing that Harrison should have intervened in the pickling process, implied that Nicholson and the crew had quite properly preserved 'food…dearly bought,' and hence obviated as much as possible the need for another killing. The implication was that Harrison's detachment was improper, and that he had failed to distinguish true barbarity from civilized, Christian, behavior.[25]

In 1711 Captain Jasper Dean found himself in unfortunate circumstances comparable to Harrison's. Like Harrison, Dean was reluctant to condone cannibalism. Unlike Harrison, Dean debated 'the lawfullness and sinfulness on the one hand, and absolute necessity on the other' before 'submitting to the prevailing arguments of our craving appetites.' Supported by the 'prayers and intreaties' of the crew, Dean, who opposed cannibalism, prepared the 'carcass' of the ship's carpenter by removing the skin, head, feet and bowels, quartering the remainder, and cutting, washing and drying thin strips of meat. Thereafter he controlled access to this 'food supply.'[26] These events did not escape the attention of the Puritan divine Cotton Mather, but, in Mather's exegesis, Captain Dean escaped censure.[27]

Of course the men on board the *Peggy* were contemplating the execution of a living human being rather than the consumption of one already dead. Harrison is at pains to point out that it was the crew, particularly Archibald Nicholson, who first proposed the drawing of lots. The crew used the argument that it was better that one die in order that the others might live, and that, if necessary, they should die separately rather than together. Harrison would have the reader believe that this was barbarous, but these were positions which had both direct and indirect Biblical support. The drawing of lots gave God's Providence the widest variety of possible interventions, and, although on the surface barbarous, could be instructive. In such a situation, each man, as he awaited the drawing of the lot, would have to consider whether he was 'deserving.'[28]

In other words, the *Peggy*'s crew's proposals may well have been sympathetically understood as legitimate. On the other hand, Harrison's response—shock followed by world-weary detachment—had far less standing within 'civilized' custom. Almost by his own admission Harrison had shown an imperfect grasp of the language, and law, of command. Control over provisions was absolutely central to the majesty of command, and maritime law clearly assigned responsibility for the control and distribution of food to commanders. As William Wellwood had it, in a seventeenth century abridgement of sea-law, the captain as the 'ordinary ruler' of his 'kippage and company' held the responsibility for keeping crew 'in peace as long as they eate his bread.' He was liable to be punished for negligence or sloth, 'especially' with regard to 'corn, victualls and such like goods.'[29] Huddled in the sternsheets of the *Bounty*'s launch, on the long voyage to Timor, that connoisseur of good captaincy, Captain William Bligh scribbled observations designed to impress upon future judges his own good seamanship. He congratulated himself on the rigor with which he controlled access to food. He wrote that his singular resolution, 'perhaps does not admit me to be a proper judge on a story of miserable people like us at last driven to the necessity of destroying one another for food, but if I may be allowed, I deny the fact in its greatest extreme.'[30]

Many readers of Harrison's narrative would have concluded that he was weak commander; the *Gentleman's Magazine* certainly implied as much. But this cannot account for the breadth of attention the narrative received, or the shallowness of commentary upon it. This is not a tale about mutiny or incompetence, it is fundamentally about cannibalism. My contention is that the events on board the *Peggy* became a cause celebre because journalists, editors, and readers believed that cannibalism had occurred while at the same time remaining largely unconvinced by Harrison's account of his actions. Harrison's account fascinated because it pointed to a much deeper and more subversive dereliction of duty and, indeed, called into question 'duty' itself.

Harrison's *Melancholy Narrative* is an account of failure and a failure as an account. In the narrowest 'sense it is describes the failure of an individual to prevent the commission of deeds which he claims to find almost unbearably distressing. More broadly, the narrative attempts to translate a failure of resolve into a triumph of piety. Several moments in the narrative undermine this endeavour. The most damaging concerns Harrison's account of the meeting with the potential rescue ship on 25 December. Much of Harrison's narrative hinges on this moment, and yet he admits that there might have been 'dexterity' in 'Captain B''s decision to 'cast off' the *Peggy*.[31] Why would it occur to Harrison that there might have been 'dexterity' in abandoning the *Peggy*? The men of the *Peggy* might have been at their most demoralized around 25 December, that is before they had eaten cat, dog, pigeon or man. The ship's cargo was liquor, upon which the crew were, apparently, reliant. When their eventual rescue ship, the Susannah, hove to, *Peggy's* mate, Archibald Nicholson, proposed that the men drink a 'cann of joy.' Harrison specifically notes that he opposed this motion because he believed that if the crew appeared drunk they might not be taken on board. On 25 December Harrison retired to his cabin and would not have been present to object had a similar motion been put to the crew. In any case, 25 December was a feast day, when even otherwise sober crews might drink to excess. In short, the unknown ship *Peggy* encountered on Christmas Day would have confronted a group of survivors who were, in all probability, drunk, desperate, and by Harrison's own admission, not under duly constituted authority. Apparently even Harrison thought it might have been 'dexterous' under the circumstances to refrain from introducing such a rabble into a healthy ship. But if readers adjudged Captain B's actions as a matter of debatable morality, they could not serve the purpose Harrison assigned them in the text. For it is Harrison's contention that there would have been no need of cannibalism had it not been for the refusal of the strange ship to aid the *Peggy*.

Even sympathetic commentary implicitly doubted Harrison's version of events here, by calling on him to name the ship and the captain. The *Gentleman's Magazine*, drawing on Harrison's own admission that there might have been 'dexterity' in the decision of Captain B not to aid the *Peggy*, went further. It denounced Harrison's refusal to name Captain B in language which is worth quoting at length:

> Captain Harrison, from some principle which he thinks laudable, and upon which, therefore, it is laudable in him to act, has suppressed the name of the man by whom he was treated with unprovoked and unrelenting barbarity. But, surely, to screen such a wretch from universal detestation and infamy, a punishment by no means disproportionate to his crime, except that it should have been greater, if greater could have been inflicted, has a tendency directly contrary to all laws and institutions that have been made by the wisest and best of mankind, for the benefit of society. We are, indeed, commanded to *love our enemies, and to do good to those that hate us and despitefully use us*. But this injunction taken literally would operate directly contrary to the spirit and intention of Christianity by precluding all punishment, and, consequently, encouraging every species of wickedness by which human nature can be made infamous or miserable. Not to punish the guilty, except where there are alleviating circumstances, which would make '*right too rigid harden into wrong*' is eventually the worst cruelty, and the most flagitious misjustice. It is cruelty to forgive a murderer, because it is laying another bosom open to the knife, and encouraging another hand to strike. It is also unjust, because it is withholding from society a benefit which it has a right to claim for every individual, as far as the individual has power to bestow it. It is therefore to be hoped, that for the sake equally of justice and mercy, to deter others from contracting the same guilt, and preserve others from being deserted in the same distress, that Captain Harrison will hang up at least the name of this offender, lest after suffering by his barbarity, he should be deemed, in some sense, a partner of his crime.[32]

Why was the *Gentleman's Magazine* the only periodical to damn any part of Harrison's narrative in such terms? Why did this journal reserve its fiercest condemnation for what might be considered a comparatively minor moment in the text?

In its account of the last night spent aboard the *Peggy* before rescue, the narrative scores its one tremendous success: an effect so powerful as to account for its widespread dissemination. By the very omissions in the narrative, Harrison invites the reader to contemplate, and reject, a ghastly chain of logic.

Two people were condemned to death on board the *Peggy* and both of them were connected to the captain. Harrison wants to the reader to see this as evidence of how personally distressing the voyage must have been for him. Yet Harrison is open to suspicion as a man who possibly hoards food rather than share it, who sanctimoniously tries to dissuade the crew from indulging in a desperate but time-honored and 'civilized' strategy for survival, and then, by sins of omission and perhaps commission, secures the death of precisely those two men who he is most duty-bound to protect—the slave Wiltshire and loyal David Flatt. He hints that the crew behaved barbarously toward Flatt by insisting that his life be forfeit, but it is the crew who attempt to comfort the unfortunate sailor. When Flatt falls 'deaf,' Harrison's response is a rather callous sense of expectation met, coupled with the fear that the crew might now kill him in Flatt's place. (The reader can almost hear Harrison's train of thought: if 'they' refused to eat Campbell because Campbell was mad, now that Flatt's reason was tottering they pass up their intended victim in favour of more trustworthy 'meat'.) Can the reader help but reflect on the justice of these fears? If Harrison had acted 'properly' the crew would not have thought of substituting him for Flatt. Harrison has shown himself to be ineffectual, uncooperative, and possibly actively duplicitous. He has, in a craven and cowardly fashion, sacrificed men towards whom he had unusual obligations to placate a crew for whom he has no respect, and in whose eyes he has no authority. Harrison, to cite the language of denunciation developed in the *Gentleman's Magazine*, is a monster liable to expose bosoms to knives. He has cheated a Georgian public of the exemplary punishment afforded criminals. Within this logic, if the crew had to make some assessment guided by rationality and morality of who among them had to die that the others might live, Harrison's name, almost by his own account, would at the top of the list. He deserved to receive the ultimate in vengeance. He deserved to be eaten, that more efficient and rational members of the crew might survive and save the ship and its cargo.

We might argue that very few eighteenth century readers would have followed this chain of logic to its end. However, that is precisely my point. Each link in the logical chain outlined (or travestied) in the preceding paragraph was implicitly or explicitly available for readers. Readers were directed, implicitly by Harrison, and explicitly by editors, down this logical road. Doubts were expressed about some or most of Harrison's conduct. His conduct was violently censured. But my point is that, whether by design or accident, by inviting the reader to speculate on his feelings on the eve of a second murder, by placing the reader in his shaking shoes, Harrison ultimately secures a validation of his conduct because he plays on fear of being eaten 'unjustly': he trades on fear of savage cannibalism. Parts of Harrison's conduct might be reprehended but no comment was made on the whole. Why? Because the subtext of the narrative runs: 'suppose, dear reader, I was a weak man, suppose my crew were more rational, were better seamen, did I deserve to be killed and eaten by them against my will?' Harrison's narrative set two notions of rationality and justice against one another. It asked contemporary audiences, (and answered for them), the question 'what punishment is worse than hanging?' That was why it was distressing—and reprinted.

To return briefly to my starting point. Harrison's narrative was published in the context of a continuing American and European rediscovery of savagery and Cannibalism. Even when Enlightenment-inspired English language accounts of 'savage cannibals' 'explained' to readers that Cannibalism proceeded from motives of vengeance and deterrence, rather than from that taste from human flesh attributed to monstrous races, their general effect was to argue for the rationality of the civilized North Atlantic peoples. If Maoris had reasons for eating people, then Europeans could have none outside pathology. The English legal code might be vengeful, but, unlike the Maori, it could be amended from within. Other accounts of 'civilized' cannibalism were circulated in the aftermath of Harrison's admission that 'civilized' people could, and had, killed humans to eat. Where such accounts describe events on land they seem, by stressing the fears of the weak, to uniformly lead the reader to assume pathology on the part of the strong.[33] The strong, wrongly, eat the weak. But maritime distress was a setting which resisted the attribution of barbarity and inhuman pathology to the custodians and beneficiaries of progress, even and especially in circumstances of extreme material crisis. Until 1892, a man could admit to surviving shipwreck by killing a crewmate without fear of legal proceedings. This is because even, or especially, within the citadel of rationality—sailing lore—the polarity between civilized and savage was unstable.

Notes

1.   'The Memoirs of John Elliott', in Christine Holmes (ed.), *Captain Cook's Second Voyage: The Journals of Lieutenants Elliott and Pickersgill*, (London, Dover NH: Caliban Books, 1984), p. 22.

2.   Michel de Certeau, *Heterologies: Discourse on the Other* (trans. Brian Massumi; Manchester: Manchester University Press, 1986), esp. chap. 5.

3.   *New York Mercury,* 22 July 1765; *Weyman's New-York Gazette,* 22 July 1765.

4.   David Harrison, *The Melancholy Narrative of the Distressful Voyage and Miraculous Deliverance of Captain David Harrison of the Sloop Peggy* (London, 1766). Harrison's narrative is hereafter cited in short form as *Melancholy*.

5   *Melancholy*, pp. 9, 10.

6.   *Melancholy*, pp. 11, 15. Harrison seems to have brokered the deal with Captain B.

7.   An article in the *London Evening Post*, 18-20 March 1766, which appeared after Harrison's story had broken, gave out the 'further information' that Harrison had named the commander 'Captain B.'

8.   Harrison, *Melancholy*, p. 22. This reaction to the exhaustion of tobacco supplies may have had roots in custom. For example, John Nicholl, in similar circumstances praised tobacco, 'which did nothing at all nourish us; yet it tooke away the desire of hunger,and

saved us from eating one another', John Nicholl, *A Houre Glasse of Indian Newes* (London, 1607), p. 26.

9.   *Melancholy*, p. 22.

10.   *Melancholy*, pp. 23-24. *The London Magazine* has Harrison reflecting 'I was by no means able to repel force by force' at this point, June 1766, p. 316.

11.   *Melancholy*, p. 25.

12.   *Melancholy*, pp. 25-26.

13.   *Melancholy*, pp. 27-29.

14.   *Melancholy*, p. 30.

15.   *Melancholy*, pp. 30-31.

16.   For early, bald, accounts of Harrison's voyage written by correspondents in Plymouth see *Lloyd's Evening Post and British Chronicle*, 19-21 March 1766; *London Evening Post*, 11-17 March 1766. Notices appeared also in the *Public Advertiser*, 14 March 1766; *St. James Chronicle*, 18-20 March 1766.

17.   Harrison's case was briefly noted in *Lloyd's Evening Post and British Chronicle*, 19 March 1766; *London Evening-Post*, 18 March 1766; *St. James's Chronicle*, 18 March 1766; *Public Advertiser*, 14 March 1766; *Pennsylvania Journal*, 22 May 1766, *Maryland Gazette*, 29 May 1766. Indications of the dissemination of the narrative: in June 1766 excerpts were offered in the *London Magazine*, pp. 315-18, *Gentleman's Magazine*, pp. 265-69, and *Annual Register*. The narrative was lengthily summarised in *Maryland Gazette*, 12 June 1766; *Virginia Gazette*, 6 June 1766; *Providence Gazette*, 20 September 1766; *Georgia Gazette*, 29 October 1766. For examples of Harrison's appearance in subsequent anthologies, see, [Charles Garnier] *Voyages imaginaires, romanesques, merveilleux, allegoriques, amusans, comiques et critiques. Suivis des songes et visions et des romans cabalistiques*, (22 vols.; Amsterdam, 1787), see esp. vol. 13; Anon. [Matthew Carey], *Narratives of Calamitous and Interesting Shipwrecks; With Authentic Particulars of the Sufferings of the Crews* (Philadelphia: A. Small, 1810); James Stanier Clarke, *Naufragia; or, Historical Memoirs of Shipwrecks, and the Providential Deliverance of Vessels* (2 vols.; London: J. Mawman, 1805); Archibald Duncan, *The Mariner's Chronicle. Being a Collection of Narratives of Shipwrecks, Fires, Famines, etc.* (4 vols.; Philadelphia, 1806). Edgar Allen Poe drew on Harrison's account in *The Narrative of Arthur Gordon Pym*.

18.   The possibility that the narrative was a Grub Street invention cannot be discounted, but the fact that the New York newspapers noted the *Peggy's* departure, and that neither the British Consul nor the Lord Mayor of London denied meeting Harrison suggests otherwise. As will become clear, this essay does not take Harrison's narrative as being accurate in every respect.

19.   James Janeway, *Mr. James Janeway's Legacy to his Friends: Containing Twenty-Seven Instances of God's Providence in and about Sea-Dangers* (London, 1675), pp. 1-9, citation 3, *passim*; 'Shipwreck Suffered by Jorge D'Albuquerque Coelho Captain and Governor of Pernambuco,' in C.R. Boxer (ed.), *Further Selections from the Tragic History of the Sea* (London: Cambridge University Press, 1968), esp. 147-48; Nicholl, *An Hour Glass of Indian Newes*, *passim*. Harrison was not the first commander to directly attest to 'civilized' sailors committing cannibalism. In 1711, Captain Dean of the *Nottingham Galley* described in print how members of his crew had resorted to eating human flesh to survive famine caused by shipwreck. See John Dean, Jasper Dean, and Miles Whitworth, *A Sad and Deplorable, but True Account of the Dreadful Hardships and Sufferings of Captain John Dean and his Company* (London, 1711). It is significant that some of the surviving crew members disputed their captain's construction of events and published their own account, [Christopher Langman], *A True Account of the Voyage of the Nottingham Galley* (London 1711).

20.   In 1764 the snow *Eagle*, out of Antigua, capsized and turned turtle in the Atlantic.

After three days the ship's carpenter died. The remaining survivors removed the entrails from the body and ate its 'meat'. This incident was reported in the *Georgia Gazette*, 15 November 1764; *Pennsylvania Gazette*, 15 November 1764; *Weyman's New-York Gazette*, 19 November 1764; *Boston Post-Boy*, 26 November 1764; *North Carolina Magazine or Universal Intelligencer*, 30 November 1764; *Providence Gazette*, 8 December 1764. In the spring of 1766, Harrison's narrative would have competed for space in American newspapers with accounts of events on board an unnamed sloop commanded by a Captain Jones. The sloop, carrying slaves, was battered into a wreck. The crew, 'in want of provisions,' 'were put to the necessity of eating one of the dead negro children, which so exasperated the negroes on board that they fell upon the crew.' For reports see *Pennsylvania Journal*, 1 May 1766; *Newport Mercury*, 5 May 1766; *Pennsylvania Gazette*, 8 May 1766; *Weyman's New-York Gazette*, 12 May 1766; *Virginia Gazette*, 23 May 1766. In 1767 newspapers on both sides of the Atlantic detailed the wreck of the French frigate Modeste whose captain, Jules Guyet, claimed he successfully dissuaded his crew from cannibalism, and the loss of the *Fanny*, under Captain Henderson, whose crew did commit cannibalism. On the Modeste see *Providence Gazette*, 7 February 1767, 6 March 1767; *Weyman's New-York Gazette*, 12 January 1767; *Public Advertiser*, 6 November 1766; *Annual Register, 'Chronology'*, 1766; *St. James's Chronicle*, 1 November 1766. For reports of the *Fanny* see *Providence Gazette*, 4 July 1767; *Public Advertiser*, 9 July 1767; *Annual Register*, June 1767, p. 105; *Pennsylvania Gazette*, 18 June 1767.

21.   *Melancholy*, pp. 1-2.
22.   *Lloyd's Evening Post and British Chronicle*, 19-21 March 1766.
23.   *Gentleman's Magazine*, June 1766, p. 267.
24.   *Gentleman's Magazine*, June 1766, p. 267.
25.   Harrison's account of the crew's drunkenness is equally unsatisfactory. He was 'concerned' by the 'continual course of execration and blasphemy' which accompanied their drinking, *Melancholy*, p. 10. But in describing how he developed an aversion to wine, he once again leaves himself open to a charge of inappropriate squeamishness. Harrison: 'imbibed the strongest aversion imaginable to wine; the complicated disorders under which I laboured induced me to abstain from it at first, and as the men were perpetually heating it in the steerage the smell of it became so offensive to the last degree; so that I subsisted entirely on the dirty water which [the crew] had forsaken, half a pint of which, together with a few drops of Turlington's Balsam being my whole allowance for four and twenty hours.' *Melancholy*, p. 18. Why were the crew perpetually heating wine if not to reduce its alcohol content? What was this 'dirty water' if not urine, or bilge contaminated from the heads?

    On the employment of urine, Phillip Hanger, adrift in a dinghy for over three weeks, pissed in his shoe and drank his urine when cool. He thought it much healthier than sea-water. He also noted that many of the sailors would not follow his example and drank sea-water even though it quickly led to 'distemper.' Phillip Hanger, *A True Relation How Eighteen Men were Castaway at Sea* (London, 1675), p. 6. See also *A Narrative of the Marvellous Escape of Captain Inglefield, and his Pinnace Crew, after Quitting her Majesty's Ship Centaur* (London, 1783), and descriptions of the wreck of the *Fanny*, *Public Advertiser*, 9 July 1767; *Providence Gazette*, 4 July 1767.

26.   [Jasper Dean?], *A Narrative of the Sufferings, Preservation and Deliverance of Captain John Dean* (London, 1722).
27.   'An affecting story,' Mather wrote, 'capable of being improved unto many purposes of piety.' Mather drew out some of the implications for mariners: ' were you in favour with God, what a friend would you have! A friend who can rescue you in the worst and last extremities…a friend who can turn your disasters into benefits.' 'The Great God,' he continued, 'can pursue you with his horrible temper. He can starve you to death in a ship laden

with provisions. He can sink the strongest vessel in the ocean…Yea, he can burn you in the midst of the water!' Cotton Mather, *Compassions Called For. An Essay of Profitable Reflections on Miserable Spectacles* (Boston, 1711), pp. 58, 60.

28.   The biblical support was adduced from Jonah and John II. For an example of the instructive interpretation of lot-drawing see the tale of Major Gibbons in *Mr. James Janeway's Legacy to his Friends*, pp. 1-9, esp. pp. 4-5. See also Increase Mather's recitation of Gibbons' tale, *An Essay for the Recovery of Illustrious Providences* (Boston, 1684), pp. 15-16.

29.   William Wellwood, *An Abridgement of All Sea-Lawes* (London, 1636), pp. 86-87, 99. See also Marcus Rediker, *Between the Devil and the Deep Blue Sea: Merchant Seamen, Pirates, and the Anglo-American World, 1700-1750* (Cambridge: Cambridge University Press, 1987), esp. pp. 222-23. (A cynical reader might have construed Harrison's reluctance to participate in the lottery as an indication that the *Peggy's* starving crew were not eating of Harrison's bread.) On the qualities of command see Greg Dening, *Mr. Bligh's Bad Language: Passion, Power and Theatre on the Bounty* (Cambridge: Cambridge University Press, 1992), esp. pp. 101-105. Castaway aboard the *Bounty's* launch, determined to show his qualifications for command, Captain Bligh returned again and again to the rigour with which kept control of the distribution of rations. 'My situation,' he wrote, 'became burthened with more than mere bodily distresses, for besides what will readily be believed (with respect to me) such as directing and pointing out the route we were to go, I had to oblige every one to drag on a lingering life with a miserable allowance of support, and to find repeatedly the melancholy request of "give us more bread" combatting a neccessary resolution of refusal. This I so sacredly stuck to that I brought eleven days allowance in with me…' Owen Rutter (ed.), *The Log of the Bounty* (2 vols.; London: Golden Cockrell Press, 1937), II, p. 207.

30.   *The Log of the Bounty*, II, p. 229.

31.   Harrison concluded his description of the *Peggy's* encounter with the unknown ship thus:

> the inexorable captain pursued his course without regarding us, and steel'd,
> as he undoubtedly must be, to every sentiment of nature and humanity,
> possibly valued himself not a little upon his dexterity in casting us off.

Melancholy, pp. 14-15. Elsewhere Harrison states that the ship's were only within hailing distance. Is 'cast off' metaphorical here, or were the ships in fact briefly roped together?

32.   *Gentleman's Magazine*, June 1766, p. 266. [Emphases in original].

33.   'The Man Eater', *New York Weekly Museum*, 31 March 1792, is a gruesome example wherein one Janvier, a trapper, preys upon snowed-in cabin-mates. See also the story of eight men who escaped from Maquarie Harbour, Tasmania in 1822, Robert Hughes, *The Fatal Shore* (New York: Knopf, 1986), pp. 219-26. For an example of this gloss being applied to cases at sea, see descriptions of the wreck of the *Morris*. Its survivors spent 32 days in distress, during 'the latter part of which they were so reduced that any one of them was afraid to go to sleep for fear they should fall sacrifice to the pinching wants and necessities of the others,' *Pennsylvania Gazette*, 4 January 1783.

Radicals and Reformers

Louis J. Kern

'STUDENTS IN THE LABORATORIES OF THEIR OWN BODIES': THE (RE)CONSTRUCTION OF MALE SEXUALITY AND THE MALE SEXUAL BODY IN VICTORIAN FREE LOVE LITERATURE

> For out of the strife which woman
> Is passing through today,
> A man that is more than human
> Shall yet be born, I say;
> A man in whose pure spirit
> No dross of self will lurk,
> A man who is strong to cope with wrong
> A man who is proud to work.
> A man with hope undaunted,
> A man with god-like power
> Shall come when he is most wanted,
> Shall come at the needed hour.

> Ella Wheeler Wilcox, *The Coming Man* (1894)

> That the Woman Question involves the Man Question, or the human
> race question, is demonstrably true, since without women there would
> be no man.

> Moses Harman, *Plain Words on the Woman Question* (1901)

1. Free Love and the Movement from Private to Public Discourses on Sexuality

Advocates of free love in late-nineteenth-century America provided the radical voices in the Victorian discourse on sex and sexuality. If, as Michel Foucault has argued for an earlier historical period, the dominant voices in the dialectic of sex constructed the 'economy of pleasures' through an 'objectification of the sexual relations' (and specifically of the conjugal relation) that 'continued to leave the question of conjugal sex in the shadows',[1] free lovers challenged the conventional silences on the physical and emotional experiences of sex and problematized the pleasure-power nexus. While they sought to extend the boundaries of what it was possible to say about sex in a public forum, free lovers saw an expanded sexual discourse as a means to social regeneration. The goal of sex radicals was a simultaneous liberation of instinct coupled with the management of sexual behavior that sought to offset self-fulfillment with self-renunciation. The discursive production of the free lovers linked unprecedented freedom of emotional expression with an unorthodox rationale for a reenforced regulation of sexual behavior in a strategy for 'constituting oneself as the ethical subject of one's sexual behavior'.[2]

In his treatise on 'scientific propagation', John Humphrey Noyes (1811-86), founder of the Oneida Community and one of the most daring popular sexologists of his day, made clear both the challenge posed by free love theory to conventional social and moral sensibilities and its fundamentally ethical and reformatory objectives. In all aspects of the consideration of marriage, sexual intercourse, conception, and childbirth, he argued, 'discussion ought to be set free', with the end of the 'radical improvement of humanity'[3] in prospect. Alternative medical practitioners, like Marx Edgeworth Lazarus and Thomas Low Nichols, cast the regenerative function of free love in a more secular and political light, arguing that it represented a new revolution that would fulfill the promise ('pursuit of happiness') of the American Revolution, a revolution of 'Passional and Social Liberty'.[4] But moral free lovers realized that the subtextual voices of both conventional monogamy and counter-cultural free love sustained male domination in the social, political, and economic spheres and validated male lust. Free love discourse, therefore, was consciously framed to appeal only to those seriously interested in a social-scientific experiment in sexual practice as a means to social reformation; it explicitly sought to exclude profligate male libertines by prescribing the disciplining of sex as a prerequisite to the practice of free love. John H. Noyes acknowledged this limitation on free love discourse when he noted that although his pamphlet *Male Continence* (1866) had been issued in four editions by 1872, distribution had remained private—copies were sent only upon the receipt of a personal request. He had avoided a widespread public discussion of his unusual sexual system, he tells us, out of 'the fear that bad men might avail themselves of our sexual theories for licentious purposes'.[5]

The physiology and hygiene of sex were volatile subjects in Victorian America, and even more ostensibly technical and scientific expressions of free love ideas, like Thomas Low Nichols' *Esoteric Anthropology* (1853) had to adopt a rhetorical strategy of indirection. Remarkably, in the preface to this aptly titled work, Nichols declared that 'I have no public'. The book was not offered for sale through any bookseller, but was available on a 'private and confidential' basis to individual subscribers. 'This is', he concluded, 'no book for the center-table, the library shelf or the counter of a bookstore. As the name imports, it is a *private treatise* on the most interesting and important subjects.'[6] The context of free love discourse, for Nichols, then, was 'a STRICTLY CONFIDENTIAL PROFESSIONAL CONSULTATION BETWEEN PHYSICIAN AND PATIENT, in which the latter wishes to know all that can be of use to him, and all that the former is able and willing to teach'.[7]

Even in the more public forum of the lecture hall, the fiction of an individual professional consultation was preserved. The sex education and physiology training that Mrs. Orson S. Fowler (widow of the 'Practical Phrenologist', who had written on 'Love, its Laws [and] Power') provided an audience restricted to 'men only' in the Music Hall in Boston in 1901 is a case in point. The quite literal *ad hominem* direction of her remarks clearly underscores the focus of much free love literature and discourse on male sexual behavior, its impact on individual women, and its role in the spread of social corruption. Mrs. Fowler succinctly demonstrated to her auditors how destructive unbridled male passion was, even within the bounds of traditional monogamy, and concluded that 'ignorant and ungoverned passion destroys the health and happiness of wives and causes them to become the mothers of imbeciles and criminals, defeating also the selfish enjoyment of the ignorant and recklessly irresponsible husband'.[8]

Male free lovers were acutely aware of the irresponsibility of male sexual desire, which they tended to identify with what they considered the unnatural practices of exclusive monogamy; but they were also conscious (and their opponents left them no chance to forget) that their own preference for 'varietism' (a plurality of sex partners), while often maintained only on a theoretical level, left them open to charges that free love was merely a flashy new sartorial disguise for the coarsely fleshy old body of masculine lust. They were scrupulously careful, therefore, in differentiating their form of sex radicalism from conventional monogamy and institutional repression on the one hand and polygamy and libertinage on the other. In his analysis of the sex problem of the age, Thomas Low Nichols found its seat in the 'civilized' sex relations as practiced under monogamy. He saw monogamy as the most dangerous social disease, which, from one perspective, 'makes men and women sick, by amative exhaustion, far more exhausting when divorced from love', and from another, through its suppression of the natural sexual instincts, 'fails to provide for the wants of thousands; more, it interposes insuperable barriers. It is thus a violation of the laws of nature; a crime of so grave a nature as to demand universal reform'.[9]

But polygamy, the institutional marital form that apparently stood diametrically opposed to monogamy, was, if anything, even more obnoxious to free lovers. Ezra Heywood (1829-90) reprinted in his journal *The Word*, under the title 'The Opposition —The Claims of Polygamy', an article by Brigham Young maintaining the moral and physiological superiority of polygyny. From Heywood's point of view, the Mormon patriarch had accurately diagnosed the evils of legalized monogamy, but had established an even more immoral alternative—sacramental polygyny. Young's argument is worth quoting at length since it serves as a boundary marker to help us position free lovers along the spectrum of the contemporary discourse. Legal monogamy, he argued,

> virtually invests the husband with the control of the wife, sexually, as well as otherwise,[and] is a great outrage upon the wife, since it frequently so happens that a man of large amativeness is married to a woman in whom it is almost wanting ...She finds herself legally bound to a man whose sexual demands her constitution cannot stand, and she gradually sinks into a hopeless decline, unless the husband recognizes the condition and resorts to prostitution to save her...[But polygamy] recognizes that there are different sexual natures and provides for them. In polygamy no wife is ever known to suffer from the sexual abuse of her husband, while in monogamy it prevails everywhere; indeed is the curse which is rapidly settling over the race like mildew.[10]

Unlike radical male free love advocates, who typically sided with the abused female trapped in a legalized sexual servitude, Young clearly identified with the sexually frustrated male, and had created a system of sexual relations that eliminated any need for the male to control the expression of his sexual drive or to forgo sexual gratification out of consideration for his wife's health. Basing his system on the widely accepted notion that the sexual needs of males and females were widely disparate, Young upheld a form of plural marriage that suited its practice to male needs.

From a free love point of view, such polygamy was male sexual domination writ large; it remained deaf to the needs of women as well as blind to their social and ethical value in the sexual sphere. As practical sexologists, free lovers saw women as victims, trapped between the physical limitations of gender demographics and the institutional restrictions on sexual intercourse. In both instances, they identified strict monogamy as the primary cause of the physical suffering and emotional privation they saw as characteristic of conventional sexuality. As Thomas Low Nichols put it, 'one of the hideous evils of our marriage system is the unnatural celibacy that it forces upon vast numbers'. According to the census of 1850, there were nearly twice as many women as men in the state of Massachusetts which, Nichols argued, 'condemned' thousands to 'perpetual celibacy—to the starvation and immolation of the affections—the deprivation of all the happiness connected with love, and to all the miseries of its deprivation'.[11]

And yet, was not such erotic desiccation preferable, for woman, to the vulgar brutalities she must endure in legalized marriage? Nichols certainly thought so, and expressed the pervasive sense of revulsion free lovers felt towards institutionalized marriage by analogizing it to socially condoned sexual violation. 'The crime of RAPE, or forcible violation', he argued, 'comes of the repressions and false conditions of civilization, and is one of its common brutalities.' Rape outside marriage, he maintained, was much less common than conjugal rape, and the law provided severe penalties for the ravishment of unmarried women. But 'when a few words have been said by the priest, not only does the law justify the outrage, but she [the wife] is severely blamed by a virtuous society for not submitting to the man, to whom her person, her whole being forever belongs!'[12]

Apart from its tyrannical legal enslavement of the female sexual body and its consequent oppression of the female spirit, free lovers believed traditional marriage was both uncivilized and unhealthy. Social reform and the progress of the race demanded the suppression of 'civilized' marriage. Writing in 1882, and echoing the words of the 1860 Republican Party platform, Ezra Heywood declared that his pamphlet *Cupid's Yokes* (1876) 'still lives to demand the abolition of that *relic of male barbarism*, Marriage, and [to] inculcate New Morality, a new Social Faith coincident with the highest teachings of Science and sanctioned by the wisest exponents of Spiritual Intelligence'.[13] A correspondent to Moses Harman's *Lucifer* underscored the social and biological retrogression inherent in conventional conjugal relations. Under the heading 'Save the Mothers', the writer maintained that

> there is no female brute on the face of the earth that is so abused by their [sic] mates as thousands and millions of wives are by their husbands, who

professed to love them and be kind to them after marriage and then,
when the knot was tied, falsified their promise and made them victims
of sexual abuse. There are no brutes on the face of the earth that can
commit that crime on their females.[14]

The best that could be said of 'civilized' marriage, from the perspective of the sex radicals, was that it hopelessly confused the social and economic processes of production with the biological and social imperatives of reproduction. T.L. Nichols, for example, stated the problem in sociological terms. Among middle class women, offsetting the sexual abuse of the married state, their revenge for unremittent physical servitude was their negative drain on the sum of familial economic productivity. By imprisoning women within the sphere of the home, men made them into 'toys of luxury', engines of relentless consumption that, for Nichols at least, were 'expensive, luxurious…extravagant and useless'.[15] In a kind of inverted Marxism, males became the primary means of production, servicing women's economic compulsion to consume; the average husband in this reductionist, functional model of matrimony becoming a romanticized wage slave, 'a mere money-making machine, on whose round of toil there never falls one ray of happiness'.[16]

Conversely, the radical approach to sexuality also maintained that the same unnatural, mechanistic quality of 'civilized' sexual relations reduced women, in their emotional lives, to sex slaves. R.T. Trall, in his physiological analysis of contemporary society, emphasized the pathologies of conventional sexual relations. 'In the sensuous world around us', he wrote, '…no propensity is more abused and abnormal, as the world is now constituted, than that of amativeness, and as sexual intercourse has become in married life, with most persons, a habit to be indulged whenever the man feels the inclination, it follows that women must be degraded to a mere machine in all that pertains to her highest interests and holiest aspirations.'[17]

The radical critique of mainstream Victorian sexual practice, then, stressed its dehumanization of both sexes, its repression of instinctual life, its starvation of the emotional needs, and its legitimation of the abuse of women. It saw monogamic marriage as unnatural and deviant, not from the point of view of established social institutions, but from the higher standpoint of the biological, physiological, and psychological requirements of the human race. Social redemption could only come about through a thoroughgoing reformation of sexual morality that would provide the foundation for 'a true union of the sexes'.[18] Social redemption was synonymous with sexual redemption. Only the pruriency of a perverted society vulgarly attributed such negative connotative terms as 'animal passions', 'lower propensities', and 'brutal lusts' to the natural emotional needs of men and women. It was not the sexual instincts themselves, but the abuses attendant upon their repression that constituted the true 'social problem'. Prostitution and the sensuous excesses that stained the marriage bed would, it was argued, 'almost entirely disappear if proper attention were paid to the physiological education of the young'.[19] Indeed, the primary burden of much of free love literature was sex education.

In the period after 1873, all of the most outspoken sex radicals were the targets of censorship campaigns, and many ran afoul of the notorious defender of public decency, Anthony Comstock. The pages of free love periodicals are filled with reports of those who were persecuted and prosecuted on account of the frankness of their discussion of sexual matters. Their denunciations of a society that condoned Comstockery were understandably bitter. Perhaps no victim of organized prudery expressed his reaction more powerfully and confrontationally than physical culturist Bernarr Macfadden. In a 1900 editorial, he proclaimed that 'Prudes are Criminals!'

> Not against the laws of pigmy man, but against the laws of Nature, against the laws of God. To them the body is something vulgar, not to be mentioned...They live in this atmosphere of impurity and narrowness. It stamps its influence upon their features. They have no mind or opinions of their own. Their standard is based on what Mr. or Mrs. So-and-so will think, not upon a clear comprehension of what they consider to be right or wrong. They go through life mental and physical slaves. Their children are taught what a shameful thing the body is. They grow up with these perverted, narrow ideas, and must often wonder how a pure mind can possibly exist in such a vulgar habitation. All this is a perversion of the natural, and is criminal in character.[20]

The key to the liberation of erotic life, then, was the reconstruction of social attitudes towards the body. Given their conclusions about the depraved and diseased state of conventional sexual relations as well as their acceptance of certain pervasive popular truisms about sexual physiology, it is not surprising that free love advocates came to focus on the male sexual body as the locus for the transformation of sexuality. They became students of the psychology and physiology of male sexuality in order to establish a basis for the redemption of the individual male body and thereby for the collective transformation of society. The inquisition of the male sexual body problematized male sexual dominion and inaugurated a discursive strategy that simultaneously legitimated the ventilation of sexual frustrations and grievances and valorized liberationist sexuality.

2. The (Re)construction and Inquisition of the Male Sexual Body

The radical construction of the male sexual body was grounded in a thoroughly conventional understanding of sexual physiology. Free lovers routinely accepted the proposition that males had a more powerful sex drive than females; that, as Thomas L. Nichols put it, a 'powerful desire for the sexual union [is] active in most men', whereas 'most women are capable of sentimental love; few in this country are controlled by passion, and a vast majority, never feel the sexual desire as a controlling motive; perhaps we may say with truth that a large proportion never feel it at all.[21] Ezra Heywood problematized male sexuality for sexual liberals, arguing that 'man's love is naturally ferocious', is pervaded by a 'consuming passional heat' and too often manifests itself in 'the repulsive evidences of sexual depravity in men [that] indicate the savage use, now made of animal force, which is capable of beneficent expenditure'.[22]

The unique burden of the male sexual body lay in the physical imperative of male lust. And that imperative rested on fundamental male physical and psychological differences from the female. Following the lead of phrenology, that located the sex drive, 'amativeness', in the cerebellum, Victorian sexology maintained that, under the influence of external stimuli, 'the organ of amativeness stimulates the action of the secreting or sperm, producing organs, the testicles. The presence of the seminal fluid in the seminal vesicles reacts upon the brain, and the mind glows with voluptuous ideas.'[23] Although a similar link between the mind and body operated in the female system, the libidinous forces were more potent in the male body for two reasons. First, in regard to their respective generative functions, the male is physically constituted differently from the female. In the male, from the onset of puberty, the 'action of the testes is uninterrupted. Whatever restraints he may have must be moral for they are not, physiological, like woman's.'[24] Then, too, the female cerebellum, the seat of amativeness, is 'always smaller than [in] the male'.[25]

Sexual conservatives concluded from these premises that male sexual desire was an irresistible force that could only be regulated by institutional restraint, but radicals rejected this conclusion as pernicious and defeatist. They contested the notion that there was any natural 'law' of male 'physical necessity', and saw the impressment of women into sexual service as a marital duty as a gross imposition of a male 'monster of lust, who profanes her life with disgusting debaucheries'.[26] Male free lovers tended to identify with the female victim of selfish and reckless husbands, and the pages of their publications are replete with illustrative tales of the inhuman brutality of unchecked male sexuality. One example will suffice. Ezra Heywood reprinted, under the heading 'Tyranny of Lust', an account of one woman's marital adversity. Speaking of her former husband, she cried,

> Oh!...[his] death is such a relief, he was so amative; I could never talk to him on any subject, or lie one moment in the morning, without his becoming excited. I submitted to it all, because I thought...it a woman's duty to submit to what I conceived to be man's right. When I think of my suffering during child-bearing and nursing, when I look on a life of force and violation, I must say...[his] death was a relief.[27]

Despite an unequivocal sympathy for the female and a reprehension of such erotomaniacal husbands, free lovers remained conflicted about the male sexual body. Their attitudes towards the penis and the generative organs suggest an ambiguity about male sexuality, a simultaneous awe and dread of masculine potency. In his physiological discussion of the 'Male Organs of Generation', for instance, Thomas T. Nichols writes: 'The penis is, in many respects, a remarkable organ.' It is, in the transition to the erectile state, almost autonomous, since 'the change from one state to another occurs in a moment, at a word, a thought, or a touch'.[28] The analogous female organ, the clitoris, is described by Nichols as 'a miniature, imperfect penis, capable of erection', but female sexual responses is not on such a hair trigger as that of the male.[29] There is a remarkable discussion in Ezra Heywood's *Free Speech* (1883), in which he finds the source of all religions in the synecdochical use of the symbolic representation of the sexual organs to represent the creative power. There is, however, a significant difference in the figurative resonance of the male and female organs. The female organs were revered as symbols of generative power, i.e., were maternally encoded; while the male organs, for Heywood, were as intimately as possible linked with the godhead—divine paternal connection. 'The idea of the Trinity', he asserts, 'originated in the same way, the male privy member and the adjacent right and left testes making the triad or triune Creator, the penis.'[30]

Though the superordination of the male sexual body in a cultural as well as a physiological sense is clearly reflected in these passages, it is equally clear that male free lovers, in their reverential awe for the penis, their pride in their elemental maleness, saw the elevation of the male organ as the logical outcome of a natural system of restored sexuality that would overthrow the repressiveness and shame of 'civilized' relations between the sexes and reestablish a joyous, playful attitude toward the sexual body. In the relation of the male sexual body to the female sexual body the sexual instincts were redeemed, the pride in the physical representation of erotic power awakened. Ezra Heywood made these connections explicit in his address to the court in the course of his final trial for obscenity. 'Gentlemen', he intoned,

> if there is anything better on earth than the body of man it is the body
> of woman, your mother, sister, daughter, wife or lady-love…what object
> on earth or in Air surer to wake all the potent beneficence of man's being
> than woman's person! Accursed is the man with idiotic indiscretion who
> is ashamed of his passion for woman! What emasculated fool is this who,
> as the flame of manly heat goes up through his body house comes down
> in charred ruins on penitent knees to apologize for and be ashamed of
> his passional vigor, his generative rectitude!…Gentlemen, I am amazed at
> the shame-facedness with which some men meet their own nature; at
> their witless weariness, if not perverse puerility in the presence of the
> divine potencies of these our body forms![31]

However, free lovers' validation of unabashed passion and the liberation of the sexual body presented them with a sobering dilemma: if conventional sexual relations and conjugal reproductive sexuality were, as they had argued, unnatural, depraved, and even criminal, how could they prioritize the pleasurable sexual body, improve the mental and physical quality of offspring, and still guarantee the health and safety of their alternative system of sexual behavior for both partners, but more particularly for the female? The resolution of this problem necessitated the separation of the pleasurable from the strictly reproductive functions of the sex act for the male, the practice of some kind of contraception, and the practice of a self-conscious system of eugenics. In resolving these issues, free lovers engaged in a conscientious reconstruction of the male sexual body. That reconstruction involved a probing of the nature of orgasmic experience for both sexes and of the neurological and physiological aspects of sexual experience.

Sex radicals consistently maintained that 'sex force is the motor power of the universe and that reproduction is only one and that not the primary use of the sexual act, and that the sexual embrace for the renewal of life and happiness differs very much in character...'[32] But given that pleasure was the essence of human sexual experience, the differences between male and female sex organs and sexual response became critical. Male experience was generally understood in the free love literature as physically uncomplicated, but female orgasm was problematical. Male sex radicals were fundamentally conflicted about the juncture between their understanding of female physiology and the social construction of female sexual experience. Their acceptance of conventional Victorian dogma on the imperious ardency of the male sex drive was matched by a stereotypically bipolar view of female sexual response— that women were either under-sexed or insatiable. The frigidity model did not mesh well with the emphasis in free love theory on sexual pleasure, and concern for inti-macy and mutuality in relationships, while female hypersexuality threatened cherished traditions about male sexuality. The conflict between these two conceptions of female sexuality was decided in favor of a hearty feminine libido, but a residue of ambiguity and even trepidation remained to distort male sex radicals' perceptions of female sexuality.

Radical physiologists argued that 'in a healthy condition, the pleasure of the female is longer continued, more frequently repeated, and more exquisite than that of the male'.[33] Unfortunately, however, such heightened female sexual sensibility was potentially dangerous, both to the woman herself and to her sex partner as well. Multiple-orgasmic women were beyond control; they were seen as diseased and deviant, threatening to exhaust their male lovers. The sense of physical apprehension about the 'over-sexed' female was most clearly expressed by Thomas L. Nichols under the heading '*Furor uterinus*'. Women who suffered deranged sexual response, he wrote,

> go further than is possible with men. A man is usually limited by the amount of semen his testicles can secrete...With a full emission, a man, unless greatly excited, cannot be prepared for another under an hour, and two or three are the extent of his powers...but a woman, who loses no semen, and simply expends a certain amount of nervous force, will have six or seven orgasms in rapid succession, each seeming to be more violent and ecstatic than the last. These may be accompanied with screams, bitings, spasms, and end in a faint langour, that will last many hours.[34]

Free love sexology, dominated by male voices, was uncomfortable with what threatened to be an anarchic female sexual body and some way of neutralizing female sexual superiority needed to be found. Male free lovers blended aspects of conven-tional sexual practice and alternative cultural theory with a more thorough under-standing of the psychology and physiology of sex to create a system of sexuality that effectively brought a potentially debilitating (for the male) female under rational (male) regulation.

Free lovers accepted contemporary medical advice that urged cessation of intercourse during menstruation, pregnancy, and lactation and generally rejected (in their personal sex lives) as unnatural all forms of 'artificial' birth control.[35] Ironically, all of these behavioral restrictions were elements of a sexual praxis that profoundly distrusted erotic pleasure and that posited reproduction as the only legitimate rationale for sexual intercourse. Radical sexual theory, though, denied an exclusive-ly generative legitimation of intercourse and maintained, as Thomas L. Nichols put it, that 'there is no physiological foundation for this belief. The desire for the sexual union is not adapted to, or governed by, this result in man or in woman—especially in man.[36] The radical rationale for the acceptance of conventional restraints on intercourse thus shared the premises but not the conclusions of conventional Victorian sexology. But that did not mean that sex radicals freely embraced a liberated pleasure principle in matters of sexuality. Although their doctrines priori-tized pleasure in the legitimation of the sex act, free lovers remained deeply ambi-valent about erotic self-realization.

Free love, as an ideological construct, stood for temperate, natural, restrained pleasure in the sex act. As Ezra Heywood described its effects on sexual ethics, 'free love tends [not] to unrestrained licentiousness, [nor] to open the floodgates of passion and remove all barriers in its desolating course; but it means just the opposite; it means the expulsion of animalism, and the entrance of reason, knowledge, and continence'.[37] The fear of unrestrained animal passion figured prominently in free love doctrine, and was grounded in two opposed physiological concerns. The first was the need to protect women against the excessive sexual demands of their brutal male partners. The second was a fundamental fear of the potential for physical and neurological enervation (for both partners, but especially for the male) resulting from erotic excesses.

Moderated pleasure was the answer to this dual problematic. Excesses upset the physical and psychological balance of the natural system. Heywood argued, for example, that intercourse, if 'escapes control… exhausts both persons, admonishing them to keep within the associative limit, which is highly invigorating, and not to allow themselves to gravitate to the propagative climax'.[38] The basis for both pleasure and the fear of pleasure in sex revolved around the application of neurological and physiological doctrines derived from the spiritualist movement and popular medical advice to the alternative sexual ethic and practices of the free love movement. From Emanuel Swedenborg and the nineteenth-century Spiritualist movement, sex radicals adopted the idea that physical energy was sustained by a nervous fluid, that served as the connecting link between the body (matter) and the spirit (soul). Though popular medical belief maintained that the most serious sexual danger for the male lay in excessive loss of semen—the 'spermatic economy' theory—many free lovers were equally concerned about the orgasm's potential for producing nervous debilitation. Their concern found its most straightforward expression in concerns about mas-turbation.

If pleasure were the legitimate end of sex, why did sex radicals share the conventional fears of masturbation? The most comprehensive answer is that while they made a sharp distinction between the procreative and the pleasurable aspects of the sex act, they had no desire to completely suppress its reproductive potential. In a more limited technical sense, however, theoretical considerations revolving around the maintenance of a balance of nervous energy, an equilibrium of corporeal magnetism, assumed preeminence. 'Solitary indulgence', as T.L. Nichols explained, 'is far more exhausting than social'. But when two persons, loving each other and adapted to each other, come together in the sexual embrace, nature has provided that a portion of the nervous energy of each goes to strengthen the other, and there is comparatively but little loss. In a union without love, or where all the enjoyment is on one side, the loss is greater, for there is less compensation. A mere sensual union is destitute of spiritual and magnetic compensations; but where there is the simple, artificial, and utterly unnatural excitement of the orgasm, without reciprocity, compensation, or use, the result is only evil.[39]

The inherent danger of masturbation, then, was self-absorption, the selfish orgasm that scorned the social warmth of the sexual embrace. Its fruits were male impotence and premature ejaculation and female frigidity and barrenness. For the female the effects were perhaps more serious, since hyperstimulation of the clitoris supplanted what medical literature considered the legitimate seat of the female orgasm—the vagina. T.L. Nichols expressed this concern most directly, writing that 'from the continued excitement of the clitoris and the labis, the seat of sensation is wholly transferred from the vagina and womb to those external organs, and even in them the sense of pleasure is finally exhausted'.[40] When such a woman 'comes to be married, she receives the warm embraces of her husband with indifference, and perhaps with disgust or absolute pain. She is cold amid his ecstasies, yields only to his commands, and turns from him with repugnance.'[41]

The male free lover, then, was caught in a particularly vexatious predicament. If he followed the selfish, lustful inclinations of his own body, with no concern for the desires and welfare of the female, he could be accused of violating or prostituting his wife or sexual partner; if he sought to satisfy the selfish desires of the woman who was clitoral, multiple-orgasmic or both, he risked sexual debilitation and genital anæsthesia of the female. Such was the male dilemma in a system of sexuality that stressed the necessity to intercourse as a means to bodily health and a conduit of mutual pleasure. Clearly, given the potential for the abuse of pleasurable sex, some means had to be found to domesticate the orgasm, to manage and direct its power.

Sex radicals proposed three alternatives to conventional sexual behavior that more or less met their standards for a balanced sexual experience by separating sex as pleasure from sex as reproduction—Henry Martyn Parkhurst's Dianism, Albert Chavannes' magnetation, and J.H. Noyes' male continence. Dianism proposed 'sexual satisfaction from sexual contact' that stopped short of penile penetration. Exchange of passional energy or bodily magnetism would issue in sexual equilibrium and pleasure. Chavannes maintained that magnetic satisfaction required orgasm, but seems to have believed that male orgasm was possible without ejaculation. The most comprehensive and well-integrated of alternative systems of sexual ethics and sexual behavior was Noyes' 'male continence'.

Noyes' system required a radical reconstruction of the male sexual body and a thoroughgoing reconstitution of heterosexual sexuality. It was grounded in his discovery of a revolutionary physiological insight. 'The amative and the propagative functions of the sexual organs', he declared, are distinct from each other, and may be separated practically…But if amativeness is…the first and noblest of the social affections…we are bound to raise the amative office of the sexual organs into a distinct and paramount function…The sexual conjunction of male and female, no more necessarily involves the discharge of semen than of the urine. The discharge of the semen, instead of being the main act of sexual intercourse…is really the sequel and termination of it. Sexual intercourse, pure and simple, is the conjunction of the organs of union, and the interchange of magnetic influences, or conversation of spirits, through the medium of that conjunction.[43]

Such a physiological construction of the male sexual role made possible the practice of a form of free love—pantagamy ('complex marriage') at Noyes' Oneida Community (1848-79) as well as eugenic reproduction—'stirpiculture' from 1867 to 1879. It also signalled in its very name—'male continence'—the central role assigned the male sexual body in creating and sustaining the physical and social conditions for the control and management of sexual pleasure.

3. The Dynamics of Liberation:
Repression in the Control and Purification of the Male Sexual Body

The male sexual body was, as we have seen, at once a source of pride and guilt. The erect penis symbolized both the shame and the glory of masculine sexuality; governed by brute instinct and lust it was an engine of destruction, but guided and regulated by reason it was the glory of man. The male sexual body was popularly but falsely believed to be uncontrollable; sex could be liberated from the prison of lust through the subordination of the body to moral obligation. The key to a renovated male sexual body, then, lay in mastery of the penis, in sensible moderation, in 'sexual continence'.[44] Ezra Heywood expressed the delicate balance of freedom and repression that free lovers' sexual moderation required. 'Vice', he wrote,

> does not consist in the judicious gratification of sexual desire. Health, temperance, self-control, and native graces are developed by intimate exchange of magnetisms, and both sexes are thereby fitted for parentage. The progress of civilization is marked by the degree of freedom and intimacy between the sexes.[45]

'LOVE REFORM' necessitated the elevation of 'domestic ethics' and the dedication of the male sexual body to a 'true affectional intercourse'.[46] Free love principles did not issue a man a license for lechery. 'Relieving one from outer restraint', Heywood wrote, 'does not lessen, but increases his personal accountability; for by making him free, we devolve on him the necessity of self government; and he must respect the rights of others, or suffer the consequences of being an invader'. Lovers are constrained 'to hold their bodies subject to reason'.[47]

As J.H. Noyes made clear, while his sexual system gloried in 'allowing them [varietist free lovers] all and more than all of the ordinary freedom of love (since the crisis always interrupts the romance)', the renunciation of the male orgasm it required assumed that 'Male Continence in its essence is [male] self control'.[48] In separating the amative from the propagative function in the male's role in intercourse, Noyes provided a powerful new vision of the regenerated male sexual body. He described the new sexual man in terms of millenarian rationalism. The glory of the male physical body would be realized in the subjection of the procreative crisis, the seminal emission, for the propagative element of male sexual response was not an involuntary physical reaction, but was 'subject to enlightened voluntary control'.[49] 'It is', Noyes cried, 'the glory of man to control himself, and the Kingdom of Heaven summons him to self-control in ALL THINGS.' Indeed, 'the seeds of the final supremacy over nature lie in the full subjection of man's own body to his intelligent will'.[50] Noyes saw the system of 'male continence' he had instituted at the Oneida Community as 'an unfinished experiment in social science', an experiment in the physiological and psychological effects of sexual self-denial on the bodies of its male members.

A critical visitor to the Oneida Community, writing for a mainstream publication, argued that the sexual experiment had enjoyed considerable social success, but only at severe personal cost. He believed that male continence 'must cause much suffering in its application, and that it will defeat its own end, by omitting from these unions all deep personal emotion'.[51] Significantly, Noyes did not deny the effects of his system on the emotional lives of community members; instead he stressed the general moral health of the Community and the physical and neurological health of its men.[52]

Control over the body and mastery of male sexuality provided a foundation for a broader reconceptualization of masculinity among sex radicals. They created a new ideal of maleness, a model for the character of the 'true man'. Free lovers shared the nineteenth-century faith in female moral superiority, and argued that masculine character must be raised to a level equal to that of women. The ideal radical male would be motivated by elevated sexual sensibility, by his desire to maintain 'his own personal and continual attractiveness',

> And as he will constantly, habitually, and all his life, endeavor to make himself attractive, and worthy of those to whose affection he will naturally aspire; so he must as sedulously avoid everything that can make him repulsive. Such vices as uncleanness, slovenliness, uncouth actions, and degrading habits, as the use of foul language, ardent spirits, or tobacco, and all the unseemly and repulsive practices of civilization would cease, by virtue of this single charm.[53]

These brutal and swinish signifiers of maleness were expressions of a gendered depravity that permeated all social institutions. Ezra Heywood echoed this concern about the pollution and degradation of the male body in his consideration of the claim to suffrage. 'Not the ability to drink', he cried, '[to] chew, smoke, lie, steal and swear, votes—though election day too often indicates these vices to be important conditions of membership in the male body politic—but intellect, conscience, character are supposed to vote.'[54]

Popular gender psychology in the Victorian era held that the kind of self-control required of temperate free lovers was more common to females; that, as one writer put it, 'women govern themselves much more easily than men'.[55] Men could only achieve the desired level of self-control through the social and sexual submission of their bodies to 'true women'. The result of the manly subjection of the sexual body to 'Cupid's Yokes', of 'temperance and self-possession in sexual intercourse', would be the elevation of male social character.

For the male sex radical, as Ezra Heywood pointed out, 'if he 'holds his body subject to reason', 'keeps his body under', as St. Paul and Free Lovers urge, this revival of sexual energy in him will make him more of a gentleman...'.[56] The ideal of the temperate gentleman would guarantee physical and emotional health as well as gender equality. Free love sexology condemned the 'amative excesses' of the sexual body (including the habitual digital stimulation of the clitoris to arouse the female), because it was thought that they led to total absorption of lovers in one another's bodies. Such obsessive couples, 'loving, absorbed in each other, actually eat each other up; with no variety in their lives, nothing but the one passion, to which all their force is turned, [and] this vital force is soon exhausted.[57] Mutual continence would avoid such excesses, thus preserving the health and conserving the nervous energy of both partners.

The ideal of sexual behavior that sustained the ideal social character of maleness was most pointedly expressed by Ezra Heywood:

> To say that every one should be free, sexually, is to say that every one's person is sacred from invasion; that the sexual instinct shall no longer be a savage, uncontrollable usurper, but be subject to thought and civilization...[I affirm] that lovers' exchange, in its inception, continuance, and conclusion, can be made subject to choice; entered upon, or refrained from, as the mutual interests of both, or the separate good of either, requires.[58]

Radical reconstruction of maleness emphasized the importance of a romantic attitude, a Victorian version of the courtly-love tradition as the only viable basis for a regenerated relationship between male and female. The ideal sexual relationship for free lovers was that of courtship, wherein

> each man is an individual sovereign, each woman the owner of herself, and the controller of her own actions; each independent of the other, drawn together solely by the charm of a mutual attraction, coming from a mutual fitness and adaptation to the spiritual and material loves, or passional desires of each other—such a union seems to us to constitute the true marriage of mutual love in perfect freedom.[59]

In their romantic enthusiasm, free lovers were almost retrogressively adolescent. Ezra Heywood evoked the image of the callow swain to explicate the nature of the irreducible emotional tie between the sexes. 'Is it not', he argued, 'rather the memory of equality, of the hour when he, a glad suppliant, courted her, a free intelligence, able to accept or reject his proposals?'[60]

John H. Noyes stated his ideal as sexual love 'in friendship and freedom, without selfish possession'.[61] Male continence, he argued, while a transcendence of the flesh, also '*vastly increases*…[sexual] pleasure'.

> Ordinary sexual intercourse (in which the amative and propagative functions are confounded) is a momentary affair, terminating in exhaustion and disgust. If it begins with spirit, it soon ends in the flesh; i.e., the amative, which is spiritual, is drowned in the propagative, which is sensual. In contrast with this, lovers who use their sexual organs simply as the servants of their spiritual natures, abstaining from the propagative act, except when procreation is intended, may enjoy the highest bliss of sexual fellowship for any length of time, without satiety or exhaustion; and thus marriage life may become permanently sweeter than courtship or even the honeymoon.[62]

Such a romantic ideal of sexual behavior had social and political ramifications that posed a radical challenge to the conventional matrimonial rights of husbands and their foundation in a prescriptive female subordination to male-dominated institutions. The romantic model of courtship provided the typology of sexual character— for the female, 'virgin liberty'; for the male, 'continent deference'. The possibility of maintaining an ideal maleness and femaleness in practice depended on a revolutionary social reformation that would accord to woman (regardless of her marital condition) in her sexual relations with man the 'power to decline or even defy his advances'.[63]

The broader implications of this position involved a direct frontal assault on patriarchal power as the cause of both social degeneration and sexual perversion. A piece entitled 'Sex laws', for instance, that appeared in *Lucifer*, argued that the 'laws made by man, and made with the selfish desire to control and own women in sex slavery, have been the cause of producing every known phase of so-called immorality.[64] Ezra Heywood was characteristically blunt in his denunciation of patriarchy. In legalized marriages, too many wives were forced to 'grind in the prison-house of his [the husband's] selfism. By whose decree is one immortal being insphered within, and made a martyr to the private interest of another?'[65] The answer, for Heywood, was self-evident. For woman, 'the prejudices against her function which makes her an independent, thoughtful, self-sustaining being is excited by narrow and despotic selfishness. We have created antagonism by establishing a *privileged male class*.'[66] With metonymic economy, Heywood condemned the macho tyranny of patriarchy, observing that 'this booted, spurred and whiskered thing called government is a usurpation, and men choose to have it so'.[67] The very symbol of that gender-suborned polity, 'liberty, is not the golden goddess we read of, but male, incontinent, libertine when not overwhelmed by an intelligent moral sense'.[68] 'A just man', he concluded, 'blushes to look into the statute book, so often does he find himself judged and sentenced by the acts of his sex.'[69]

Heywood was proposing a revolutionary sexual politics or, alternatively, was politicizing sexuality. He and other free lovers constituted a male fifth-column movement in support of 'Woman Insurgent'. They conceived the moral and physical progress of the race (and most especially of its masculine element) as indissolubly linked to the social, economic, and political elevation of woman. Heywood issued the clarion call to all sex radicals of the age:

> We must count it, therefore, the first and chief of man's rights to undo, without asking this injustice to woman; for in so far as he deprives her of vigor and scope does he maim himself.
>
> Since in correcting wrong we enact right, men's actual influence will not only not be lessened, but vastly increased, by abolishing the despotic and irresponsible power they now wield. If authority is natural and beneficent the votes of a world united cannot overthrow it; if it is usurped, the quicker it falls the better.[70]

Sex radicals, like Heywood, who stood out boldly against patriarchy, frequently ran afoul of defenders of the phallocentric order like Anthony Comstock. Though in their own construction of the sexual body they typically opposed the use of artificial means of contraception, they nevertheless widely advertised and promoted books and pamphlet written by others as well as such devices as contraceptive syringes. Heywood himself ran a provocatively offensive advertisement for a feminine hygiene appliance in his periodical *The Word*. He called it the 'Comstock Syringe'. When Heywood was charged with violating the obscenity laws by virtue of running this notice, he responded with a characteristically *ad hominem* acerbity:

> Since Comstockism makes male will, passion and power absolute to impose conception, I stand with women to resent it. The man who would legislate to choke a woman's vagina with semen, who would force a woman to retain his seed, bear children when her own reason and conscience oppose it, would waylay her, seize her by the throat and rape her person.[71]

Male power, for free lovers, was illegitimate because it vested authority over sexual mores in the hands of those who were demonstrably unable to control their own sex drives. Their system of alternative sexuality sought to empower women for the express purpose of reenforcing and sustaining the male venereal will. Free lovers consistently urged that women be accorded full and unintermitted sovereignty over their sexual bodies: that they be granted an absolute veto power over the sexual advances of the male; that if they agreed to an amorous relationship their desires and sensibilities would determine the degree of sexual intimacy allowable; and that they be completely free to accept or reject motherhood. Some male sex radicals also accepted the idea that women should take the lead in initiating sexual relations. But a woman's fundamental bodily sovereignty inhered in her personal control of her conception.

'Compulsory child-bearing', Thomas L. Nichols warned, 'is one of those hideous wrongs which cannot be too often denounced—a wrong so unnatural, such a violation of all principles of right that every clear-minded man must shudder at its existence; yet it is a wrong which pervades our whole society; and the marriage institution rests upon it'.[72] John H. Noyes, whose separation of the amative and the propagative aspects of the sex act had provided a practical basis for avoiding unwanted and intrusive conception, was even more direct in his condemnation of male conduct that entailed the imposition of pregnancy. That man, he wrote,

> who under the cover of social intercourse, commits the propagative act, leaves his child with the woman in a meaner and more oppressive way, than if he should leave it full born in her apartments; for he imposes upon her not only the task of breeding and providing for it, but the sorrows and pains of pregnancy and childbirth...it is not to be wondered at that women, to a considerable extent, look upon ordinary sexual interchange with more dread than pleasure, regarding it as a stab at their life, rather than a joyful act of fellowship.[73]

The logic of free love sexuality was based on a liberated instinctual mutualism. The arbitrary and repressive 'invasive heism' that was sustained by patriarchy was tantamount to socially sanctioned mass rape.[74] The only way for love to be free would be to require mutual consent in all sex acts, to liberate sexual choice for both genders. In a system of freely elected associations and freely granted sexual favors, 'woman will have every opportunity to bestow herself upon the man worthy of her choice'.[75]

T.L. Nichols summarized the free love support for women's sexual autonomy best. 'The right of a woman to herself is the first and the highest of woman's rights, and includes all others; and among these is the right to bestow herself in love according to her attractions; in other words, to choose the father of her child.'[76] It was the duty of men to submit the male sexual body to control by the female in order to liberate the female sexual body and to elevate the sexual relations. The social effects of the subordination of male desire to the requirements of female health and sexual equality were clear. In the romantic tones that free lovers typically used to describe the instinctual life of the sexes, Nichols provided a summation of the extensive social effects of sexual reform. Under a regime of liberated sexual mutualism, he declared,

> It is the part of woman to accept or repudiate; to grant or refuse. It is her right to reign a *passional queen*; to say thus far shalt thou come and no farther! It is for her nature to decide both whom she will admit to her embraces, and when; and there is no despotism upon this earth so infernal as that which compels a woman to submit to the embraces of a man she does not love; to receive even these, when her nature does not require them, and when she cannot partake in the sexual embrace without injury to herself and danger to her offspring...If a woman has any right in this world, it is the right to herself; if there is anything in this world she has a right to decide, it is who shall be the father of her children. She has an equal right to decide whether she will have children, and to choose the time of having them.[77]

4. *Embattled Patriarchy, Eugenics and the Ideal of Female Sexual Autonomy*

In the context of the broader Victorian sexual discourse, free lovers were considered a radically subversive voice, dedicated to the overthrow of established sexual institutions and mores. Their support for the 'emancipation of woman from sexual slavery', of her right to the 'control of her own person, within wedlock as well as out of it', provided the individual basis for the more sweeping demand for institutional change—'the utter ABOLITION of marriage'.[78] Their celebration of the sexual body, coupled with their insistence on control of the instincts, offended both the prudish and the licentious. Their publications were repeatedly suppressed and their major spokespersons were imprisoned. Despite official censorship, however, sex radicals constituted an important strain in the general discourse on sexuality. While their specific ideas on the male sexual body, the sexual and political emancipation of women, and a liberated sexuality did not produce substantial change in conventional attitudes and behavior in their own time, we can recognize the roots of a modern sexual sensibility in certain of their ideas. In the short-term, the influence of free love thought flowed into two channels that became important elements of the popular health creed of late-nineteenth and early twentieth-century America—eugenics and the physical culture movement.

The link between free love principles and eugenics was an integral one. John H. Noyes had pioneered in the practical application of eugenic principles in the Oneida Community, where he instituted a system of 'scientific propagation' or 'stirpiculture' in 1873. Through the system of 'male continence' (*coitus reservatus*), so intimately bound up with the doctrine of the rational control of the male sexual body, Noyes provided both the means and suggested the desirability of eugenics. Given the emphasis sex radicals placed on the individual physical body and the health of the collective social body, when the female made her choice of a mate, it was presupposed that, she would select the best biological and moral specimen that presented himself. Since acquired characteristics (including behavioral and psychological ones) were believed to be eminently transmissible and genetically heritable, free lovers, who saw themselves engaged in a grand program of the perfection of the male sexual body and the purification of male sexual attitudes and behavior, adopted a eugenic stance as a means of quite literally reproducing reform. Cultivation and control of the sexual body in an environment of erotic liberation came to constitute the primary qualification for parenthood. As Ezra Heywood expressed it, 'until lovers, by pregood sense, become capable of temperance and self-possession in sexual intercourse, it is an outrage on children to be begotten by them'. And eugenics, in championing the rights of the unborn, provided, by refraction, additional support for sex radicals' critique of conjugal exclusivity. If the fundamental question was—'what clearer right has a child than to be well-born?', it logically followed that 'no woman or man should have a second child by his marital partner, when there is another person, willing to assume the relation, by whom he or she can have a better child'.[79]

Though free love eugenicists did not discount the hereditary contribution of the female and the power of uterine ecology, or the traditional beliefs about the ambient external environment (the folk belief that the mother's experiences during gestation 'marked' the foetus), they tended to place more emphasis on the hereditary and reproductive role of the male. Noyes was quite blunt in his treatise on 'scientific propagation', for example, in maintaining that 'suppressing the poorest and breeding from the best' required the exercise of 'a very stringent discrimination in selecting males'.[80] Refining Noyes' concern with selection of fathers, and filtering it through the lens of free love temperance, Dr. E. P. Foote, Jr. argued that the male could enhance and mold his genetic contribution to conception. For the male, he argued, the 'paternal impressions' by which 'he becomes born again in his child',

> may be greatly modified for better or worse by his own course of life. Has he dissipated his patrimonial endowment of vital force, or augmented it by right living? That will determine whether he has or has not properly prepared himself for conferring a potential impression upon an embryo which will give it a place among the 'well-born'.[81]

Eugenics, then, made the male reformation promoted by free lovers even more critical. It also reenforced the central importance of the female's autonomy over her sexual and reproductive body by constituting the choice of the father of her child as the most critical one of her life, for it would affect not only her initial pregnancy, but the entire course of her subsequent reproductive life. Foote maintained that 'the male element has an influence on the female organism over and above that of ferti-lization...her first impregnation has literally a double result'. The male element combines with the female to produce the embryo, but the sperm continues to act on the womb, and 'afterwards modifies...[the intrauterine influences] of the mother'.[82] The critical responsibility of female selectivity was clear:

> Here is the double reason why women should be more particular as to who they accept in marriage, for if, through pity for or propinquity with some mongrel male or puny specimen, he is accepted as 'number one', and dies leaving her with a few unfortunate reminders of his deficiencies, then if she should attract a better specimen as 'number two', she may be disappointed to see this finer stock mongrelled by the persisting paternal impressions of her first mistake.[83]

For eugenics advocates, then, just as for free lovers (but with greatly intensified consequences for misjudgments), the pivotal role for women lay in opting for motherhood and in choosing the father of her children. For male self-control and self-cultivation, the qualities of an ideal free love masculinity, comprised the essential prerequisites for selection for eugenic reproduction. In tones that echoed the earlier admonitions of J.H. Noyes and Ezra Heywood, young men were warned against 'going astray and dissipating their vital endowments, [and] robbing, to some extent, their own progeny of that vitality which is essential to longevity and health'.[84]

5. The Pursuit of the Perfection of the Male Sexual Body
and the Promise of a Regenerated Masculinity

Free lovers had long maintained that 'health is beauty, energy, purity, holiness, happiness'. T.L. Nichols had claimed that

> there is no part of the human figure where the best condition for use is not, at the same time, the condition of the highest beauty, and both together are synonymous with health. Consequently, every deformity, every ugliness, every departure from the standard of the highest beauty of its kind, is a consequence and a symptom of disease.[85]

Eugenics and the physical culture movement evolved out of the free lovers' concern for personal reformation and breeding from the best stock. Nichols had already brought these ideas together in the 1850s: 'Weakness, mental or passional or physical, is a sign of disease, as it is a consequence. It is want of development, or exhaustion, or hereditary taint, or acquired morbid condition, or all together, one producing the other.'[86]

Bernarr Macfadden (1868-1955), the apostle of 'Body love' and editor of *Physical Culture* magazine, was in many ways a direct intellectual descendant of the sex radicals of the late Victorian era. Like them, he was harassed and arrested by Comstock, and like them, his advocacy of physical culture was rooted in an evangelical sensibility. The masthead of his periodical bore the motto 'Weakness is a sin, don't be a sinner.' Like the free lovers, too, he valued the natural over the artificial productions of a degenerated civilization. He held 'that health and strength of a high degree is the natural condition of man, and it is otherwise only when one's life does not conform to nature's laws'.[87]

The goal of the physical culture movement was to bring the body into temperate accord with the imperatives of natural law. For the male, cultivating and modelling his physical and specifically sexual body meant avoiding 'becoming intemperate in his desires and in his exercises…[for] the results often work serious injury to that higher state of physical health, the development of which all physical culture should strive to improve'.[88] Macfadden felt that 'the prudishness of the average individual about matters appertaining to sex is to be deplored'.[89] Sex was essential to the fullest culture of the body. 'The highest degree of attainable physical perfection can certainly never be acquired unless this condition [marriage] is entered at the proper period of life'.[90] Indeed for Macfadden, as for the free lovers, intercourse promoted health and was a natural imperative of the human body:

> if you are a man, a woman, in every sense, with the power of body and mind which accompanies this state of maturity, with all the faculties fully alive, with all the emotions tingling, with the intensity of their strength, with the glory and ripeness of life, of health, and of strength, stirring your senses, *you will be committing a crime if you do not marry.*[91]

Macfadden also shared the concern of the sex radicals for the transmission of physical perfection. 'Worse than theft and well nigh as bad as murder', he argued, 'is the bringing into the world, through disregard of parental fitness, individuals full of diseased tendencies.'[92] We must accept the biological fact that 'man is an animal—and in order to enjoy the happiness and success of this life, he must first be a fine, strong, wholesome, beautiful animal'. 'The Gospel of Health', then, Macfadden concluded, 'is of far more importance than any religion. *It is a religion.*'[93]

The free love crusade had been a jeremiad against patriarchal depravity; it sought to evangelize the male sexual body to physical and moral renewal, through a cycle of conversion, repentance, and regeneration. The 'fearful superabundance of manhood depravity'[94] would be atoned by the subjection of the male sexual will to the female, through the grace of liberated love. Through rational control of the sexual instinct and enlightened reproduction, the covenant of regenerated masculinity would pass to the physical bodies of the next generation. But the key to the regeneration of the male sexual body was the emancipation of women, for:

> the fact remains that woman, incarnating love, has ruled and will rule man, for better or for worse, just in proportion as she is assured or denied a right to herself...for nature has a seriously honest intent in creating a woman as in creating a man. If he makes badness a necessity and bribes to silence her moral sense, designed to call him to order, why may not the 'weaker vessel' plot to upset the stronger?[95]

To secure male salvation and to secure domestic tranquility, then, free lovers sought to insure that 'Intelligent Mutualism prevails in sexuality'.[96] The male ideal they advocated demanded a delicate passional balance. 'When man loves woman intelligently', Ezra Heywood advised, 'what is now consuming passional heat, will make him a genial, civil, and serviceable being.'[97] Man would be, then, an athlete of his passions, training his sexual body to obedience to his will in subjection to the social and sexual needs of woman, and would be by his own love redeemed. Through the sexual redemption of men and the sexual, reproductive and social liberation of women, sex would he restored to its natural purity as the sovereign of the passions.

The *sine qua non* of the reformation of sex life, as free lovers clearly realized, was the exposure of the depraved practices and the withered emotional life of Victorian America. Their discursive strategy was confrontational, their diction direct; they aimed to shock and to shame their contemporaries into social reformation. They attacked 'obscenists' and prudes wherever they found them as enemies of the gospel of natural sexual relationships (in both the sexual and social sense). Angela Heywood summed up the discursive strategies of the free love movement as well as anyone. 'Why not', she asked,

> make voyages of discovery into our body-selves, study attractive, fruitful lessons in Moral, Sexual Physiology? Why blush or be shamefaced in Stirpiculture more than in Agriculture, Horticulture, Floriculture, or amid iron-clad steel bright, golden-pure wonders of Mechanics? Are not the Penis and Womb as native, handsome and worthy in use as pivot and

socket, pistil and stamen, pollen and ovule? What rioting debauchery, what rotting disease, what stroke of moral death or stark idiocy is upon men that they are less intelligent, respectful and orderly with their own body-selves than with the mental, wooden or vegetable manifestations of form and power? Not the voting question merely, but the Sex Question, calls for discovery and Conversation; in dark, hidden ways men legislate on the use and destiny of women's bodies,—when we may or may not conceive; whether we shall have syringes to take an injection, enema, or for other cleansing purposes, and Citizens are imprisoned for daring to ask the reason why![98]

The inquisition of the male sexual body, of the patriarchal domination of the female sexual body, and of the appropriate principles for a systematic, scientific reproduction informed the sexual discourse of free lovers, and their sexual politics marginalized them in Victorian America as sex radicals. But they were hardly cranks, or representatives of some socially deviant lunatic fringe. Their 'Conversation' on the 'Sex Question' was an honest and an earnest one, and it provided a pointed public discourse on many aspects of the troubled relationship between the sexes and several of the most fundamental social problems stemming from that relationship that still remain unresolved today. Male free lovers took a strong public stand against the privileges of patriarchy and staunchly supported the political, economic, sexual, and reproductive liberation of women in the name of the progressive future of the race. Their credo was 'Good Generation'—'Its central thought is Natural Selection through Freedom of Motherhood, the Self-ownership of Women in the Realm of Sex and Reproduction—Intelligent and Responsible Parenthood. Woman first, Man second.'[99] Though the practical application of their principles on an experimental basis was not able to compass it, they envisioned a gender neutral world.

> Absolute maleness or absolute femaleness is simply an abstract conception of the mind. There is no such thing anywhere in the universe as an embodiment of life purely female or purely male…Sex, in itself suggests the union, the interaction of two complementary forces—forces so necessary to each other one can have no existence without the other. The man and the woman are indeed one![100]

Modern feminist critics have recognized that even under the most repressive patriarchal regimes there may be male dissenters, who identify more closely with the oppressed and repressed feminine than with the hegemonic masculine power structure. Building on the theoretical insights of Luce Irigaray, they have asked,

> 'what can be said about a *male* sexuality 'other than the one prescribed in, and by phallocentrism?' That is, it is not enough to locate woman on the other side of a maleness that is assumed to coexist with patriarchy. For there is at least the possibility that maleness exists in a relation to patriarchy as a third term of gender discourse, whose terms are woman, man, and patriarchy'.[101]

Maleness as constructed by radical free lovers was opposed to the domination of patriarchy. Male free lovers attempted to establish a mutualist dynamic of sexual relations, and enthusiastically supported women's rights in the sexual and reproductive sphere, championed woman suffrage, and upheld women's right to equal pay for equal work.[102] In approaching their maleness, they asked, why can't a man be more like a woman? And yet, they remained at bottom ambivalent towards both their own and women's sexual bodies. They were the first generation of what we would recognize today as feminist men, who stood between the female body and phallic sexual oppression and patriarchal sexual politics. That the love they 'freed' did not give access to a realm of unalloyed erotic pleasure, but issued rather in a rough gender equality in limitation of instinct by the will, and in temperate intercourse, should not detract from the significance of their efforts to place the pleasure principle at the center of sexual life. Nor should the ambiguity of their ideas about the respective male and female roles in the sex act and in reproduction—they were socially feminist and sexually masculinist—be allowed to obscure their undeniable commitment to a feminist perspective. Male free lovers were dissenters from and critics of the orthodox sexuality of their day; theirs were the 'other' voices in the Victorian discourse on the sexual body.

Notes

1.   Michel Foucault, *The Care of the Self* (New York: Pantheon Books, 1986), p. 165. The phrase quoted in the title of the paper is from Ezra Heywood, *Cupid's Yokes; or, The Binding forces of Conjugal Life. An Essay to Consider Some Moral and Physiological Phases of Love and Marriage, Wherein is Asserted the Natural Right and Necessity of Sexual Self-Government* (Princeton, MA: Cooperative Pub. Co., 1877), p. 18.

2.   Foucault, *Care of the Self*, p. 240.

3.   John H. Noyes, *Scientific Propagation* (Oneida Community, 1877), pp. 23-24.

4.   The phrase is quoted from Marx Edgeworth Lazarus, *Love vs. Marriage* (1852) in Thomas Low Nichols and Mary Gove Nichols, *Marriage: Its History and Results; Its Sanctities and Its Profanities; Its Science and Its Facts. Demonstrating Its Influence as a Civilized Institution; or, the Happiness of the Individual and the Progress of the Race* (Cincinnati, OH: Valentine Nicholson, 1854), p. 187.

5.   John H. Noyes, *Male Continence* (Oneida Circular, 1872), p. 4.

6.   Thomas Low Nichols, *Esoteric Anthropology* (Port Chester, NY: Author, 1853), p. 5. This work was actually the first technically descriptive marriage manual (with detailed diagrams of the male and female reproductive anatomy) published in the US

7.   Nichols, *Esoteric Anthropology*, p. 5.

8.   Mrs. Fowler's remarks reported in *Lucifer, the Light bearer* V, 2 (26 January 1901), pp. 21-22. Orson Fowler's most straight forward physiological text was *Creative and Sexual Science* (1870), which was available only by subscription and was sold discreetly by private publisher's agents. See O.S. Fowler, *Creative and Sexual Science; or, Manhood and Womanhood and Their Mutual Interrelations* (repr.; ed. Adelaide Hechtlinger; Chicago: Follett Pub. Co., 1971 [1870]), Introduction, n.p.

9.   Nichols, *Marriage*, pp. 101, 178.

10.   *The Word*, III, 5 (September 1874), p. 1. That Young's defense of polygamy had

touched a sensitive nerve among free lovers was suggested by the fact that Heywood quoted the piece at secondhand. It had originally appeared in *Woodhull and Claflin's Weekly*.

11.   Nichols, *Marriage*, pp. 178-79.

12.   Nichols, *Marriage*, pp. 337 and 102 respectively.

13.   *The Word* 7 (November 1882), p. 4. My emphasis. The reference here is to the 'twin relics of barbarism'—chattel slavery and Mormon polygyn cited in the Republican Party platform of 1860.

14.   *Lucifer*, NS, XI, 33 (9 November 1891), p. 1.

15.   Nichols, *Marriage*, p. 180.

16.   Nichols, *Marriage*, p. 180.

17.   R.T. Trall, *Sexual Physiology and Hygiene; or, The Mysteries of Man* (New York: L. Holbrook & Co., 1885), pp. 279-80.

18.   *Bible Communism; A Compilation from the Annual Reports and Other Publications of the Oneida Association and its Branches; Presenting in Connection with Their History, a Summary View of Their Religious and Social Theories* (repr.; Philadelphia: Porcupine Press, 1972 [1853]), p. 41.

19.   Trall, *Sexual Physiology*, p. 344. The phrases quoted above are from p. 304.

20.   Macfadden, *Physical Culture* III, 4 (July 1900), p. 180.

21.   Nichols, *Marriage*, pp. 82-83.

22.   Heywood, *Cupid's Yokes*, p. 9.

23.   Nichols, *Esoteric Anthropology*, p. 151.

24.   Nichols, *Esoteric Anthropology*, p. 150.

25.   Nichols, *Esoteric Anthropology*, p. 134.

26.   Nichols, *Marriage*, p. 85. The phrases on 'physical necessity' are from *Lucifer*, XI, 48 (22 March 1895), n.p. (badly deteriorated copy). See also Nichols, *Esoteric Anthropology*, p. 130.

27.   Heywood, *Cupid's Yokes*, p. 245n.

28.   Nichols, *Esoteric Anthropology*, pp. 50-51.

29.   Nichols, *Esoteric Anthropology*, p. 56. In a diagram of the female sexual organs (fig. 25, p. 56), the analogy is made even more pointedly, when Nichols delineates a '*Prepuce* of the clitoris, around the *glans* clitoris'. Emphasis mine.

30.   Ezra H. Heywood, *Free Speech: Report of Ezra H. Heywood's Defense Before the United States Court in Boston, April 10, 11, and 12, 1883; Together with Judge Nelson's Charge to the Jury* (Princeton, MA: Cooperative Pub. Co., 1883), p. 26.

31.   Heywood, *Free Speech*, p. 24.

32.   'Sexual and Social Science', *Lucifer* (November 1894?) n.p. (deteriorated original).

33.   Nichols, *Esoteric Anthropology*, p. 153. See also p. 132 under the discussion of masturbation. R.T. Trall, less radically inclined than Nichols though he argued that some women never experienced orgasm during intercourse, nevertheless conceded that other women enjoyed an orgasm 'fully as intense as that which accompanies ejaculation in the male'. Indeed, he asserted that 'most writers of the present day admit' that women experience a uterine ejaculation during orgasm. See his *Sexual Physiology*, p. 155.

34.   The term *furor uterinus* was in common usage until the middle of the present century as a medical euphemism for nymphomania. A modern reader will recognize nothing excessive or certainly nothing specifically nymphomaniacal about the sexual experience described here. This is simply a frankly clinical description of a quite normal female multiple orgasm. Nichols maintains that there is a range of male hyper-sexuality that stretches from once to three times a day, which corresponds to the physical limits of male capacity. He says nothing here about the threat that male hyper-sexuality poses to the health and lives of wives and sex partners. Concern about loss of semen was an article of faith of the nineteenth-

century sex doctrine of 'spermatic economy', which claimed that male physical energy and creative force inhered in the sexual secretion, and that males ought to husband it so as to insure a stable reserve of energy over the long term. In sexual practice, this put a premium on never 'wasting' the seed.

35.   For restrictions on times of intercourse, see: Nichols, *Esoteric Anthropology*, p. 150, and *Marriage*, p. 185; and Trall, *Sexual Physiology*, pp. 153-54. On the rejection of standard methods of contraception, see: Heywood, *Cupid's Yokes*, p. 20; and John H. Noyes, *Male Continence*, p. 7.

36.   Nichols, *Marriage*, p. 365.

37.   Heywood, *Cupid's Yokes*, p. 19.

38.   Heywood, *Cupid's Yokes*, p. 20.

39.   Nichols, *Esoteric Anthropology*, p. 399. For further discussion of magnetism, see: *Bible Communism*, p. 48; Noyes, *Male Continence*, p. 20; and Moses Harman, 'Men More Merciful Than Women', *Lucifer* III, 2 (14 January 1899), p. 13.

40.   Nichols, *Esoteric Anthropology*, pp. 402-403.

41.   Nichols, *Esoteric Anthropology*, p. 403. See also, pp. 269-70.

42.   For a description of these sexual systems, see: Taylor Stoehr, *Free Love in America: A Documentary History* (New York: AMS Press, 1979), pp. 55-59. See also *Lucifer* XI, 3 (10 August 1894), p. 1, and XI, 32 (October 1894), p. 1 for magnetation and Dianism, respectively.

43.   *Bible Communism*, pp. 47-48.

44.   Heywood, *Cupid's Yokes*, p. 19.

45.   Heywood, *Cupid's Yokes*, p. 19.

46.   The phrases are drawn, respectively, from: *Cupid's Yokes*, p. 9, *Uncivil Liberty*, p. 11.

47.   Heywood, *Cupid's Yokes*, pp. 4 and 3 respectively.

48.   Noyes, *Male Continence*, pp. 9, 20.

49.   *Bible Communism*, p. 49.

50.   Noyes, *Male Continence*, pp. 9-10; and *Bible Communism*, p. 49, respectively.

51.   Thomas Wentworth Higginson in the *Woman's Journal*, reprinted in Noyes, *Male Continence*, p. 23.

52.   Noyes, *Male Continence*, p. 24; and *Essay on Scientific Propagation with an Appendix Containing a Health Report of the Oneida Community by Theodore R. Noyes, M.D.* (Oneida Community, 1877), pp. 30-32, which effectively denies that Oneida sexual practice was productive of nervous disorders among its male population.

53.   Nichols, *Marriage*, p. 359. See also Heywood, *Uncivil Liberty*, p. 7.

54.   Heywood, *Uncivil Liberty*, p. 7.

55.   Nichols, *Esoteric Anthropology*, p. 154.

56.   Heywood, *Cupid's Yokes*, p. 20; and *Free Speech*, p. 28, respectively.

57.   Nichols, *Esoteric Anthropology*, pp. 270-71.

58.   Heywood, *Cupid's Yokes*, p. 19.

59.   Nichols, *Marriage*, p. 289.

60.   Heywood, *Uncivil Liberty*, p. 12.

61.   *Bible Communism*, p. 88.

62.   Noyes, *Male Continence*, p. 14.

63.   Heywood, *Uncivil Liberty*, p. 12. The terms cited above are also found on this page.

64.   'Sex Laws' (excerpted from *Occultism*), *Lucifer* (1894?, n.p., badly deteriorated original).

65.   Heywood, *Uncivil Liberty*, p. 17.

66.   Heywood, *Uncivil Liberty*, p. 13. My emphasis.

67.   Heywood, *Uncivil Liberty*, p. 8.

68.   Heywood, *Uncivil Liberty*, p. 23.

69.   Heywood, *Uncivil Liberty*, p. 5.

70.   Heywood, *Uncivil Liberty*, pp. 15-16. The phrase 'Woman Insurgent' is the title of one of the sections of *Uncivil Liberty*, pp. 6-8. It is interesting to note that Heywood, who stood in the forefront of those sex radicals advocating woman suffrage, endorsed the notion of an ancient, worldwide matriarchal order 'based on the ground of absolute female superiority'. Modern societies, he believed, resulted from male flight and revolt against the original gynocentric order. See *Cupid's Yokes*, p. 7n.

71.   Heywood, *Free Speech*, pp. 17-18.

72.   Nichols, *Marriage*, pp. 181-82. See also pp. 286 and 306-307.

73.   *Bible Communism*, pp. 52-53.

74.   The phrase is from Heywood, *Free Speech*, p. 17n. The term 'invasion' was a typical euphemism for rape. In a discussion of the question of a young girl's culpability in a case of statutory rape, for example, Lillian Harman (Moses' daughter) wrote that 'she does not invade him…there is but one criminal in the case, and that is the invader, the man', 'Age of Consent Symposium', *Lucifer* XI, 48 (22 March 1895), p. 1.

75.   Thomas Low Nichols, *Woman, in All Ages and Nations. A Complete and Authentic History of the Manners, Customs, Character, and Conditions of the Female Sex, in Civilized and Savage Countries, From the Earliest Ages to the Present Time* (New York: H. Long & Brothers, 1849), p. 25.

76.   Nichols, *Marriage*, p. 309. For the connection of the sexual and reproductive self-possession of women and a range of other women's rights issues, see also: *Marriage*, p. 52; and *Woman*, pp. 212-15; and Heywood, *Uncivil Liberty, passim.*

77.   Nichols, *Esoteric Anthropology*, p. 151. See also Heywood, *Free Speech*, pp. 16-17, *Uncivil Liberty*, p. 12, and *Cupid's Yokes*, p. 21.

78.   The first phrases quoted are from Jonathan Mayo Crane, 'Reproduction of the Unfit', *American Journal of Eugenics* I (July 1907), p. 17. The final phrase is from Col. William R. Greene, 'Anti-Marriage', *The Word* III, 6 (October 1874), p. 3.

79.   Heywood, *Cupid's Yokes*, pp. 20 and 17 respectively.

80.   Noyes, *Essay on Scientific Propagation*, pp. 15, 12.

81.   E.B. Foote, Jr, 'Paternal Impressions', *American Journal of Eugenics* I, 1 (July 1907), pp. 11-12.

82.   Foote, 'Paternal Impressions', p. 14.

83.   Foote, 'Paternal Impressions', p. 14.

84.   Foote, 'Paternal Impressions', p. 13.

85.   Nichols, *Esoteric Anthropology*, pp. 227-28.

86.   Nichols, *Esoteric Anthropology*, p. 230.

87.   *Physical Culture* I, 2 (April 1899), p. 35. For an extended biographical and critical discussion of Macfadden, see: Robert Ernst, *Weakness is a Crime: The Life of Bernarr Macfadden* (Syracuse, NY: Syracuse University Press, 1991); and William R. Hunt, *Body Love: The Amazing Career of Bernarr Macfadden* (Bowling Green, OH: Bowling Green State University Popular Press, 1989).

88.   'The Development of Energy, Vitality, and Health', *Physical Culture* I, 1 (January 1899), p. 7.

89.   *Physical Culture* I, 1 (January 1899), pp. 39-40.

90.   'Can the Highest Degree of Attainable Physical Perfection be Acquired if Absolute Continence is Observed?', *Physical Culture* I, 2 (April 1899), p. 37.

91.   'Can the Highest Degree', pp. 40-41. Italics mine.

92.   Alice B. Stockham, 'Marriage of the Unfit', *Physical Culture*, I, 5 (July 1899), p. 134. The inclusion of this article by Stockham indicates a clear tie with the traditions of Oneidan 'male continence' and 'stirpiculture' because Stockham was a popularizer of Noyes's sexual technique, whose book describing its practice, *Karezza: Ethics of Marriage*, had been published in 1896.

93.   *Physical Culture* I, 7 (September 1899), p. 199.

94.   Heywood, *Free Speech*, p. 17.

95.   Heywood, *Free Speech*, pp. 16-17.

96.   Heywood, *Free Speech*, p. 21.

97.   Heywood, *Cupid's Yokes*, p. 9.

98.   Angela Heywood, *Leaflet Literature*, quoted in Heywood, *Free Speech*, p. 27.

99.   'Good Generation', *American Journal of Eugenics* IV, 1 (January-February 1910), p 48.

100.   Paul Tyner, 'Sex in Social Evolution', *American Journal of Eugenics* I, 4 (October 1907), p. 199.

101.   Luce Irigaray, *This Sex which is not One (Le sexe qui n'en est pas un)*, quoted in Laura Claridge and Elizabeth Langland (eds.), *Out of Bounds: Male Writers and Gender[ed] Criticism* (Amherst, MA: University of Massachusetts Press, 1990).

102.   The classic statement of free love 'feminism' is Ezra Heywood's *Uncivil Liberty: An Essay to Show the Injustice and Impolicy of Ruling Woman against her Consent* (Princeton, MA: Cooperative Pub. Co., 1871). The pages of *The Word* and *Lucifer* also offer numerous examples of feminist perspectives and proposals.

Margaret Jones

WOMAN'S BODY, WORKER'S RIGHT:
FEMINIST SELF-FASHIONING AND THE FIGHT FOR BIRTH CONTROL,
1898-1917

In an early short story for the New York radical magazine *The Masses*, feminist author Helen Hull portrays a woman doctor who feels unable to aid her patient to have an abortion.[1] 'You must make the best of it', the doctor tells this working-class mother tied to a violent husband by unwanted pregnancies, 'for the children':

> The woman stared, her face wrinkling slightly, as if fanned by a hot wind.
> 'The children?' Her lips moved over the words. Then she relaxed,
> slumping into a heap, her face in the angle of her arm. 'Oh, the children:
> the children'.[2]

In a time of laws which made the giving of birth control information a crime, the miseries inflicted upon working-class women by restrictions which upper-class women were usually able to circumvent were, not surprisingly, a concern of feminist reformers across a wide political spectrum. Given, however, that the majority of birth control activists of the period were drawn from the middle classes, it seems worthwhile to examine a complementary term which not infrequently accompanies the middle-class woman reformer's concern with reproductive rights—that of feminist 'self-fashioning'.[3]

Between 1890 and 1910, for the first time in US history, women attended colleges and received higher degrees in large numbers. Between 1900 and 1920, the numbers of women awarded PhDs nearly doubled.[4] During roughly the same period, the demand for readily available cheap labour in an expanding industrial economy brought native-born and immigrant women flooding into the tenements and factories of rapidly growing US cities. The pressures and tensions engendered by the ensuing shifts, however slight, in women's roles, forced women cultural critics, writers and activists to re-evaluate their representations of femininity—even to re-evaluate their conceptions of the possible future path of woman's biological evolution.[5]

It was in the early 1900s that the term 'feminism' first became current in the United States. It is a term whose usage was promoted largely by Greenwich Village feminists—women like Henrietta Rodman and Ida Rauh, men like poet and novelist Floyd Dell.[6] Instrumental too in the wider dissemination of the concept of feminism was the leftist–feminist magazine *The Masses*. The magazine, published in Greenwich

Village between 1910 and 1917, was notable for, among other ideological positions, its pro-feminist stance in articles and poetry.[7] Some of the verse, in particular, merits quotation in the present context for what it illustrates of how literally the ideal of feminist self-fashioning might be taken. In this context it is worth considering, for instance, the radical revision of self and of self-definition envisaged in a poem like Jean Starr Untermeyer's 'Zanesville', in which the poet invokes the name of her native town to express her refusal to be shaped by Man into 'vases and cups of an old pattern'.[8] She will be her 'own creator,/ Dragging myself from the clinging mud', to mould herself into 'fresh and lovelier shapes'.[9] It is surely no accident that the poet envisages her self-reconstruction in the medium which, for the Judeo-Christian-Islamic traditions, has represented in mythic terms the very stuff of bodily existence—clay. For, as I shall argue shortly, feminist self-fashioning in this turn-of-century period of medical innovation and radical political ferment, is frequently conceived of as the reconstruction of femininity not only in sociopsychological but, quite literally, in biological terms.

Two poems by Helen Hoyt in *The Masses* are representative in this respect.[10] Hoyt's 'Menaia' may be said to address and contest a particularly repressive social construction of femininity, in its celebration of the biological processes involved in the socially tabooed subject of menstruation. For Hoyt, the monthly biological cycle represents a surrender to benign cosmic powers, the linking by poetic analogy of the human body to the gravitational pull of the moon on the tides:

> Always returning
> Comes mystery
> And possesses me
> And uses me
> As the moon uses the waters.[11]

While clearly couched in the anti-rational language of religious mystification, the poem nonetheless, in its celebration of a female biological process, represents a defiant and radical challenge to hegemonic patriarchal ideals of women's supposed 'purity' and 'spirituality'. 'Menaia' by implication firmly rejects turn-of-century shame and secrecy about women's physiology, of the kind which entitled a contemporary medical authority to write ponderously of 'the reverberations…of woman's physiological emergencies'.[12] Or which caused the anthropologist and social critics Elsie Clews Parsons (about whom more in due course) to protest that the menstruation taboo caused women to act furtively and secretively in order to disguise the fact that they were menstruating. In so doing, Parsons contended, a woman 'spreads the impression of being generally unreliable'.[13]

Biological 'otherness' is also the theme of Helen Hoyt's poem 'Comparison', in which a woman compares her body with that of her male lover. At first she does so in terms which seem to valorise male physiology, describing the male body in images which identify it with the phallus: 'the shaft of a strong pillar,/ Or brawny tree-trunk, firm and round and hard'. 'How frail I look next thee!' the poet exclaims. By the poem's conclusion, however, she has come to regard her own and other women's bodies as superior in design to those of men:

> And yet I think I like my own self better:
> What has thy body lovely as my breasts ?[14]

The assertion of female biological superiority represents a defiant reversal of centuries of masculinist and sexist denigration of female physiology, and of contemptuous and negative stereotyping of femininity in general.[15]

Two issues emerge as of particular centrality in the context of turn-of-century feminist discourse—those of the social construction of gender, and of racial and gender evolution. A further question is that of their connection with the advocacy of the rights of working women to control their own fertility.

A strong anti-militarist strain appears in the work of the leading advocates of birth control—no doubt in response to the rhetoric of 'family planning' opponents whose racist doctrines of 'race suicide' laid emphasis on the duty of upper-class Anglo-Saxon women to reproduce for the sake of the virility of the national stock.[16] This anti-militarism is partly a function of the liberal and radical positions held by many prominent feminists—Elsie Clews Parsons a leftward-leaning liberal; Margaret Sanger (at least in her early days of activism) a socialist; Emma Goldman an anarchist. But it also represents a response to the pervasive national chauvinism of much anti-birth control discourse, of the fears of so-called 'race suicide' of the Anglo-Saxon race.

Emma Goldman as birth control campaigner articulates the rhetoric of anti-militarism particularly forcefully. As with Parsons and with Sanger,[17] a clear strain of feminist self-fashioning runs throughout her autobiographical and other texts. As an integral part of her anarchist and feminist creed, Goldman believed that a woman could only find full liberation by 'refusing the right to anyone over her body', but also by refusing to religious institutions, the family, patriarchy or the State, the right to determine her life choices.[18] Goldman's own supreme moment of self-fashioning, if so one may term it, seems, in her own eyes at least, to have resided in her conscious decision not to undergo surgery which would have made it possible for her to bear children. In Goldman's own words, she had resolved to 'serve completely' her recently-found ideal of anarchist radicalism: 'To fulfil that mission I must remain un-hampered and untied…I would find an outlet for my mother-need in the love of all children…'[19] Even more marked, though, in Goldman's position on birth control, is her anti-militarism. Her stand in this regard is perhaps nowhere better exemplified than in her speech of 1916 to a New York court, when on trial under Section 1142 of the New York penal code which forbade distribution of contraceptives or of contraceptive information. The question of birth control, Goldman told the court, was 'largely a working-man's question, above all a working-woman's question'. In a country where 300,000 children died annually of malnutrition, parents, unlike the entrepreneur or the politician, who might require quantities of factory or cannon fodder, clearly had no vested interest in producing large families for their own sake. (The judge, unimpressed by Goldman's prediction that women, given choice, would increasingly refuse to 'go on like cattle breeding more and more', sentenced her to fifteen days in jail.) For Goldman, the fight for free access to birth control information was only one battle against capitalism and the state for 'a seat at the table of life'.[20] The double oppression suffered by working-class women—the fight for access to birth control as a blow struck for the working-class—is more clearly fore-grounded in Goldman's recorded statements than in those of either Parsons or Sanger, to be considered in due course.

A number of middle-class birth control activists display both a concern for working-class women's reproductive rights, and concern for the evolution of woman-hood in general. An interest in eugenics broadens from a focus on individual self-fashioning to what might be called a preoccupation with collective self-fashioning—and, ultimately, of the re-fashioning of the human race. Probably the best-known examples of faith in the possibilities of women's collective evolution are to be found in Charlotte Perkins Gilman's *Women and Economics*, where Gilman envisages new social roles for women as possessing the potential eventually to bring forth a female sex biologically superior to its predecessors. In *Herland*, which posits a world entirely peopled by women, this evolutionist speculation takes the form of a fable in which women have outgrown the childishness which still characterises the behaviour of those men who stumble into the women's domain.

A year before *Herland* appeared, another, less known, work of feminist science fiction was published by Inez Irwin, fiction editor of *The Masses*.[21] *Angel Island* (1914) offers a symbolic representation of the processes whereby women at the turn of the century were attaining the liberation of their intellectual and creative potential—but it also embodies an interest in feminist progress as a function of evolutionary change. In *Angel Island* a group of men shipwrecked on a desert island discover a nearly-extinct race of women—an evolutionary variation on the more common human biological form—who possess the power of flight. The men capture the women, cut off their wings and, in the name of the dictum, 'God never intended women to fly', try to subdue and domesticate them. The male ideal fails when a girl child born on the island turns out to have wings—and the women resolve to teach her both to walk and to fly, in order to reach her fullest potential. When, at the novel's close, a male child is born with the power of flight, the women have passed on their enhanced potential to the entire human race. The novel may be read as an allegory of collective self-fashioning—but also as an assertion of women's right to control over their own bodies.

I now wish to examine, as framed within the personal experience of two repre-sentative individuals, Elsie Parsons and Margaret Sanger, two specific explorations of the meaning to turn-of-century feminists, of 'self-fashioning'.

Elsie Clews Parsons, best known today as an anthropologist, was also a cultural critic, a feminist, and an encourager and active supporter of contemporary workers for reproductive rights.[22] Margaret Sanger devoted the better part of her life exclusively to the single issue—which for her came to constitute the main issue—of women's control of their fertility.[23]

Elsie Clews Parsons was the daughter of a wealthy New York banker and a Southern society belle. She was an anthropologist in the field, travelling unaccom-panied in Ecuador and New Mexico when her female contemporaries shrank from a car journey with a male acquaintance, unless another woman were present.[24] She was one of the first lecturers at the New School for Social Research, and the first

woman to be elected president of the American Anthropological Association.[25] She
became a leading authority on the native Pueblo culture of the American Southwest.
She also found time for active involvement in work for woman suffrage, for women's
reproductive rights, and for anti-militarism.

From childhood Parsons was a rebel against constraints imposed on her by her
class and gender, playing in the New York parks with working-class children against
the admonitions of adults; refusing to dress conventionally or to restrict herself to the
pursuits thought appropriate for women of her day.[26] In a concrete definition of the
term 'feminism', Cynthia, Parsons' fictional character in *The Journal of a Feminist*—a
character closely modelled on the author herself—explains:

> When I would play with the little boys in Bryant Park, although you said
> it was rough and unladylike, that was feminism. When I took off my veil
> or gloves whenever your back was turned…that was feminism…When I
> would go to college, in spite of all your protests, that was feminism.[27]

As an adult, Parsons continued to define her own conception of her social role
and to contest the gendered social expectations of her culture—walking hatless in the
street, sitting smoking with the men after dinner instead of 'retiring' with the women;
going in bathing on a fashionable Rhode Island beach without the stockings called
for by turn-of-century notions of feminine 'modesty'. Her ideals for social behaviour
were premised on what she called a 'love for personality'[28] and a resistance to prescriptive social constructions of human identity. Nowhere are these ideals clearer than
in her discussions of gender, and of gender socialisation. She is, for instance, to my
knowledge, the first feminist thinker to address the questions of the role of language
in gender socialisation. As she wrote in *The Old-Fashioned Woman* (1913): 'Are not…
"lovely", "darling", "sweet", "horrid", "mean", peculiarly girls' adjectives, and
"bully", "fine", "jolly", "rum", "rotten", "bum", peculiarly boys'?'[29]

Though never completely escaping the heterosexual biases of her day, Parsons
all the same expressed her opposition to pejorative terms such as 'tomboy', 'mannish',
or 'bachelor maid' when applied to women who failed to meet prescribed contemporary norms for heterosexual femininity.[30] She deplored the influence of European
mores on the practices of transvestism among the Zuni pueblo peoples of New
Mexico. (Transvestism, after all, calls into question rigid European-derived definitions of gender.) In *The Journal of a Feminist* Parsons has her fictional narrator
describe what one may take to be her own feminist ideal:

> This morning perhaps I may feel like a man; let me act like one. This
> afternoon I may feel like a female; let me act like one. At midday or at
> midnight I may feel sexless; let me therefore act sexlessly.[31]

In an anticipation of the cultural feminism of the early 1970s, Parsons' narrator
Cynthia writes:

> It seems to me that women are just as unemancipated as ever they
> were…Hitherto feminists have been so impressed by the institutional

> bondage of women...that questions of inner freedom have rarely
> occurred to them. That is why many of the objective customary signs of
> the lack of it have not troubled them, checks upon going about alone,
> clothes that hinder movement, endless little sex taboos.[32]

Another area in which Parsons asserts women's rights against the claims of a patriarchal society is that of women's control over their own reproduction. A majority of US birth control advocates entertained a preoccupation with birth control as an adjunct or accessory of eugenics which many today would find highly controversial, as in Parsons' protest at legislation which prevented educated women from breeding. Parsons is very much of her time in her interest in eugenics—and unfortunately, while democratic and egalitarian in much of her thinking, imbued in her thought on eugenics with some of the elitism of that movement. One of her reasons for deploring the childlessness of unmarried women teachers, for example, is that she believes such women 'belong to a superior [intellectual] stock; to penalize marriage and childbearing for them is a crime against eugenics'.[33] In a more enlightened vein, Parsons maintained that so-called 'race suicide' would be infinitely preferable to 'an only child custom or a flourishing system of foundling asylums'.[34] In her firm insistence that women's rights to control their own reproduction should take precedence over all other considerations, she shows herself at her most committedly feminist.

Awareness of and concern about the legal bans on disseminating birth control information made of Parsons an activist on reproductive rights issues. She was among a group of supporters who defended the birth control advocate Margaret Sanger—in 1915 and again in 1916—when Sanger was prosecuted for giving birth control information to working-class patients in her New York clinic. At a pre-trial dinner at the Brevoort Hotel, it was Parsons who proposed that twenty-five women who had themselves used contraceptives should stand up in court with Margaret Sanger and declare themselves guilty of breaking the law. (Only one, however, volunteered.)[35] In *The Journal of a Feminist* Parsons' narrator Cynthia advocates a similar strategy in connection with the abortion issue, proposing that a doctor should be found who is willing to challenge the law by performing abortions for women in need, and that a group of concerned citizens be formed to back them, during the inevitable ensuing prosecution. A medical practitioner with whom Cynthia raises this idea is understandably reluctant to take Cynthia's advice, given the stiff criminal penalties, not to mention the professional stigma, such a stand would incur. Instead, he expresses a wish that the American Medical Association or similar professional body would interest itself in the abortion and birth control issues.[36]

Quite as much as Margaret Sanger or Emma Goldman, both of whom were directly involved in agitation and propaganda for birth control, Parsons shows herself aware, in her writings at least, of how reproductive rights issues affected society's working-class majority. Access or lack of access to an abortion constituted, as she argues in *The Journal of a Feminist*, 'the crassest of class distinctions', since poor women were unable to gain assistance which upper-class women obtained relatively easily.[37]

Margaret Sanger's ('ghosted') *Autobiography* is less imbued with irony than Parsons' autobiographically based, if fictional, *The Journal of a Feminist*. In its own way, however, it reveals a comparable preoccupation with self-fashioning. In this connection it seems less than accidental that Sanger's narrative makes much of the fact that her father was not only an advocate—if a somewhat inconsistently practising advocate—of feminism[38]—but also an artist and a sculptor by profession. Sanger shared her father's uncritical faith in phrenology. In the autobiography she quotes with approval his dictum: 'Nature is the perfect sculptor; she is never wrong.'[39] Yet, as we shall see, this interest in and belief in nature's ability to 'sculpt' the human personality, stamping upon it its unalterable physical features, was not inconsistent with an individualist faith that a determined personal will might actually be capable of re-fashioning the original clay.

Writing—or rather, being ghost-written—with hindsight from the perspectives of 26 years on—Sanger tells of her decision to devote her life to the cause of birth control advocacy as the discovery of a vocation. Seen from this point of view, her autobiography offers its readers a religious conversion narrative. The tale of conversion begins with Sanger's early years as an organiser for the Socialist Party—a mission which afforded her a degree of personal satisfaction but left her frustrated, Sanger was later to claim, that many of the party's leaders—at least in her view—seemed unaware of the sufferings of working-class women overburdened with child-bearing and child-rearing. (One might wonder why, if the indifference she describes were really as pervasive as she maintains, she felt able to call on so many left-wing publications for subscriptions to start her birth control periodical *The Woman Rebel*.)[40]

Sanger tells how she went to work as a nurse on New York's Lower East Side as if attracted there by destiny, 'as though I were being magnetically drawn there by some force outside my control'.[41] She details the 'recurrent nightmare' of her visits to a slum district in which she heard 'the story told a thousand times of death from abortion and children going into institutions' or of the suicides of women driven to end their lives by inability to cope with the twin burdens of poverty and parenting. These experiences, events happening to women she knew as patients and as friends, haunted her: 'One by one worried, sad, pensive and aging faces marshaled themselves before me in my dreams, sometimes appealingly, sometimes accusingly... My own cozy and comfortable family existence was becoming a reproach to me.'[42]

Possibly not without the skilled assistance of the unknown ghost-writer, the narrative's next paragraph pointedly and dramatically foregrounds the specific moment of conversion in its opening phrase: 'Then one stifling mid-July day of 1912...' Sanger goes on to tell of her summons on this fateful day to the sick-bed of a patient, Sadie Sachs, close to death from septicemia, the aftermath of a botched self-induced abortion. When Sanger felt unable to offer birth control advice, despite her patient's desperate pleas for assistance, Sadie Sachs became pregnant again three months later. This time, her second attempt to perform an abortion put an end to her life.[43]

The final section of this chapter of the *Autobiography* recounts how Sanger 'walked and walked and walked' through New York's night-time streets, then stood awake all night before her bedroom window, while all the 'pains and griefs' of the city 'crowded in' upon her. Her vision of child labour, of 'six-year-old children with pinched, pale, wrinkled faces, old in concentrated wretchedness...making lamp shades, artificial flowers', is a vision of the exploitation of their labour into which children were driven by parental inability to control the size of their families. The scenes, writes Sanger, 'piled one upon another on another. I could bear it no longer'.

Fittingly, symbolically, with the dawn comes revelation, an answer to the narrator's anxious quest. 'It was the dawn of a new day in my life also', Sanger relates. '[N]o matter what it might cost, I was finished with palliatives and superficial cures; I was resolved to seek out the root of evil, to do something to change the destiny of mothers whose miseries were vast as the sky'.[44]

Elsewhere in the autobiography, Sanger tells of the titanic personal struggles of her adolescence, to 'sculpt' and refashion her own being to her greater satisfaction. Having defined her psychic identity as split between a 'wilful and emotional' self, and a self she identifies as more 'rational'—'the head Me'—Sanger describes how she set herself 'the task of uniting the two by putting myself through ordeals of various sorts'—braving her fear of the dark, or forcing herself to jump from heights. One of these self-imposed tests nearly cost her her life.[45] In her adult experience, she was to turn such exercises in empowerment of the will to good use by forcing herself to give birth control lectures, despite her terror of speaking in public. During her first of these lectures, to a large audience in Pittsburgh in 1916, she spoke, she says, 'in fear and trembling', and with her eyes closed.[46] Sanger attributes her timidity about public speaking to a Victorian ideal of respectable middle-class womanhood: 'My mother used to say a decent woman only had her name in the papers three times during her life—when she was born, when she married, and when she died'.[47] Insofar as she became a public figure—and indeed insofar as she re-fashioned herself in the image of a turn-of-century progressive activist, Sanger had, at least in the autobiographical fiction of self she offers us, to discard a late-Victorian construction of feminine identity.

In Sanger's autobiography, there is also consciousness of a popular image of the social activist as celebrity to which the narrator fails to approximate. Sanger recalls her sense of inadequacy when larger, more robust, women were mistaken for her in public gatherings where she herself would be overlooked. At such moments she felt herself to resemble 'a hungry flower drooping in the rain'.[48] For a brief period, according to her own account, she tried to make herself 'seem more competent-looking by wearing severe suits...'—a practice which she claims finally to have abandoned only because of lack of money to maintain the necessary wardrobe.

Above all, Sanger expresses an interest in the effect of public life on the shaping of her own personality. She vividly recalls, for instance, the speculations of a Portland, Oregon, chairwoman, in introducing Sanger's birth control lecture. The chairwoman wondered aloud what public life would make of Sanger after ten years. 'Most movements', the chairwoman said, 'either break you or develop the "public figure" type of face—hard and set through long and furious battling'. Sanger quotes the speaker as adding, 'I should like to see how she [Sanger] comes out of it.' Sanger comments, 'I have thought of this many times—how, if the cause is not great enough to lift you outside yourself, you can be driven to the point of bitterness by public apathy and, within your own circle, by the petty prides and jealousies of little egos which clamor for attention and approbation.'[49] Sanger's commentary here simultaneously refutes the importance of individual self-fashioning, and exalts it.

With the possible exceptions of Sanger and of Goldman—that both worked as trained nurses seems hardly accidental—the middle- and upper-class women who in their activities advocated reproductive choice for working-class women lived lives more or less removed from the experiences of those for and about whom they wrote. Their concern for reproductive freedoms—freedoms which, by and large, women of their class already enjoyed de facto, was intimately involved with their interest in individual self-fashioning. A corollary interest lay in feminist projects which envisaged collective female evolution as one possible outcome of 'family limitation' and of the experimentation in eugenics such practices seemed at least potentially to empower. This is not to suggest that turn-of-century birth control advocates were hypocrites— or even that they were exclusively bourgeois individualists, unmotivated by an authentic concern for working women's situations. But they were not working class, after all, and could hardly be expected to understand working-class experience at first hand. Their means of finding, or making, common cause with the needs of working-class women was to focus on an issue which in crucial if differing respects at least could be said to concern women of all classes—that of birth control. In this arena they served working-class women in an incidental manner, by first considering themselves.

Notes

1.   Helen R. Hull (1888-1971). Best-known as a novelist and author of short fiction, for her pioneering early feminist work: *Labyrinth* (New York: Macmillan, 1923); *Islanders* (New York: Feminist Press, 1988 [1927]). Hull's first short stories were published in *The Masses*. See Patricia M. Miller's excellent Afterwords to the recent editions of *Islanders* and *Quest* (New York: Feminist Press, 1990 [1922]). For biographical notes on Hull see: Stanley J. Kunitz (ed.), *Authors Today and Yesterday* (New York: Wilson, 1933); Margaret C. Jones, *Heretics and Hellraisers: Women Contributors to 'The Masses'* (Austin: University of Texas Press, 1993).

2.   Helen Hull, 'Till Death…', *The Masses*, January 1917, p. 6.

3.   My use of 'self-fashioning' is appropriated, of course, from the Renaissance context in which it has been employed by Stephen Greenblatt. See *Renaissance Self-Fashioning from More to Shakespeare* (Berkeley: University of California Press, 1980).

4.   See Nancy Cott, *The Grounding of Modern Feminism* (New Haven: Yale University Press, 1987).

5.   In this connection, the writings of Charlotte Perkins Gilman and Inez Irwin are of particular interest—Gilman's *Women and Economics* (New York: Harper & Row, 1966 [1898]) and *Herland* (ed. Ann J. Lane; London: Women's Press, 1979 [1915])—and Inez Irwin's *Angel Island* (ed. Ursula Le Guin; New York: New American Library, 1988 [1914]). See also n. 21, below.

6.   A useful source on Rauh and Rodman and their intellectual and social milieu is Judith Schwartz's *Radical Feminists of Heterodoxy: Greenwich Village 1912-1940* (Lebanon, NH: New Victoria Publishers, 1982).

7.   As associate editor and poetry editor of *The Masses* Dell exercised a significant ideological influence over the magazine's content. Although *Homecoming*, his autobiography

of 1933, expresses fairly reactionary views on gender roles and gender relations, at the time of his editorship Dell's ideas on sexual relations and on woman suffrage placed him in the avant-garde of feminist intellectual activism. (*Homecoming: an Autobiography* [New York: Farrar, 1933]).

8.   Jean Starr Untermeyer (1886-1970), poet and translator. See her *Love and Need: Collected Poems, 1918-1940* (New York: Viking, 1940). For further biographical data on Untermeyer, see Stanley J. Kunitz and Vineta Colby (eds.), *Twentieth Century Authors: First Supplement* (New York: Wilson, 1955).

9.   Untermeyer, 'Zanesville', *The Masses*, October 1916, p. 20.

10.   Helen Hoyt, poet, and associate editor of *Poetry*. See *Who Was Who among North American Writers, 1921-1939* (Detroit: Gale, 1976)—also Jones, *Heretics and Hellraisers*, pp. 6, 17, 18, 19, 177, 189 n.7.

11.   Hoyt, 'Menaia', *The Masses*, September 1915, p. 16.

12.   Quoted by Floyd Dell, 'Adventures in Anti-Land', *The Masses*, October-November 1915, pp. 5-6.

13.   Elsie Clews Parsons, writing in *The Old-Fashioned Woman: Primitive Fancies about the Sex* (New York: Arno Press, 1972 [1913]), p. 9. Parsons was a prolific writer of such works of social criticism as *Fear and Conventionality* (New York: Putnam's, 1914); *Social Freedom* (New York: Putnam's, 1915); *Social Rule: a Study of the Will to Power* (New York: Putnam's, 1916), as well as of her better-known work on the cultures of native Americans and on Afro-American folklore. There exist two thoroughly researched biographies of Parsons: *A Woman's Quest for Science* by her great-nephew Peter Hare (Buffalo, NY: Prometheus, 1985); and Rosemary Levy Zumwalt's *Wealth and Rebellion* (Urbana and Chicago: University of Illinois Press, 1992). Parsons' previously unpublished *The Journal of a Feminist* has recently been published. (ed. Margaret C. Jones; Bristol: Thoemmes Press, 1994).

14.   Hoyt, 'Comparison', *The Masses*, September 1915, p. 16.

15.   Gilman's *Herland*, which imagines a society exclusively composed of women—and women who exhibit greater maturity and intelligence than men—makes a similar gesture. (See n. 5, above.)

16.   In this connection, see the remarks of Henry A. Wise Wood, president of the Aero Club of America to a congressional committee on woman suffrage, in which he called it 'a damnable thing' to 'weaken ourselves by bringing into the war the woman, who has never been permitted in the war tents of any strong, virile, dominating nation' (Quoted in William L. O'Neill, *Everyone Was Brave: A History of Feminism in America* [Chicago: Quadrangle, 1969]).

17.   A particularly useful source on the contributions of Emma Goldman and of her lover Ben Reitman to birth control activism—contributions called into question by Margaret Sanger, who believed that Goldman had merely jumped on an already rolling popular bandwagon set in motion by, among others, herself—is to be found in Linda Gordon's *Woman's Body, Woman's Right: A Social History of Birth Control in America* (New York: Grossman, 1974).

18.   Goldman, *Anarchism and Other Essays* (Port Washington: Kennikat, 1969 [1910]), p. 217.

19.   Goldman, *Living My Life* (New York: Knopf, 1931).

20.   'Emma Goldman's Defense', *The Masses*, June 1916: p. 27.

21.   Inez Haynes Irwin (Gillmore) (1873-1970). Fiction editor of *The Masses*, and a prolific novelist in her own right, Irwin is probably best known for her history of the militant woman suffrage movement in the United States, *The Story of Alice Paul and the National Woman's Party* (Fairfax, VA: Dellinger's, 1921). Her novels *Gertrude Haviland's Divorce* (London: Harper, 1925) and *Gideon* (New York: Burt, 1927) are worth reading also—in particular for their

feminist exploration of possible definitions of the 'New Woman'.

22.   In this connection see, for example, Parsons's *The Journal of a Feminist*, pp. 82-83.

23.   See Margaret Sanger's 'ghosted' autobiography, discussed below.

24.   An attitude satirised in *The Journal of a Feminist*, pp. 101-102.

25.   Zumwalt is particularly interesting on the struggles and triumphs involved in this achievement of Parsons in a male-dominated scientific community. See in particular pp. 13-14 of *Wealth and Rebellion*.

26.   An amusing impression of the startling effect of Parsons' contempt for convention upon her immediate social circle is given by Clarence Day in a 1919 tribute, 'Portrait of a Lady', published in the *New Republic*: 'Every now and then her neglect of some small ceremonial sets the whole tribe to chattering about her, and eying her closely, and nodding their hairy coiffures or their tall shiny hats, whispering around their lodge fires, evenings, that Elsie is queer' (*New Republic*, 23 July 1919, pp. 387-89).

27.   *The Journal of a Feminist*, p. 86.

28.   *Fear and Conventionality*, p. 217.

29.   *The Journal of a Feminist*, p. xviii.

30.   *The Journal of a Feminist*, p. xxv.

31.   *The Journal of a Feminist*, p. 91.

32.   *The Journal of a Feminist*, p. 45.

33.   Parsons, 'Penalising Marriage and Childbearing', *The Independent,* 18; January 1906, pp. 146-47.

34.   'Penalising Marriage and Childbearing', p. 146.

35.   Margaret Sanger, *Autobiography* (New York: Norton, 1938) p. 189.

36.   *The Journal of a Feminist*, pp. 81-82.

37.   *The Journal of a Feminist*, pp. 82-83.

38.   For a revealing account of some of these inconsistencies, see the first chapter of Sanger's *Autobiography*: 'Father took little or no responsibility for the minute details of the daily tasks. I can see him when he had nothing on hand, laughing and joking or reading poetry. Mother, however, was everlastingly busy sewing, cooking, doing this and that. For so ardent and courageous a woman he must have been trying, and I still wonder at her patience...Father's devotion to mother, though equally profound, never evidenced itself in practical ways' (p. 16).

39.   *Autobiography*, p. 19.

40.   'They were still subject to the age-old, masculine atmosphere compounded of protection and dominance' (*Autobiography*, p. 109). Sanger then goes on to explain how she collected 'several hundred subscriptions' to the *Woman Rebel* by advertising in '*The Masses, Mother Earth, The Call, The Arm and Hammer...*' (p. 109). All of these, with the exception of Emma Goldman's anarchist publication *Mother Earth*, were socialist in their ideological perspectives.

41.   *Autobiography*, p. 86.

42.   *Autobiography*, p. 89

43.   *Autobiography*, p. 91.

44.   *Autobiography*, p. 92.

45.   *Autobiography*, pp. 25-26.

46.   *Autobiography*, p. 193.

47.   *Autobiography*, p. 192.

48.   *Autobiography*, p. 204.

49.   *Autobiography*, p. 205.

Configuring the Body
at the Turn of the Century

Barbara Will

NERVOUS SYSTEMS,
1880–1915

'It's this wild hunt for rest that takes all the life out of me', Waymarsh complains to his companion Lambert Strether in the opening pages of Henry James's *The Ambassadors*.[1] Suffering from a case of 'prostration', the American Waymarsh has been sent on a rest cure to Europe in order to be distracted from 'the stress of occupation, the strain of professions'. As Waymarsh comes to realize, however, attempting to elude 'a general nervous collapse'[2] has itself become a stressful 'occupation', a 'wild hunt' staged in a 'Europe' with its own aggressive social ethic of consumption and pleasure. Rather than being freed from the worry of capital gain, investment, risk, and savings, the nervous American abroad must work doubly hard to safeguard his thrifty values which are threatened by the very consumption-oriented rest he is hunting for. Strether himself suffers from the nervous 'distraction' of safeguarding the most valuable investment of the absent Mrs. Newsome, her son Chad. As he puts it when pressed about his 'failure to enjoy' the European setting: 'I'm always considering something else; something else, I mean, than the thing of the moment. The obsession of the other thing is the terror'.[3] It is already interesting to note that this novel plots a decidedly late Jamesian transformation of 'Europe' from a seductive and elusive social space for Americans to the site of 'terror' and 'wild hunt[s]'. What is striking, however, is that for James's Americans, the adverse reaction to 'Europe' and its pleasures is written on the body—in a physical 'exhaustion' and 'distractedness' which encodes a complex national ethos.

The 'disease' from which both Waymarsh and Strether suffer, and with which James himself was engaged in a private battle, was the turn-of-the-century physiological condition called 'nervousness' or 'neurasthenia'. Introduced to the general American public in the early 1880s by its most ardent popularizer, the New York physician George M. Beard, neurasthenia, also known as *The American Disease*, was defined as a peculiarly American condition of 'nerve deficiency' or 'nerve weakness', afflicting those who had exhausted their store of 'nerve energy' through tiring, reckless, or sexually profligate behavior.[4] Henry, William, and Alice James were among the thousands of men and women at the turn of the century who claimed to be 'neurasthenics', and who sought relief in a veritable industry of practitioners devoted to its diagnosis and cure; others included Theodore Roosevelt, Owen Wister, Thorstein Veblen, Henry Adams, Charlotte Perkins Gilman, Theodore Dreiser, Edith Wharton, Emily Dickinson, and Charles Chesnutt. With such a burgeoning crisis within the ranks of the productive elite, 'nerve specialists' sought to find cures for nervousness by focusing on the body as the primary locus for the 'disease', by searching for a lesion or wound which would link nervousness to a physiological disorder. Yet such investigations into the ætiology of neurasthenia were invariably stymied by the failure of the nervous body to signify its own organic processes, to *signify itself* as a contained or bounded materiality. Multiply signifying, the nervous body nevertheless eluded the scientific gaze, 'readable' rather only as a physical *effect* of changes in the national landscape. It is as if the elusive 'disease' of nervousness and its symptoms underscore what Mary Ann Doane has recently argued in another context: that the body always becomes visible as a model for something else.[5]

In focusing here specifically on the ways in which doctors constructed interpretations of the disease, and on the implications of these interpretations within turn-of-the-century American literature produced by and about neurasthenics, we shall see that 'nervousness' is from the beginning understood in *both* physiological *and* metadiscursive and textual terms—as a disease at once seemingly 'grounded' in a stable and concrete referent—the body—and as a currency which enabled other social discourses to circulate. It is this latter aspect of nervousness which precluded medical discourse from wholly perceiving the nervous body as a material object of empirical analysis. In the first place, while doctors attempted to 'ground' conclusions about the nervous body in terms of physiological or metabolic propensities and deficiencies, they found themselves confronted with a series of physical symptoms which invariably failed to eventuate in any organic illness. In addition, physicians writing on the condition were continually drawn toward larger social issues with which neurasthenia was finally seen to be inextricable. Thus for many, 'nervousness' came to be seen less as a physiological condition or neurological disorder, than as what enabled the discursive 'reading off' of overdetermined social abstractions as material or corporeal effects.

Thus, for example, the constitutive bodily imbalance between 'excessive' behavior and exhaustion, of which Beard and others imagined nervousness as the effect, was never simply a physiological problem but was always already perceived as both a national trait and a sign of national difference, emerging as a physiological complement to American imperialist ideologies at the turn of the century. In *The Ambassadors*, for example, 'nervousness' is thematized less in terms of a specific malady than as a general *façon de vivre*—as what, ironically, subtends the ambassadorial office itself. If to be an 'ambassador' means to keep alive and potent an absent national *épistème*—whether American capital and its values as represented by the town of Woollett, Massachusetts, or phallic maternal authority as embodied in the figure of Mrs. Newsome—then it is equally, for James, either to transform a violent national ethic of literal-mindedness and 'hard work' into a death drive, as with Waymarsh, or to suffer, as Strether does, from 'distraction', a simultaneous identification with and resistance to the Other. In either case, the obeisance to this absent and terrifying 'other thing' only intensifies the physical symptoms which one had hoped to elude temporarily or even to cure in the flight abroad. Unwilling ambassadors on failed rest cures, Waymarsh and Strether cannot escape from the iron cage of their national nervousness, for to do so would be ironically to lose their very constitutive difference from a Europe which holds out the possibility of their 'cure'. Published in 1903, the year in which President Theodore Roosevelt introduced a stringent immigration act designed to 'purify' the American race, *The Ambassadors* clearly thematizes the relation between claims to American national difference and the constitutively nervous American body.

This double-edged aspect of neurasthenia—as a debilitating disease and as the very condition of the modern American subject—informs countless other contemporary discussions of the phenomenon, discussions which were themselves richly encoded with not only nationalist ideologies but also those pertaining to gender, class, and race. For the progressivist George Beard, nervousness was considered to be the evolutionary outcome of 'civilization'—of which he considered America the shining example—and was thus seen primarily to afflict those occupied with 'the modern'—writers, artists, commerce-oriented 'brain workers' and upper-class women. Beard clearly links the weakness of the neurasthenic not only to the national but equally to the social development of 'the civilized, refined, and educated...of women more than of men': nervousness is less 'debility' than 'sensibility'. In comparison, Beard's contemporary and rival spokesman for the disease, the Philadelphia physician Silas Weir Mitchell, saw neurasthenia as a pathology linked to a demasculinized internal constitution, a physiological aberration which need to be purged from the upper-class American body in order for the nation to assume its power over threatening primitives within a rapidly expanding world. For both writers, the national dimension of nervous illness was inextricable from concerns over class, race, gender and the changing roles of men and women, as from the possibility and danger of 'modernity' itself.

As Tom Lutz has recently argued, neurasthenia was, 'most succinctly, a sign of modern life'.[6] In fact, it is precisely as a sign of 'the modern', as a 'modern sign', a sign marked by no necessary correspondence between signifier and disease, and signified and body, that 'nervousness' within turn-of-the-century American culture functioned as a term of equivalence, as what enabled homologies to be drawn between different levels of social meaning. While medical discourse provides us with one instance of the interpretive challenge posed by the emergence of the phenomenon of 'nervousness' within turn-of-the-century American culture, what is striking indeed—and as yet relatively unseen by contemporary historians—is the insistence with which scores of writers, cultural critics, capitalist entrepreneurs, politicians, as well as doctors, appropriate 'nervousness' as a central trope within their individual discourses: as a crucial character trait within turn-of-the-century literature such as *The Ambassadors*, as the sign of a new organization of gender within medical discourse, as a metaphor for the logic of the American marketplace within the emerging science of economics, as the mark of American national 'effeminacy' or of national strength and superiority within certain political discourses. Thus when considering the question posed by many nerve doctors of the day—'what is nervousness?'—we might begin by tracing the circular logic in which the signifier 'nervousness' is implicated, looking less for what the nervous body can reveal to us than for what was produced on and around this body.

Asymptotic Symptoms

If it was physicians who produced the first definitive accounts of the 'disease' of 'nervousness', then these accounts were at the same time always already implicated in the literary, in textual questions of signification and interpretation. At a moment when the line between 'doctor' and 'author' was being blurred, an investigation into the disease of neurasthenia was at the same time conceived as a confrontation with the fragmentary and slippery nature of the modernist text itself.

Beard, himself a neurasthenic, claimed credit for having given a label to a series of symptoms baffling in its very lack of physiological coherency or reliability. At one point in his 1881 text *American Nervousness*, Beard presents a two-page list of 'typical' neurasthenic symptoms, among them:

> insomnia, drowsiness, bad dreams, cerebral irritation, dilated pupils, pain, pressure and heaviness in the head, tenderness of the scalp, changes in the expression of the eye, increased blushing, desire for stimulants and narcotics, sweating hands and feet with redness, impotence, hopelessness, ticklishness, writer's cramp, fear of lightning, or fear of responsibility, of open places or of closed places, fear of society, fear of being alone, fear of fears, fear of contamination, fear of everything [7]

What is amusing to contemporary readers looking back through a post-Freudian lens is the familiar landscape of neurosis, of unconscious processes scrawled arbitrarily on the surface of the body. What is interesting historically is the sense, for Beard and other neurasthenia specialists at the dawn of psychoanalysis, of being faced with an enormous, arbitrary juxtaposition of physiological and psychological symptoms—symptoms which precisely in their variety and logical inconsistency at once demanded and defied interpretation. What frustrated the doctor confronted with these symptoms was at once the need and the difficulty of finding any direct physiological cause, or 'lesion', for the sickness. In Anson Rabinbach's terms, neurasthenia was a condition prone to misdiagnosis, marked by its capacity to signify other illnesses, by its 'incessant orchestration of analogies to other maladies'.[8] Precisely in its signifying excess, the disease threatened to overwhelm the interpretive powers of the physician, even to produce its own 'neurasthenia-effect', as Beard himself writes: 'the magnitude, multiplicity and imminence of the phenomenon of American nervousness overawe[s] and wear[ies] us…'[9]

The pursuit of a diagnosis in the face of neurasthenia's literally exhausting ('nerve-depleting') uninterpretability pertains to the peculiar textuality of its symptamotology. Charcot described the neurasthenic as '*l'homme de petit papier*',[10] referring to the tendency of literate neurasthenics to write down their symptoms before appearing at the doctor's office. Not only did the neurasthenic patient with his written list of symptoms demand diagnosis, but it was precisely the test put to the authoritative powers of the physician which so fascinated prominent members of the medical community—many of whom, like Weir Mitchell and William Dean Howells, were already published novelists and poets of some repute. Doctors confronted with the neurasthenic body felt they were entering into unknown territory, and they perceived this journey into the signifying body as a problem of interpretation, representation, and textuality.

In his 1895 *Studies on Hysteria*, Freud describes the problem of the patient suffering from nervous exhaustion as being in inverse proportion to the 'tirelessness' of neurasthenic language, to 'the indefiniteness of all the descriptions', in short to the very generative power of the signifiers 'expressing' this condition:

> When a neurasthenic describes his pains…he is clearly of opinion that language is too poor to find words for his sensations and that those sensations are something unique and previously unknown, of which it would be quite impossible to give an exhaustive description. For this reason he never tires of constantly adding fresh details, and when he is obliged to break off he is sure to be left with the conviction that he has not succeeded in making himself understood by the physician…[11]

While elsewhere Freud had described neurasthenia largely in terms of exhaustion or 'willllessness', here the language of the neurasthenic, or neurasthenic language, is marked by excess and proliferation, by a metonymic tendency to elude final signification. This at once posed a problem to interpretation, and illuminated the peculiar failure within the neurathenic setting of a doctor-patient relationship which would later be called transferential. At the same time, the problem of neurasthenia marked out a new field of linguistic expression, a textual field which echoed the endlessly symptomatic nervous body, continually suggesting yet failing to result in any organic disease. Like a modernist text, furthermore, the language which emerged to 'speak' the nervous body gestured toward but ultimately defied the closure of any final interpretation or diagnosis.

The Writing Cure

For Silas Weir Mitchell—like Beard and many other nerve doctors, a neurasthenic—the slipperiness of neurasthenic symptoms and 'the indefiniteness of all the descriptions' of the nervous body strongly influenced his famous and elaborately gendered 'Rest Cure', which Freud himself was to praise for its ability to 'overcome…severe and long-established states of nervous exhaustion'.[12] Reading neurasthenia in terms of the failure of a natural and national organization of the sexes, an interpretation also forwarded by his close friend Theodore Roosevelt, Mitchell demanded that his patients' fragmented bodies be 'made whole' again through a treatment based on rest, isolation, and the encouragement in his male subjects—and denial in his female ones—of creative expression.[13] While he held equally deep scorn for the effeminate, neurasthenic urban brain worker as for the tiring, weepy, nervous 'lady', Mitchell also conceived of the disease of neurasthenia as a kind of bodily resistance to modernity and its inherent effeminacy, a wordless physical cry for the loss of individuality, personal liberty, and the entrepreneurial values of an older masculine America. In his 1871 text *Wear and Tear: Or, Hints for the Overworked*, Mitchell appeals to something 'authentic' in the patient suffering from nervous exhaustion, something which signifies not the future, but the past, a kind of nostalgia written on the body which his Rest Cure promised to respond to.[14] This 'authentic' element was seen as being available to his male patients precisely through the act of writing, while for the female neurasthenic under Mitchell's care, 'she who, for months, and wisely, read no newspapers, and who asked another to open and read all her letters and telegrams',[15] any textual engagement was deemed inextricable from the onset of nervousness.

Mitchell's Rest Cure is best known today through its damning portrayal within Charlotte Perkins Gilman's 1892 short story, *The Yellow Wallpaper*, where the bored and restless female narrator suffering from a prolonged bout of nervousness is warned by her physician husband that 'if I don't pick up faster he shall send me to Weir Mitchell in the fall'.[16] The story is usually read autobiographically, focusing on the fact that Gilman herself underwent a Rest Cure, after which she was advised by Mitchell to 'Live as domestic a life as far as possible', and 'never [to] touch pen, brush, or pencil again'.[17] This and other such statements expose the threat within Mitchell's prescriptions for women, articulated again and again in his various roles as private physician, public lecturer, and novelist. In the first place, Mitchell argued, women were not only physically weak, but their bodies manifested a psychological weakness as well; a theory which informed the quite simple (and often wrong) assertion that 'you cure the body and somehow find that the mind is also cured'.[18] Second, for Mitchell, women had a 'natural' tendency to mental excitation, only exacerbated by such things as education; women's minds were in a sense more active or more capable of transgressing normative boundaries than men's, and as such sorely tested the authority of the physician:

> The terrible patients are nervous women with long memories, who question much where answers are difficult, and who put together one's answers from time to time and torment themselves and the physician with the apparent inconsistencies they detect.[19]

Finally, Mitchell was no Freud, fearlessly venturing beyond the science of physiology into the far reaches of the female psyche; sensing the 'transgressive' possibilities of the unbounded and 'indefinite' signifying economy of neurasthenia, Mitchell's response was to reassert the doctor's power over the literal and the 'definite':

> To those still actually nervous…a word or two of sustaining approval, a smiling remonstrance, or a few phrases of definite explanation, are all that the wise and patient doctor should then wish to use…To read the riot act to a mob of emotions is valueless, and he who is wise will choose a more wholesome hour for his exhortations.[20]

In a powerful reversal of Mitchell's prescriptions, Gilman claimed to have written *The Yellow Wallpaper* as a way of curing herself of the injury of Mitchell's Cure; she recognized that in writing the story and thus in 'recovering some measure of power' she had proved Mitchell's ideas about women and writing wrong.

The narrative energy in *The Yellow Wallpaper* devolves from the sort of zero-degree state of nervous exhaustion; as the story opens, the artistic young female narrator asks herself, 'And what can one do?'[21] Gilman's story develops with a bitter awareness that women denied access to the public sphere risk turning their energy inward, toward a dissection and dissemination of the bounded self, caged by a female body and literally confined within the nursery of a country house. A symbol of pure consumption in her constant ingestion of food, the narrator of *The Yellow Wallpaper* 'does' the only thing that is left to her, turning her surroundings into a scene of writing, into the text of her boredom and despair. This is far from the 'stenuous' theory of writing which will otherwise subtend Mitchell's advice to his male patients, for in the prison of Mitchell's Rest Cure writing spends, rather than strengthens, a woman's nerve force. Here writing signifies the sickness itself (she refers to her journal, which chronicles her disease, as 'dead paper'), rather than a means to a cure.

In such a reading, *The Yellow Wallpaper* represents a woman's terrifying fall into madness, and as representation offers an unrelenting critique of patriarchal and bourgeois treatments of the female body. But there is as well a utopian element within Gilman's text. The narrator's nervousness is at once the cause and the effect of her confinement—an impossible double bind, but one that also signifies a crucial textual break in Gilman's æsthetic, with implications beyond the act of representing a woman's emprisonment. For Gilman's supposedly autobiographical story, in a sense, proves Mitchell's fears about the relation between nervousness and women's 'transgressive' creativity to be *right*. It is precisely Gilman's break with a representational imperative which stages a scene of recognition between the language of neurasthenia and that of the fragmentary or disruptive text of high modernism. Ending with the fragmentation of perspective and the breakdown of narrative coherency, *The Yellow Wallpaper* figures neurasthenia as the cause of the transition from 'realist' to 'modernist' representation. As though exemplifying Freud's description of the neurasthenic, the text imagines the narrator's 'neurasthenic consciousness' as resistant to a 'realist' ordering of language—precisely the type of resistance Mitchell hoped to erase from his female patients' consciousness by denying them access to pen, brush, or pencil. Either way we read the ending of this story, therefore—as Gilman's autobiographical projection of madness away from herself onto a fictional character, or as the liberation of character itself into a new 'modernist' textual landscape—the nervous female body proves an intractable textual problem to the authority of the attending physician.

But Gilman tells only half the story of the Weir Mitchell Rest Cure. Where *The Yellow Wallpaper* creates an implicit analogy between female neurasthenia and the modernist æsthetic, the texts produced by Mitchell's male patients figure the rejection of the neurasthenic subject as a return to a masculine territory based on a 'natural', pre-modern order. In these latter, the nervous body and its symptomatic 'indefiniteness' is the very impetus for a rejection of modernity itself.

Mitchell's theories about nervousness were as committed to establishing the difference between male and female bodies as to providing a cure. Briefly put, in his male cases Mitchell understands physical symptoms as not being psychological in origin, precisely because the subjects are male. Rather, he saw the gradual emasculation of the American male in the face of a rapidly industrializing modern culture, especially the bureaucratic 'brain worker', as disrupting the natural balance of the male body. Unlike George Beard, who extolled the effects of brain work on American 'civilization', Mitchell saw this development as the sign of a dangerous weakening in American national powers. In this he was adding his voice to a chorus of other social critics, like John Barrett, Roosevelt's minister to Siam, who claimed that the '"rule of survival of the fittest" demanded an American "strong enough to stand the pace", not one in whom "brain-force" had vanquished "nerve-force".'[22] What was needed was a pre-industrial cultural space in which to right gender imbalances, to rediscover a 'manly' entrepreneurial spirit and thus to rescue male neurasthenics from the sphere of 'the feminine'. By 'feminine', here, I refer to appearances, actions, desires, coded by dominant social discourses and institutions as at once inherent to biological females, and as constituting the 'not-male' or the 'not-masculine', as the very negation of the masculine, to use Luce Irigaray's terms.[23]

Mitchell's gendered interpretation of the causes and cures of neurasthenia is neatly taken up and transformed within the literature of another socially-prominent Philadelphian and one of his most famous patients, Owen Wister. Along with fellow neurasthenics Theodore Roosevelt and Frederic Remington, Wister, who reinvented the Western genre for the twentieth century, was the first to conceptualize 'the West' as the proper counterpart to a consumptive, feminized East. Like Gilman, Wister—at the time a bank clerk—was treated by Mitchell for 'nervousness', and also consequently produced a literary work as a result of his cure. Unlike Gilman, who was sent to bed to cure her nervousness, Wister was advised by Mitchell to 'go West and seek rest', taking along plenty of paper and pencils in order to write or draw as much as he wished. Wister eagerly took up the challenge, envisioning an uncharted wilderness where he could be 'something of an animal and not a stinking brain alone'.[24]

As the literary outcome of his Rest Cure, Wister's *The Virginian* was published in 1903, the same year, interestingly, as James's *The Ambassadors*; but unlike the latter, *The Virginian* carves out a textual space in which the effete neurasthenic is less tragic than risible, and the identification with an imperialist 'America' less traumatic than triumphant.[25] *The Virginian* figures some imaginary American West as the site of 'masculine' identity and activity, toward which the East is its negating, decadent, 'feminine' Other. This spirit is embodied in the figure of the entrepreneurial cowboy, virile, Saxon, and thrifty, who is juxtaposed within the novel to the effeminate Eastern 'tenderfoot' narrator—a juxtaposition which Roosevelt was to appropriate in his own extremely successful public transformation from Eastern neurasthenic weakling to rough-riding champion of American imperialism. Indeed, though a 'dying breed' and thus the symbol of resistance to modernity, Wister's cowboy hero would in fact come to symbolize the virile strength of a 'progressive' American imperialist ideology at the turn of the century—not the less so in his paternalistic relations toward his Mexican farmhands. Furthermore, Wister's anti-modern cowboy is no outlaw but an able and honest homesteader with a head for business; by the end of the novel he is 'an important man, with a strong grip on many enterprises'.[26] Patently non-nervous, the Virginian is to the white, masculine values of entrepreneurial capitalism what the neurasthenic narrator is to the effeminate values of commodity capitalism. Wister's use of the figure of the neurasthenic Easterner as a contrast to the Western cowboy-entrepreneur enables the romance of a lost world of gallantry and paternalism to be thrown into relief, a world which would be in turn ideologically rehabilitated by turn-of-the-century political and economic policy.

What Gayatri Spivak has described as the process of 'Othering'[27] is effected in the manner with which the nervous body is variously encoded by both Mitchell's prescriptions for men and Wister's Westerns: as a model for the sickness eating away at the American heartland (in the threat of the Eastern Establishment, its particular capitalist organization, immigrant labor force, and feminized ideology of social reform), as well as for the excess which lies beyond American shores and which Roosevelt and his Rough Riding cowboys would attempt to contain in their 'big stick' campaign of healthy male imperialism. Yet at the same time as Mitchell and his patients were figuring the struggle over the 'health' of the nervous body as a struggle for national power and virility, alternative medical visions of the nervous body were attempting to link nervousness to the potent 'modernity' of the American nation.

Nervous Economies

In *American Nervousness*, George Beard writes:

> Neurasthenia is the direct result of the five great changes of modernity: steam power, the periodical press, the telegraph, the sciences, and the mental activity of women.[28]

In formulating neurasthenia as the effect of rapid changes in industrialization, and of the phenomenon of female intellectual power, Beard argues ultimately that neurasthenia is less a pathology to be eradicated from the national body than a necessary condition of modern 'civilization' and national character to be adjusted to. As such, nervousness is not a disease but a constitution: that which signifies a certain fitness for the modern urban space and its social and business networks.

Emerging out of the labor-saving achievements of industrialization, Beard writes, neurasthenia is endemic to a new physiological type, 'the brain worker'. Characterized by 'fine, soft hair…small bones…and a muscular system comparatively small and feeble', the neurasthenic brain worker is more physiologically adapted to 'the desk, the pulpit, and the counting-room' than to 'the shop or…the farm'.[29] Because of his physiology, the brain worker is constitutionally inclined to 'overtax' his supply of nerve force, leading to the state of 'nervous bankruptcy, from which he finds it as hard to rise as from financial bankruptcy'.[30] Beard's homology between the language of nervousness and the language of finance here underscores once more the permeability and superfluity of these discourses, as well as, for Beard, their comparable 'modernity'. In the late nineteenth century, the language of the modern American marketplace was increasingly incorporating a neurasthenic vocabulary into its conceptual framework, as though market culture were not only productive of neurasthenia, but were itself a 'nervous system'. Terms like 'depression' or 'panic', entering into the vocabulary of the market in the last two decades of the nineteenth century, echoed the symptomology of the neurasthenic body, just as the shift between excess and depletion of the capitalist business cycle was often read in terms of the typically unbalanced nervous constitution of modern individuals. As with the fluctuations of capital, therefore, the stage of breakdown and depression in the nervous body is seen by Beard as a necessary counterpart to the overinvestment of nerve energy, a sort of self-enforced rest cure during which the 'vital energy' or nervous force returns; it is because of this that Beard points to the great longevity of 'brain workers' and identifies the merits of nerve exhaustion in all its varieties, which protects the body from 'fatal, acute, inflammatory disease'.[31]

Beard's description of the typically neurasthenic 'brain worker' here has significant implications for the medical debate over the interpretation of nervousness. First, he rehabilitates the argument of Mitchell and others that intellectual labor—that of businessmen, lawyers, clergymen, financiers, clerks, scientists, as well as artists and writers—be understood as inherently pathological. 'Brain work' is simply another form of 'labor', one performed in cities rather than on farms. Furthermore, Beard's idea of the brain as a 'laboring' organism analogous to other muscles devolves from a more general late nineteenth-century effort to see analogies between the body and that most suggestive image of modernity, the machine. By making a conceptual analogy between manual labor and mental labor—both now in some way implicated in the process of mechanization and quantifiable as to value—Beard appealed to a market logic of equivalence to attempt to restore the relationship between mind and body.[32]

Secondly and relatedly, Beard stresses the centrality of this neurasthenia-producing brain work to the forward economic and imperialistic march of modern American civilization: 'activity in our higher forms of civilization, especially in modern times, is carried to a degree from which nervous diseases must be the inevitable result'.[33] Ultimately, therefore, neurasthenia is less the sign of debility than of cultural superiority, vital longevity, and innate genius; it is less the sign of a specific type of labor than of the greater value of one labor over another. Neurasthenia is 'one of the cardinal traits of evolutionary progress marking the increased supremacy of brain force over the more retarded social classes and barbarous peoples'.[34]

What is interesting in this celebratory account of the 'brain worker' as the most evolved accomplishment of natural selection is its explicit link, for Beard, to 'the mental activity of women'. For if neurasthenia is the condition of the modern urban brain-worker involved in the great technological projects of the future—if, indeed, 'brain work' is prone to excess and 'overinvestment'—then this idea at least in part emerges from the sense that 'the intellectual' in turn-of-the-century American culture properly belongs to the sphere of 'the feminine'. This is not to suggest, of course, that work which could viably be called 'intellectual labor' was in any sense the prerogative of women, nor that Beard is conceiving women's productivity in market terms. Political, economic, and academic institutions which would encourage and reward such labor were largely closed to women. And despite the numerous best-selling female authors on the market in the last two-thirds of the nineteenth century, it was precisely mass culture's association with women, in Andreas Huyssen's formulation, which marked popular texts as devalued cultural commodities, as pulp.[35]

Clearly, however, George Beard's point is that the social groups most involved with the modern—brain workers—are seen to have a decidedly feminine mental and physical constitution. In particular, the mental negotiation of modern life—the sensitivity to shocks, the response to the new, the ability to lapse into an energy-saving fatigue—was for Beard and others inextricable from the feminine. By 'feminine', here, I refer again to Irigaray's notion of the 'not-male', as to Huyssen's reference to the 'imaginary male femininity' which signifies a radical sensibility in Western literature and philosophy since the eighteenth century.[36] If the 'mental activity of women' is for Beard one of the five great changes of modernity which produces neurasthenia, then there must be something inherent in the 'feminine' constitution which is more adapted to modern life or 'civilization'. At the same time as women themselves are incapable of scaling the heights of intellectual genius, what is implied by 'femininity'—a constitution, which, when seen in men, enables a certain negotiation of the demands of modern life—lays out an important paradigm for a new, not-masculine form of subjectivity.

Beard's description of the feminized male in which nervousness is constitutional coincides with an appeal to a reactionary social Darwinism. For 'mental work' rooted in the ambiguously gendered body serves to naturalize class difference, as though such work were somehow inherent in the physiological makeup of fine-boned, soft-haired, effeminate men: 'the fine organization…is the organization of the civilized, refined, and educated, rather than of the barbarous and low-born and untrained'.[37] The masculine, patently non-nervous working classes differ in their bodily labor from feminized brain workers only in the greater 'modernity' of the latter's labor—modernity here being synonymous with refinement and delicacy.

The nervous body thus figures a new form of 'feminine' subjectivity read through bourgeois class privilege. In *The Theory of the Leisure Class*, Beard's contemporary Thorstein Veblen conceived of 'the feminine' and 'the aristocratic' as the remnants of an obsolete class system, prehensile limbs surviving within the progressive realms of market and machine culture.[38] For Beard, however, these categories subtend modernity itself. Such a problematically-gendered and vestigially-aristocratic individual type as the genius, to which Beard devotes a great deal of consideration in *American Nervousness*, is seen finally as having *the* effeminate and nervous constitution equal to the demands of modern life. The standard nineteenth-century notion of the degenerate, impotent, and effeminate genius, in being newly characterized as neurasthenic, re-emerges in turn-of-the-century public discourse as the representative modern male, capable of negotiating the pressures and 'depressions' of capitalist expansion while also, like a woman, remaining acutely sensitive to the shocks and stresses of the city.

This relationship between nervousness and a 'modern' subjectivity is clearly thematized within Theodore Dreiser's 1915 novel *The 'Genius'*.[39] Dreiser stages the artistic genius as a figure for something seemingly Other to the artist—the successful capitalist 'brain worker'—and in so doing names his nervous and feminized pro-tagonist 'Eugene', as though to underscore the relationship between the 'genius' and one who is eugenically fit to survive in the modern world. In the novel, Eugene begins life as a talented artistic 'genius', suffers a nervous breakdown, undergoes a form of Rest Cure in which he adopts the life of a manual laborer, and returns to life as a successful businessman. From the beginning of his life, Eugene's artistic capacity is linked to ill health: 'He was not very strong to begin with, moody, and to a notable extent artistic. Because of a weak stomach and a semi-anemic condition, he did not really appear as strong as he was'.[40] This initial difference from the 'vigorous, healthy manhood' of his Midwestern father eventually emerges in two distinct ways: in his art and in his inconstant relations with artistic women, whom he finds 'closest to his soul'. In his art, Eugene is a modern and a nationalist in his commitment to representing not worn images of Paris, but the new, the as-yet-unseen in the life of such great American cities as Chicago or New York; he is vaunted as an original painter of working-class life, of the common people, of railroads and tanneries and the street. Yet this is precisely the working-class world which, because of his physical weakness, he cannot or will not enter, preferring the drawing rooms of rich artistic ladies, the ones who initially proclaim him a genius. This is the company who at once launches him on his wildly successful career as an artist, but to whom the Veblenesque opprobrium of leisure, excess wealth, and sickly femininity clings. This period of Eugene's life comes to an end when he suffers a nervous breakdown.

The 'cure' for Eugene's 'excess' of nervous excitement is to be found, not surprisingly, in the manual labor of men—the kind of work which Eugene has represented in his art but in so doing kept at a distance from immediate experience. Yet, crucially, Eugene does not join the ranks of men as a fellow laborer, but appeals for work 'as an artist, temporarily incapacitated by neurasthenia'.[41] Knowing that his physical labor has no value on the railroad (which Veblen, for one, associates primarily with a masculine modernity), Eugene is nevertheless able to convince the foreman of his need for work precisely because the foreman recognizes not his unemployability but his alternative market status: 'artist-neurasthenic'. At this moment Eugene is able to escape the drawing-room and move freely among social classes: as though his nervous body and corresponding 'sensibility' give him a freedom unavailable to other forces of labor on the market. Through this hands-on encounter with the patently non-nervous working class, Eugene finally abandons the path of the artistic genius creating masterpieces and embarks on a career as a successful businessman—retaining nothing from his past but his nervous 'sensitivity' and his love of female beauty. It is the latter which ultimately fells him, while the former—his nervousness—is precisely what makes him a successful reader of the constantly shifting whims and tastes of the capitalist market.

Dreiser is here taking up and transforming a familiar turn-of-the-century discussion over genius and physiological degeneracy, encapsulated in William James's 1896 claim that the type of the genius is more prone to nerve diseases than 'any other member of the sedentary class'.[42] James's findings echo what had become common-place in post-Enlightenment discourses on genius: that genius is at once only found in a male body, but in a body prone to exhibit decidedly feminine reproductive traits of passivity, receptivity, and the power to produce 'intellectual children'. By the end of the nineteenth century, the contradictions in the gendering of genius had become acute, the innate 'femininity' of the type now seen to be pathological, linked to weakness and illness. Dreiser's genius Eugene is, as stated in the 'Foreword' to the novel, a 'pathological specimen of life', and this pathology is located in his weak and feminized body. It is interesting in this respect that Dreiser changed his plans for the title of this text after he wrote it, putting quotation marks around the word 'genius': this change in the figuration of the term clearly underscores an authorial awareness of the ambiguity of the representation itself. At the same time, however, Eugene's 'making' is caused by the social institutions and practices which appropriate his nervousness as the ideal condition, not for artistic success, but for business success. Indeed, *The 'Genius'* seems to be suggesting that the intellectual predisposition (with its implicit femininity) most suited to the labor of the nineteenth-century artistic genius has emerged in the early twentieth century as the ideal constitution for the commerce-oriented brain worker. Eugene succeeds because he is a nineteenth-century neurasthenic genius in a turn-of-the-century business suit.

From Nervousness to Stress

Dreiser's and Beard's celebration of neurasthenia—as the condition appropriate to a new organization of the gendered body in the modern American marketplace—thus works to encourage an accommodation to the cyclical excess and depletion which characterizes both the nervous physiology and the capitalist market at the turn of the century. Gilman's story offers another account of the creative and disruptively modern possibilities encoded in the nervous body, but, like James, represents these possibilities as a reaction to an external and oppressively authoritarian influence. Even Weir Mitchell's championing of 'balance', of a 'proper alternation of physical and mental labor',[43] and its literary expression, the nostalgic dream of an American West untinged by nervous blight where healthy entrepreneurs operate financially balanced farms, is simply a recognition of the power of neurasthenic modernity and its polar by-products, a strenuous life or exhaustion. Roosevelt's injunction after touring the West to 'acquire fearlessness'[44] is the statement of a perpetual neurasthenic, and a supreme oxymoron: one is either nervous, or one never has been, like *The Virginian*, and is naturally 'fearless'.

In any case, it is the signifying excess of its symptoms—and the appropriation of this signifying economy by a variety of social discourses—which most marks the nervous body as wholly a product of a particular moment of social and cultural change which I have been calling 'modernity'. A product of this moment—and pro-ductive of it, giving form to a new subjective constitution as to its imagined counter-part, as the continued currency of the term 'nervousness' throughout the first decades of the twentieth century attests to.[45] The interpretive struggles over the phenomenon of nervousness, I believe, can prove illuminating as we consider our own *fin-de-siècle* preoccupations with such physiological attributes of the postmodern body as stress, total allergy syndrome, and chronic fatigue syndrome; and as we grasp their usefulness —and slipperiness—as signifiers for shifting social, political, and economic relations.

Notes

1.   Henry James, *The Ambassadors* (London: Penguin, 1986 [1903]), p. 73.

2.   *The Ambassadors*, p. 71.

3.   *The Ambassadors*, p. 67.

4.   George M. Beard, *American Nervousness: Its Causes and Consequences* (New York, 1881).

5.   See Mary Ann Doane, *Femmes Fatales: Feminism, Film Theory, Psychoanalysis* (New York: Routledge, 1991).

6.   Tom Lutz, *American Nervousness, 1903* (Ithaca: Cornell University Press, 1991), p. 4.

7.   Beard, *American Nervousness*, p. 7.

8.   Anson Rabinbach, 'Neurasthenia and Modernity', in *Incorporations* (ed. Jonathan Crary and Stanford Kwinter; New York: Urzone, 1992), p. 179. For a longer exploration of these issues see also his *The Human Motor: Energy, Fatigue, and the Origins of Modernity* (New York: Basic Books, 1990).

9.   *American Nervousness*, p. 18.

10.   Rabinbach, 'Neurasthenia and Modernity', p. 180.

11.   These remarks were made in the context of Freud's case study of 'Fraulein Elisabeth Von R', now entitled 'Case 5' in Sigmund Freud and Joseph Breuer, *Studies on Hysteria* (London: Penguin, 1980), pp. 203-204.

12.   Freud was especially taken with Mitchell's advocacy of electrotherapy, massage, and isolation as a 'cure' for nervousness. See his 1887 'Review of Weir Mitchell's *Die Behandlung gewisser Formen von Neurasthenie und Hysterie*', in *The Standard Edition of the Complete Psychological Works of Sigmund Freud* (ed. Strachey; London: Hogarth Press, 1974), I, p. 36.

13.   For an overview of Mitchell's theories, see his *Fat and Blood: And How to Make Them* (Philadelphia: Lippincott, 1877).

14.   Silas Weir Mitchell, *Wear and Tear, or Hints for the Overworked* (Philadelphia: Lippincott, 1871).

15.   Silas Weir Mitchell, *Doctor and Patient* (Philadelphia: Lippincott, 1888), p. 130.

16.   Charlotte Perkins Gilman, *The Yellow Wallpaper and Other Writings* (New York: Bantam, 1989), p. 8.

17.   Quoted in Suzanne Poirier, 'The Weir Mitchell Rest Cure: Doctor and Patients', *Women's Studies* 10 (1983), p. 26.

18.   Quoted in Poirier, 'The Weir Mitchell Rest Cure', p. 19.

19.   Mitchell, *Doctor and Patient*, p. 48.

20.   *Doctor and Patient*, pp. 6-7.

21.   *Yellow Wallpaper*, p. 2.

22.   Quoted in Bill Maxwell, 'Owen Wister and the Imperial Wages of the West' (unpublished paper, Duke University), p. 9.

23.   See her *Speculum of the Other Woman* (trans. Gillian C. Gill; Ithaca: Cornell University Press, 1985).

24.   Quoted in Maxwell, 'Owen Wister', p. 10.

25.   Owen Wister, *The Virginian* (New York: Viking Penguin, 1988 [1903]).

26.   *The Virginian*, p. 392.

27.   See *The Empire Writes Back* (ed. Bill Ashcroft *et al.*; London: Routledge, 1989), p. 97.

28.   *American Nervousness*, p. 96.

29.   *American Nervousness*, p. 26.

30.   *American Nervousness*, p. 10.

31.   *American Nervousness*, p. 197.
32.   For a highly suggestive analysis of American 'machine culture' and its relation to discourses of the body at the turn of the century, see Mark Seltzer, *Bodies and Machines* (New York: Routledge, 1992).
33.   *American Nervousness*, p. 176.
34.   Quoted in Maxwell, 'Owen Wister', p. 8.
35.   Andreas Huyssen, 'Mass Culture as Woman', in *After the Great Divide: Modernism, Mass Culture, Postmodernism* (Bloomington: Indiana University Press, 1986), pp. 44-62.
36.   *American Nervousness*, p. 49.
37.   *American Nervousness*, p. 26.
38.   Thorstein Veblen, *The Theory of the Leisure Class* (New York: Penguin, 1979 [1899]).
39.   Theodore Dreiser, *The 'Genius'* (New York: Simon and Schuster, 1923 [1915]).
40.   *The 'Genius'*, p. 11.
41.   *The 'Genius'*, p. 311.
42.   For a general discussion of James's views on genius, see Eugene Taylor, *William James on Exceptional Mental States: The 1896 Lowell Lectures* (New York: Scribner, 1983).
43.   Mitchell, *Wear and Tear*, p. 19.
44.   Theodore Roosevelt, *An Autobiography* (New York: Da Capo, 1985 [1913]), p 54.
45.   Several recent studies have plotted the relation between neurasthenia and 'modernity' as a transcultural phenomenon. See in particular Arthur Kleinman, *Social Origins of Distress and Disease: Depression, Neurasthenia, and Pain in Modern China* (New Haven: Yale University Press, 1986); Edward Shorter, *From the Mind into the Body: The Cultural Origins of Psychosomatic Symptoms* (New York: Free Press, 1994).

Tim Armstrong

Disciplining the Corpus:
Henry James and Fletcherism

'Oh yes', she rejoined in answer to his exhibition of the degree in which
what was before him did stir again to sweetness a chord of memory, 'oh
yes, food's a great tie, it's like language—you can always understand your
own, whereas in Europe I had to learn about six others'.[1]

These are the words of the nurse Miss Mumby in Henry James's unfinished novel *The
Ivory Tower* (1917), having just fixed lunch for the novel's hero Graham ('Gray')
Fielder. Miss Mumby articulates a connection between food and language which
stresses the distinction between the natal or natural and what one acquires by dint of
education or choice. Gray, brought up in Europe, understands that 'the so many
things she had learned to understand over there were not forms of speech but
alimentary systems'. Alimentary systems, organized ways of eating which are like
ways of talking, were very much part of James's thinking as he began *The Ivory Tower*
in 1910. Formerly the famous eater-out whose large appetites embellish Elizabeth
David's cookbooks ('the eggs were so good that I am ashamed to say how many of
them I consumed…It was the poetry of butter, and I ate a pound or two of it'[2]), he
had just abandoned the austere dietary procedures recommended by the American
health reformer Horace Fletcher, which he had followed since 1904. What I want to
consider here is the nature of the link (if any) between writing and Fletcherizing in
James's work—a link which is tantalizing because it does not seem to appear in any
systematic way; because it always seems held at arm's-length by that simile, eating
being 'like' a language. The notoriously abstract late James thus seems a kind of limit
case of the connections between bodily reform and literary texts.

1. Horace Fletcher

The charismatic and influential Horace Fletcher, 'The Great Masticator', was one of
a number of American dietary reformers in the Progressive era, all of whom aimed to
maximize bodily efficiency using scientific techniques. Others included J.H. Kellogg,
with whom he had rivalrous links in the period of his greatest activity, 1903-1910,
and later C.W. Post, inventor of Grape Nuts.[3] Fletcher sold a technique: the aim of

Fletcherism was complete mastication to the point where an automatic swallowing reflex ('nature's food filter') intervened. Chewing food to a liquid would, Fletcher postulated, produce perfect digestion, 'internal antisepsis', and avoid the 'auto-intoxication' produced by food wastes lodging in organs. Fletcher's followers also aimed to eat sparingly, and minimize luxurious foods. The theory of auto-intoxication, developed in England and Europe in the 1890s by Alexander Haig and others, had quickly spread to the USA, spawning a range of techniques and products aimed at its alleviation.[4]

The most fundamental aim of Fletcherism was thus the elimination of waste. Fletcher was fond of the comparison between bodies and sewerage systems, practicing internally what Victorian hygiene campaigners had advocated externally; and was obsessed with the purity of Fletcherite fæces, which were to be so well-processed that they could cleanly be expelled into the hands and even mailed to interested parties (unlike Kellogg's bulky fibre-based diet, his dairy-rich diet aimed at minimal throughput, producing a light 'ash'). He also claimed that his techniques, as well as reducing weight, gave him immense bodily resistance, demonstrated in well-publicized strength and fatigue tests against college athletes—he always won. In maximizing efficiency and minimizing waste or toxicity, the body becomes like a scientifically-managed factory: in his *Glutton or Epicure* (1899), Fletcher compares the body to a power-plant in which the engine is the heart, the dynamo the brain, and so on; a section on 'unprofitable management' making clear his ideological convergence with Frederick Taylor.[5] As James Whorton points out, the Fletcherite body could be analysed in terms of fiscal metaphors: 'deposits of food and rest, and withdrawals of exertion and self-neglect'.[6] This way of thinking has its origins in the steady-state system of bodily energies postulated by psychologist George Beard and others, and in the writings of other physiologists (Herbert Spencer, for example, had written in his essay 'The Social Organism' that 'what in commercial affairs we call *profit*, answers to the excess of nutrition over waste in a living body').[7] But like other progressive thinkers, including William James in 'The Energies of Men', Fletcher is more optimistic than the Victorians, stressing the possibilities of boosting energy levels through efficiency and waste management.[8]

Fletcher lectured messianically to business and popular audiences. His supporters included influential progressives like John D. Rockefeller and the economist Irving Fisher (with whom he founded the Health and Efficiency League of America), S.S. McClure (of *McClure's Magazine*), and Bernarr Macfadden, the publisher of *Physical Culture*. In England Eustace Miles preached a similar dietary doctrine in his journal *Healthward Ho!*[9] Literary fans included William and Henry James, Upton Sinclair, who wrote books on fasting and diet, as well as his famous attack on the meat industry in *The Jungle*, and Conan Doyle; others like Arnold Bennett and H.G. Wells adopted related stomach-culture techniques.[10] Gertrude Stein's brother Leo was a follower, and Stein herself, a devotee of machine-age Americana, seems to have absorbed some of the doctrine.[11] Admittedly, such discipline was not to everyone's taste: the expansive Ezra Pound (before he himself succumbed to Method) registers a protest against it in a doggerel section of a letter to Marianne Moore in 1919, implicitly criticising her self-discipline (he calls her 'a

Malthusian of the intellect'): 'And the wildreness iwll not be healed/either by fletcherizing or by a diet of locusts' (sic).[12] Put on some weight there, Marianne!

James too is different from a Sinclair or Stein: for all that he struggled with recurrent constipation, his adherence to a reformist American dietary cure sits oddly beside his usual ironic distance from American enthusiasms and technological modernism.[13] Compare Gray Fielder's desire in *The Ivory Tower* to 'have, in a quiet way, the American palate without emitting the American sounds';[14] or his likening of the house he inherits in the novel to 'some monstrous modern machine'.[15] James's work does not readily encompass the mechanical, as some of the prose of later American realists and modernists does—one might recall Alfred Kazin's comments on the machine æsthetic in John Dos Passos's *U.S.A.*: 'the wonderfully concrete yet elliptic prose…bears along and winds around the life stories in the book like a conveyor belt carrying Americans through some vast Ford plant of the human spirit'.[16] On the contrary, James seems most in consonance with the other side of the equation in turn-of-the-century psychology; the parallelism which seems mind as an epiphenomenon floating free from a deterministic universe. So what did Fletcherism and its stress on bodily efficiency mean for James, and how is it connected to his writing?

2. Fletcherism and Revision

Begin with the timing. James's Fletcherism started in May 1904, as he was finishing *The Golden Bowl*, his last major novel. Extolling 'the divine Fletcher' to Edith Wharton and others, and boasting of making a small meal last almost an hour, he chewed slowly for over five years, lunching with the Great Masticator himself in 1909 (one would have liked to be a fly on that wall), and only abandoning the habit, after a change in medical advice, in February 1910. The period coincides reasonably closely with the most famous of James's late tasks, the re-writing of his corpus for the New York Edition—a project which had been in the air for some time, and was negotiated at the end of the American tour undertaken for *The American Scene*, in June 1905. The revisions were finally off his hands in the summer of 1909; by the time James abandoned Fletcher he had begun to sketch out what was to become *The Ivory Tower*.[17]

It is tempting, given this chronology, to hypothesize a *prima facie* equation between the two tasks: the complete digestion of food, and the 'chewing-over' and purification of James's corpus for the new edition; rumination in both the literal and figurative senses. Two physical tasks, since the handwritten revisions broke James's late practice of composition by dictation. Is this a link that any of the many critics writing on James's revisions have considered? The answer is no.[18] Philip Horne, in his study of the New York Edition, *Henry James and Revision*, runs through several of James's proliferating metaphors for revision implicit or explicit in James's writings without considering 'chewing-over'—those he discusses include restoring a painting (admittedly, the most pervasive metaphor in James's comments), the cosmetic beautifying of a face, re-reading, unconscious process, following one's own tracks, tidying up his 'uncanny brood' for the drawing room, revivification.[19] Anthony

Mazella's recent survey of criticism on the revisions for *A Companion to Henry James Studies* is silent on the issue—as eating should be in polite company.[20] And Hershel Parker's ringing cry in 1984 for a more detailed attention to biography and sequence mentions only James's extensive social and publishing obligations. Is something lurking behind this flagrant disregard for the alimentary? Or is the suggestion of a connection between Fletcherism and revision perverse, like the food-obsession of the anorexic?[21] What's wrong with talking about food?

For the suggestion is there. In the New York Edition preface to *The Golden Bowl*, which contains James's most extensive comments on the process of revision, he writes:

> The 'old' matter is there, re-accepted, re-tasted, exquisitely re-assimilated and re-enjoyed—believed in, to be brief, with the same 'old' grateful faith (since wherever the faith, in a particular case, has become aware of a twinge of doubt I have simply concluded against the matter itself and left it out); yet for due testimony, for reassertion of value, perforating as by some strange and fine, some latent and gathered force, a myriad more adequate channels.[22]

This 're-tasting' or rumination is consonant with Fletcherism; the channels and perforations through which is conducted (and through which 'material' is voided) are at least partly those of the digestive tract. The metaphor of eating occurs sporadically throughout the prefaces: he 'tastes again' the feel of a work;[23] he 'bites into' a character;[24] his imagination is a pot-au-feu mixing flavours;[25] writing is like making jam, or a 'residuum of admirable 'stock''.[26] In particular James expresses a Fletcherite disapproval of his younger self, suggesting incomplete digestion of material: he labours 'too greedily' for truth,[27] he takes 'too prompt a mouthful...of the fruit of the tree of knowledge' into 'so juvenile, so generally gaping a mouth',[28] he is 'fed at every pore'.[29] The pace of Roderick Hudson is 'too fast...Roderick's disintegration... swallows two years in a mouthful'.[30] Elsewhere, bodily metaphors are implicit: he comments of *The Tragic Muse* 'I delight in a deep-breathing economy and an organic form' before considering the misplacing of the girdle and waistband.[31] The same terms are also present in later essays: in the famous meditation on 'the slice of life' in 'The New Novel' (1914), for example, and in that essay's equation of 'method' with the selection, preparation and consumption of material ('matter into which method may learn how to bite').[32] In such passages, James equates perception and writing with ingestion—as, from a critical perspective, F.R. Leavis did when he accused James of a 'malnutrition' of the 'deep centre' of his being. Taking up James's own terms, critical reception of his work has centred on metaphors of taste and consumption from the beginning.[33]

3. Solitude and Hygiene

A tantalizing link is thus proposed. If we consider (as Parker suggests we should) the conditions of creation of the New York Edition, there are further links between revision and Fletcher's project. James's letters on the two share a stress on solitariness:

the Fletcherite eschewed company as conductive of bolting; the edition required the avoidance of other tasks. The letter of 25 September 1906 in which James recommends Fletcherism to Mrs Humphrey Ward is a crucial piece of evidence, explicitly linking feelings about interruptions and the technique. He begins by praising solitude and non-communication: 'The letters of life, in general, become more and more its poison, moreover, surely—and are a matter against which, for myself, my heart is rapidly encasing itself in impenetrable steel'. He then moves on to Fletcherism: 'Fletcherize hard... Am I a convert? you ask. A fanatic, I reply'. He concludes by returning to the steel bands, which are now located firmly around the dietary technique rather than writing: 'Grapple it [Fletcherism] to your soul with hoops of steel. I rejoice to know that you've begun'.[34] The 'poison' of involvement in life and letters modulates into the toxins which the Fletcherite avoids.

A later letter to Edith Wharton reinforces the point about solitary discipline. Writing of her marital problems in October 1908, James is uncertain: 'I move in darkness; I rack my brain; I gnash my teeth'. Nevertheless the teeth-gnashing— which is of course other than Fletcherite—produces some advice on emotional hygiene, the relation between inner and outer. (It also modulates Strether's famous 'Live all you can' in *The Ambassadors* into a more controlled form):

> Only sit tight yourself *and go through the movements of life*. That keeps up our connection with life—I mean the immediate and apparent life; behind which, all the while, the deeper and darker and the unapparent, in which things *really* happen to us, learns, under that hygiene, to stay in its place. Let it get out of its place and it swamps the scene; beside which its place, God knows, is enough for it! Live it all though, every inch of it—out of which something valuable will come—but live it ever so quietly; and—*je maintiens mon dire*—waitingly![35]

Patience, going through the movements, hygiene are James's literary and physical preoccupations. Dorothy Richardson noted that James's writing involved a material and physical discipline in 1924, calling his punctuation 'a spiritual Swedish Drill'.[36] We might even see here a flight from the feminine 'swamp' and from the swelling female body, which Camille Paglia sees as implicit in James's late style:

> James describes states of *waiting*. He seeks fullness, retention, rumination in the bovine sense. The unexpressed is an endemic engorgement, a male pregnancy without issue...The prose resists us with its weight and opacity...It is a large, humming, hovering mass.[37]

Mass, waiting, passivity: Paglia's terms are redolent of the 'anabolic' energy which Patrick Geddes had ascribed to the feminine in *The Evolution of Sex* (1889); and while they seem essentialist in the late twentieth century, they fit well with modernist preoccupations with the line and the 'scientific' elimination of a bulk which it often sees as feminine.

As we watch James self-consciously move between a bodily economy and a more general economy in which the world impinges too much, we see what the

discipline of Fletcherism could represent: a rationale for self-concentration and solitude. Accumulating material for his books is a matter of being abroad in the world—
as in the American dinner parties which irked him on his 1905 tour, important
though they were to his project. Revision is a different matter, a self-consuming
reformation in which, as Thomas Leitch comments, he becomes 'his own ideal
reader', dramatizing his encounter with himself.[38] To cease to write on and contemplate a shape, to turn from the big novel to the corpus and to reproduce that corpus
in a streamlined form, to adopt a solitary discipline, all these factors find a convergence in this period, and a bodily reflection in Fletcherism.

    One motivation for reformation of both corpus and body was James's fear of
death. Sir James McKenzie, the heart specialist whom he consulted in 1909, compared James's anxiety to the horrors of his ghost stories (particularly *The Turn of the
Screw*): 'it is the mystery that is making you ill. You think you have got *angina pectoris*
and you are very frightened lest you should die suddenly'.[39] Mystery can make the
heart stop, body acting in tandem with literary effects. Mackenzie recommended
continued mastication, and exercise to reduce the figure. But as James neared the end
of the process of revision, the New York edition is itself figured as a blockage to the
'corpulent, slowly-circulating and slowly-masticating' author.[40] To his nephew he
described it as a 'Nightmare', and a few months later, in August 1908, he wrote to
W.D. Howells:

> I could really shed salt tears of impatience and yearning to get back, after
> so prolonged a blocking of traffic, to too dreadfully postponed and
> neglected 'creative' work; an accumulated store of ideas and reachings-
> out for what even now clogs my brain.[41]

In voiding himself of the Edition, James could return to more productive work; to
the late autobiographies and his last two novels. And he abandoned the chewing cure.

4. Reforming the Corpus

Fletcherism thus allows us to see writing as rumination. It is unsurprising that
metaphors re-tasting, re-assimilating, and re-digesting should occur to James. He
tended to see writing in two ways. In one, it is organic, often a form of bodily
production—using 'a bellyful of fresh and nutritive impressions', for example; or
praising the sculpture of Hendrick Anderson for its sense of blood-flow 'under the
surface', of an 'internal economy' including bladder and belly.[42] He describes his
work as progeny (a 'brood'), as flowering seed, a 'living affair'.[43] Revision may thus
be a re-birth, re-tasting, or a God-like 'breathing' upon 'old wounds and mutilations
and disfigurements'.[44] Readers have often noticed a similar embodiment of James's
characters: in 1920 Gilbert Seldes commented 'always, in whatever he wrote, the
bodily presence of his characters and the effect of their presence on others are
tremendously rendered'.[45] On the other hand, James could refer to the 'veiled and
disembodied' author lying behind the central consciousness he uses to present many

of his works, with an accompanying stress on technique, manipulation, system (a 'particular degree of pressure on the spring of interest'), the working out of a 'scheme', the weaving of a carpet. This is James the calculating maker, and in this scheme reworking can be 'patch[ing] up one's superstructure',[46] the lubrication of a machine, the restoration of a picture or the tying up of loose ends. These familiar oppositions can be projected onto others in James—the distinction between writing as 'vision' (a godlike gift); versus the accumulation of material, of 'good stuff'.

Mark Seltzer, in his *Bodies and Machines*, provides co-ordinates for this opposition between the organic and the mechanical in what he calls the 'realist machine'; a discursive mode which reproduces the tensions and relays in modern society between the organic and the mechanical, between bourgeois individualism and rationalized industrial production.[47] Seltzer's terms are ultimately derived from Thorstein Veblen; in *The Theory of Business Enterprise* (1904) and elsewhere, Veblen argued that the real opposition in American society was not between traditionally-defined classes but between the engineers or managers, whose aims were science and efficiency, and the business classes for whom the perpetuation and naturalization of oligarchy and the accumulation of wealth were priorities. These opposed conceptualizations, in Seltzer's view, are constantly in tension and in relation, typically in an oscillation between ideas of self-possession and of abandonment to social process, and often involving questions about bodies and their status.[48]

A version of this opposition is constantly present in James, for whom his entry into the market is a fraught issue. James, Seltzer suggests, presents us with bodies which are 'natural' and integral while also registering their nature as artefacts. Fletcherism might also be seen as attempting to resolve these uncertainties: it is an *organic discipline*, a technique which works on the bodily self, aiming to restore a state of 'natural' hygiene. It resembles a religion—indeed, William James used Fletcher as an exemplar of 'the religion of healthy-mindedness' in *The Varieties of Religious Experience* (1902), and of 'ideas considered as dynamogenic agents' in 'The Energies of Men' (1907).[49] Yet it also makes claim as a science, its bodily engineering linked to other reform movements in the progressive era: eugenics, the body-building of Macfadden and Sandow, Boys Scouts, mass-exercise movements, calorie-counting.[50]

William James's writings on consciousness are a useful context here, since they too address the paradoxical position of the mind-body complex in modernism, at once an object of systems and science which remove its authority, and the focus of ideologies which assert its autonomy. James opposes any dualism, stressing that bodily experiences or emotions cannot be distinguished from things in the outside world: '"outer" and "inner" are not coefficients with which experiences come to us aboriginally stamped, but are rather results of a later classification performed by us for particular needs'. The body, in particular, is 'the palmary instance of the ambiguous' here: it can be thought of either as 'part of outer nature', and treated as an object; or it can be thought of as 'me', in which case 'its breathing is my "thinking", its sensorial adjustments are my "attention", its kinesthetic alterations are my "efforts", its visceral perturbations are my "emotions"'.[51] For James it is in intentional activity, in 'doing', that these categories are best resolved: the body which acts and has consequences cannot be seen in dualistic terms, it works on a world which is neither entirely nature or culture.[52]

Henry James's attitudes to his writing, and in particular the New York Edition, suggest a similar mix of idealism and pragmatism: in Leon Edel's account the Edition is a Temple of Art, the perfected version of his self; but it was also, as recent critics have stressed, what James hoped would be the instrument of his survival in late life— 'the bread of my *vieux jours*', as he put it to Edith Wharton, from which he would continue to feed.[53] The body needs food, and the work needs sales in order to achieve that; the corpus is a commodity. Yet James could also imagine a corpus which needed no food, no truck with a market, writing in 1902 that 'my work insists upon being independent of such phantasms [as a public] and on unfolding itself wholly from its own "innards".'[54] This self-consuming body is the literary self, a private rather than public entity.

As with William James, one way of resolving this opposition was to do something with the body of his work in order to represent it on the market, disciplining it both in the name of order and presentability. James's most fundamental metaphor for revision, Mazella suggests, is the 'religion of doing' described in the preface to *The Golden Bowl*:[55] 'the whole conduct of life consists of things done, which do other things in their turn', so that 'to "put" things is very exactly and responsibly and interminably to do them...these things yield in fact some of its most exquisite material to the religion of doing'.[56] The 'innards' here are the 'vast smothering boa-constrictor[s]' of proofs with which he was struggling in 1908; a self which must be set in order.[57] Fletcher's own religion of 'doing' lends weight to the sense of the 'innumerable acts' which might reform a life or a corpus, innards or proofs, bringing together technique and body.

In order to see what such a bodily technique might imply in terms of the discursive location of the *literary* corpus, it is helpful to set it in wider social perspective. Hillel Schwartz, in his fascinating history of food, fat and diets in America, *Never Satisfied*, argues that the period after 1900 saw a revolution in attitudes to body size:

> Between 1880 and 1920, gluttony (freed from its association with [dyspepsic] thiness), would be bound to fatness, fatness to inefficiency, inefficiency to lack of energy and loss of balance, and imbalance to overweight. This knot of relationships would hold as well for housewives as for dancers, and in the home as in the heavens.[58]

The aim of a variety of disciplines, including Fletcherism, fasting and thyroid-medication, was a balanced, regulated and lighter body. Fashion followed a similar course (after 1910 in particular) with lines which emulated the flowing forms of modernist design—an emphasis which Stuart Ewen links to 'an emerging ideal of mobile immateriality', evidence of the 'increasingly abstract trajectory' of capitalism itself.[59]

The modern regime of bodily self-control was thus born. Calorie-counting was pioneered by Irving Fisher, the rather crazy economist also responsible for what came to be the Consumer Price Index. For Fisher, fatness and inflation were conceptually linked, as were 'racial health' and prosperity. In *Stabilizing the Dollar* (1920) he wrote:

> Imagine the modern American business man tolerating a yard defined as
> the girth of a President of the United States! Suppose contracts in yards
> of cloth to be be now fulfilled, which had been made in Mr Taft's
> administration![60]

The 300 pound Taft—the last President (1908-12) whose size public perception
allowed to be equated with solidity, according to Schwartz—becomes an index of
inflationary (and consuming) possibilities which Fisher tries to stabilize with his
unshrinkable 'commodity-dollar', an index-linked currency whose value would
remain steady while its weight in metal was adjusted as necessary. Progressive
economic philosophy and bodily reform are linked.

The shift in attitudes to the body which Schwartz describes can be related to
the literary corpus, beginning with Elaine Showalter's contrast between the
'poisonous volume' of the *Fin de Siècle* and the Victorian triple-decker (which
Showalter equates with the solitary bachelor and the mother-father-child family
structure respectively).[61] James had written slim novellas before returning to the
sprawling final novels, with what seemed to many (himself included at times) their
over-inflated treatment of small matters. Size was a double burden, encompassing the
body and the book: *The Golden Bowl* was 'too big and the subject is pumped too dry';
the English edition was 'fat, vile, small-typed, horrific'.[62] In the project of the New
York Edition there was the possibility of reforming the corpus, pruning works,
radically recasting others, reissuing the result in a 'handsome' new form. That itself
posed problems, as Michael Anesko points out: 'with comfortable margins and
attractive type, all those hefty Victorian triple-deckers burst the seams of a one-
volume format'.[63] What emerged was thus necessarily related to the heavy ranks of
the collected editions which were James's models (Balzac, Kipling). The difference is
that the process represented a discipling of the corpus as a whole, a 'doing away' with
it, as it were, that it might be re-born. The external constraints of the format (the
Uniform Edition) are less important than its internal consistency. Peter Wollen's
version of the paradigm-shift over shape described above is useful here:

> Once the Belle Epoque look had been overthrown and women had been
> liberated from the corset, by Poiret and others, it soon gave way to the
> new look we associate with Coco Chanel and Patou, a transformation
> completed by the mid-1920s...This involved adopting a new set of
> disciplines, internal rather than external: exercise, sports and diet, rather
> than the corset and stays.[64]

Internal discipline is the point. Other writers might make minor revisions for a de
luxe Collected Edition; James would rewrite his with a thoroughness never seen
before, not even in Balzac, eliminating the unevenesses of chronology in favour of a
sense of overall balance and tone, re-creating and well as re-marketing himself. His
elimination of earlier works set in America, and others he considers poor means that
they take on the status of waste. 'By the mere fact of leaving out certain things', he
wrote to Herrick, 'I exercise a control, a discrimination, I treat certain portions of

my work as unhappy accidents'.[65] Like the Fletcherized body, the corpus thus steps out of its own history and succumbs to technique; it is re-formed according to an ideal.

5. Taste and Consumption

Many historians have argued that the period from 1880-1930 saw a significant shift in America (in particular) from an economy governed by scarcity, in which problems of production dominated economic thought, to one governed by abundance, in which consumption replaced abundance as the main term.[66] Economists like Simon N. Patten and Irving Fisher attempted to grapple with this new order of abundance; Fisher's 'goods-dollar' was an attempt to tune the currency away from the steady-state model and productivism implied by the gold standard.[67] Horace Fletcher's theories— like the emerging sexual science which might be thought of as an attempt to regulate the individual desires liberated in modern life—attempted to regulate consumption in this new age of abundance, in which eating too much was suddenly a problem.[68] Like Fisher, Fletcher proposes an internal governor that will regulate consumption: *taste*. Taste is 'the most important of all the faculties man possesses', the unfallible indicator of nutritional value which should keep us chewing pleasurably until there is no taste left and an 'involuntary swallowing' mechanism intervenes, leaving only a fibrous residue which is spat out.[69] Taste allied to chewing to the point of fatigue is thus the key mechanism of self-control, a 'sentinel' preventing waste and over-con-sumption in an economy of abundance, tuning each body to its requirements via a kind of internalized æsthetics. In terms of consumption rather than production, it operates correctively, in the manner that fatigue does in contemporary post-Taylorist studies of industrial efficiency, ensuring that bodily mechanisms are not over-taxed.[70]

In the passage which follows the remarks from the preface to *The Golden Bowl* on 're-tasting' cited earlier, James notes that in revision a writer retraces

> the whole growth of one's 'taste', as our fathers used to say: a blessed comprehensive name for many of the things deepest in us. The 'taste' of the poet is, at bottom and so far as the poet in him prevails over everything else, his active sense of life: in accordance with which truth to keep one's hand on it is to hold the silver clue to the whole labyrinth of his consciousness.[71]

Taste guarantees the process of revision, and is yielded up in a struggle with it (as in Fletcher, it is 'active'). It is central to our consumption of literature in that we prefer the novel in which the 'luxury' exists as a constant regulated demand for our atten-tion, 'when we feel the surface, like the thick ice of the skater's pond, bear without cracking the strongest pressure we throw on it'.[72] It is an index of pleasure, of 'my and your "fun"', as James put it, in which his own pleasure and sense of 'luxury' or even 'a delightful bargain' at re-reading and self-consumption (a dish of innards) parallels the reader's.[73] James's sense of revision thus shares with Fletcher's method an understanding that the mechanism of taste will regulate the flow of materials between inner and outer, preventing the malnourishment of cheap literature or the over-straining of the system.

In making himself an exemplary reader of himself, and incorporating his own consumption of his work into the scheme of the New York Edition (via the prefaces as well as the books), James creates an ideal economy of production and consumption. To that extent, the revision process can be seen as as a response to the paradigm shift towards economies of consumption outlined above, with 'taste' as a key point of mediation ('nature's filter', as Fletcher called it) between the luxury of reading and the managerial imperative which seeks to regulate the process. Yet it must also be noted that the 'fit' here between works are their consumer is solipsistic; James's actual relations with his market were notoriously fraught, and the New York Edition a bitter failure as a commodity.[74] In a market culture, 'taste' is difficult to regulate—it takes on a 'wild' character in which its is best controlled via such external mechanisms as advertising.[75]

In order to see these issues of the market, consumption and art at work, we can return briefly to the uncompleted late novel *The Ivory Tower*: the only novel for which there is a full set of working notes, a 'formula for building a novel', as Pound put it.[76] In the 'Notes' James writes of his work as a machine constructed on a series of major premises and crises:

> What I want is to get my right firm *joints*, each working on its own hinge, and forming together the play of my machine: they *are* the machine, and when each of them is settled and determined it will work as I want it. The first of these, definitely, is that Gray does inherit, has inherited.[77]

We might call this the novelist as Veblenian engineer, constructing characters and performing a social calculus on their persons—who can say of a character 'I see that I really am in complete possession of him, and that no plotting of it as to any but one or two material particulars need here detain me.'[78] The construction is described in terms of an ideal of compaction and the elimination of waste: 'my action', he reflects approvingly, 'will strain my Ten Books, most blessedly, to cracking.' Later he adds:[79]

> and what has the very essence of my design been but the most magnificent packed and calculated closeness? Keep this closeness up to the notch while admirably *animating* it, and I do what I should simply be sickened to death not to! Of course it means the absolutely exclusively *economic* existence and situation of every sentence and every letter; but again what is that but the most desirable of beauties in *itself*?

The 'economic' here signals efficiency and beauty of design rather than simply the accumulation of material ('animated compaction' is a term which Fletcher might have coined).

If the 'Notes' suggest writing as engineering, the text of the novel as we have it proposes a crude embodiment of financial status in its characters. Rosanna is fat, tasteless, has a vast inheritance, and is 'morally elephantine' in the positive sense that she has a huge reserve of moral force. On the first page of the novel we are told that she rejects 'the most expensive modern aids to the constitution of a "figure"' which she might have used. In other words, she does not diet, Fletcherize or take Thyroid extracts. Gray—whose dietary exchange with Miss Mumby began this article—is small in stature, 'light and nervous',[80] and wants to be a 'non-producer', to resist the inheritance or accumulation which has fallen his way. He represents a true cosmopolitan taste, and we are told that he may turn out to be a writer. His friend Horton is tall, fleshier, authoritative (their difference in stature is emphasized), and wants capital—to fill out his height, as it were, to give his figure the bulk it deserves and which, for mysterious reasons, has not achieved. He also generates financial waste, squandering Gray's fortune.

In this equation, the characters embody social values in which, as Seltzer puts it of Newman in *The American*, there is a perfect 'equation of interior states and economic conditions'.[81] As with the commodity, what you see is what you get—a perfect example being Gray's comment to Horton: 'Well, you're simply a figure—what I call—in all the force of the term; one has only to look at you to see it, and I shall give up drawing conclusions from it only when I give up looking'.[82] A similar algebra of appearances operates with characters like Mrs. Bradham. In this logic 'figures' are a kind of coinage; their appearance embodies a cash value or marketability. Disembodiment, on the other hand, is associated with the more etherial Gray and with the writerly consciousness which watches the machine-like plot unfold. The plot, as described in the 'Notes', was to centre round Gray's inheritance of his uncle's dubiously-acquired and modest fortune, his distaste for it, and his placing it in Horton's management—tacitly acquiescing to being swindled. In the speech which James imagines Horton making to Gray, their differences are seen in terms of the embodiment of wealth and its toxicity:

> You *mind*, in your extraordinary way, how this money was accumulated and hanky-pankied, you suffer, and cultivate a suffering, from the perpetrated wrong of which you feel it the embodied evidence, and with which the possession of it is thereby poisoned for you. But I don't mind one little scrap—and there is a great deal more to be said than you seem so much as able to understand, or so much as able to want to, about the whole question of how money comes to those who know *how* to make it.[83]

Gray is happiest within a zero-sum economy in which there is no surplus value or conspicuous consumption; he seeks to divest himself of the merely (and dubiously) accumulated. Like the progressive reformer, he is suspicious of the business world—whose foul play is, we understand, detailed in the letter lodged in the ornamental Ivory Tower which gives the novel its title. We could call the equation of excess with 'poison' Fletcherite in its desire to eliminate what the novel codes as weight. It also allows taste, to be moved away from the world of consumption—in which it is always in danger of becoming conventional and self-perpetuating, 'heavy'—towards the solitary technique and discipline of the maker, the writer who Graham will become.

In the last pages of the novel as we have it (Book 4, chapter 1), he walks around his inheritance (notice the 'joints' of the prose):

> He circled round the house altogether at last, looking at it more critically than had hitherto seemed relevant, taking the measure, disconcertedly, of its unabashed ugliness, and at the end coming to regard it very much as he might have eyed some monstrous modern machine, one of those his generation was going to be expected to master, to fly in, to fight in, to take the terrible women of the future out for airings in, and that mocked at *his* incompetence in such matters while he walked round and round it and gave it, as for dread of what it might do to him, the widest berth his enclosure allowed.[84]

There is a set of dialectical contradictions: Gray desires to be weightless, yet eschews the machine that would let him fly as an agent of modernist sexual commodification, like the aeroplane with which wins the girl in H.G. Wells's *Tono-Bungay* (1909). The house is a machine to be hated, yet the 'modern machine' is also James's well-knit novel; the Ivory Tower is both a symbol of the craft and another bauble in which a rotten secret is hidden. Machine-products, like bodies and books, are inevitably commodified; there is no place for the Veblenian engineer outside the market. The novel presents a character who who wishes to be disembodied (like those other modernist avatars, Kafka's Hunger Artist and Melville's anorexic Bartelby); to resist commodification and the work of accumulation.[85] But he exists in the novel within a bodily economy which equates the body both with capital (flesh equals inherited wealth) and with the idea of an 'animated closeness' in text, with writing itself. Similarly, James's edition can be neither the pure product of the maker, the reformed corpus, nor the a commercial entity embodying a particular commodified taste (the two poles of criticism of the New York Edition); it is condemned to expose the interdependence of the two. The 'monstrous modern machine' which is capitalist enterprise is yoked to the body which tastes and as well as the body which is organized into a tighter shape—a body which might also be a literary corpus.

5. Conclusion

This has, to be sure, been a partial case, a willful reading of James's project in terms of its 'innards'. I have said nothing about what is in the guts; the content of James's revisions. But neither do the metaphors of picture restoration and 'tidying up a brood' tell us much about that. What they reveal is James's sense of what it was to write and read. James himself commented in 'The Art of Fiction' that it was the naive reader who thought that 'a novel is a novel, as a pudding is a pudding, and that our only business with it could be to swallow it'.[86] Yet how it is made, and swallowed, and digested is a different matter, in which eating (or rumination, chewing-over) becomes a metaphor for the art of fiction and the science of criticism; for a kind of consumption which might be moderated within a discipline like that offered by Fletcherism.

If the gross materiality of eating as consumption is one aspect of its critical invisibility, a more important issue is James's involvement in a Progressive project which re-forms the body. Dana Ringuette has recently suggested that revision is for James a pragmatics in which the subject is constituted within a semiosis which is always capable of modification: 'revision…is a developmental principle revealing an expanding consciousness, constantly revealing growing relations'[87] Revision becomes a metaphor for writing itself: as William Spengemann puts it, James's later novels aim to 'burst the settled bounds of of the author's prior intentions and propel the action beyond the well-kept paths of literary intention into the unpredictable, morally ambiguous world we all inhabit'.[88] But the pragmatics of revision, I would argue, should also include the bodily engineering of Fletcherism, which seeks to discipline rather than expand, which fears the freedom of the economy of abundance, and which aims to regulate taste in the interests of an ideal of compaction. In answer to our opening question about a simile (writing being 'like' eating), it is difficult to see James's late writing as 'like' Fletcherism because in a strict sense it *is* Fletcherism— 'like' it in its self-description as 'hygiene', its elimination of waste material; but even more the thing itself in its solitary economy and self-preoccupation, its obsession with a technique which re-works the corpus. No other writer before James had undertaken what he now did, moving over an entire body of work as a whole and making it anew; eliminating some works; altering the texture of the whole in the name of a desired total shape. In the Progressive Era, the disposition of the body became a moral duty; it stepped outside of a natural plot in which it expanded comfortably with age and prosperity, suffering from the infirmities that time brings, and became forever an indicator of moral rectitude and vitality, implicated in a technological praxis.

In taking on that praxis as he revised, James reminds us that the body (like the corpus) is always the site of work, always constructed, and that its attempts to free itself from history and the marketplace are as contradictory as Gray's in *The Ivory Tower*. We began with Gray on alimentary systems, and can end with him consuming himself, ruminating and enjoying it, as his own best consumer: 'It was still beyond his dream that what everything merely seen from the window of his room meant to him during these first hours should move him first to a smile of such ecstasy, and then to such an inward consumption of his smile, as might have made happiness a substance you could sweetly put under your tongue'.[89] This is all for Gray, yet the 'you' here also suggests an audience which might share the pleasure, popping the pill of happiness. As William James put it, a 'palmary instance of the ambiguous' which is the modern body.

Notes

1.   Henry James, *The Ivory Tower* (London: W. Collins, 1917), p. 79.
2.   Elizabeth David, *A Book of Mediterranean Food* (2nd edn.; Harmondsworth: Penguin Books, 1965 [1958]), p. 31. The rather baroque passage on eggs is from James's *A Little Tour in France*.

3.   Writings on Fletcher include: Hillel Schwartz, *Never Satisfied: A Cultural History of Diets, Fantasies, and Fat* (New York: Free Press, 1986), pp. 124-31; Harvey Green, *Fit For America: Health, Fitness, Sport and American Society* (Baltimore: Johns Hopkins University Press, 1986), ch. 11; James C. Wharton, 'Physiological Optimism: Horace Fletcher and the Hygenic Ideology in Progressive America', *Bulletin of the History of Medicine* 55 (1981), pp. 59-87.

4.   The Russian biologist and Nobel laureate Elie Metchnikoff argued that aging was linked to toxins, advocating a sour-milk diet; Haig, an English physician, stressed the dangers of alkaline diets and uric acid in the bloodstream. The issue was much debated in the 1910s, and in the 1920s Fleismann's Yeast was sold in the USA as a preventative to auto-intoxication.

5.   Horace Fletcher, *Glutton or Epicure* (Chicago: Herbert Stone, 1899), pp. 41-53.

6.   Whorton, 'Physiological Optimism', p. 62.

7.   Herbert Spencer, 'The Social Organism', in *Essays: Scientific, Political and Speculative* (3 vols.; London: Williams & Norgate, 1891), I, p. 290.

8.   Anson Rabinbach, in *The Human Motor: Energy, Fatigue, and the Origins of Modernity* (New York: Basic Books, 1990), provides a brilliant survey of such ideas. On William James, see Cynthia Eagle Russett, *Sexual Science: The Victorian Construction of Womanhood* (Cambridge, MA: Harvard University Press, 1989), p. 163.

9.   See Jeremy MacClancy, *Consuming Culture* (London: Chapmans, 1992), pp. 26-31.

10.   Both followed the prescriptions of F.A. Hornibrook's *The Culture of the Abdomen*.

11.   In *Brewsie and Willie* she criticizes the GIs for preferring 'soft stuff': 'we don't except at a little meat we don't really chew'. *Brewsie and Willie* (New York: Random House, 1946), p. 78.

12.   The full text of the letter, dated 1 February 1919, was only published in *The Gender of Modernism* (ed. Bonnie Kime Scott; Bloomington: Indiana University Press, 1990), pp. 362-65.

13.   A parallel is Oscar Wilde's period of adherence to the rational-dress philosophy of Dr Gustave Jaeger—which may, Alison Adburgham suggests, have been to please his wife, but which also reinforces the connection between the art of presenting or packaging the body (Wilde's posing) and reformist techniques. Alison Adburgham, *Shops and Shopping, 1800-1914* (London: Barrie & Jenkins, 1989 [1964]), p. 185.

14.   *Ivory Tower*, p. 80.

15.   *Ivory Tower*, p. 259.

16.   Alfred Kazin, *On Native Grounds* (New York: Harcourt, Brace & World, 1942), p. 353.

17.   Chronologies for the revisions are provided by Hershel Parker, 'Henry James "In the Wood": Sequence and Significance in His Literary Labours, 1905-1907', *Nineteenth Century Fiction* 38 (1984), pp. 492-513; Philip Horne, *James and Revision: The New York Edition* (Oxford: Clarendon Press, 1990), appendix.

18.   There are flickering mentions of the metaphor of 'rumination' in Leon Edel's biography, *The Master: 1901-16* (New York: Avon Books, 1972), p. 250 and in Camille Paglia's *Sexual Personæ* (Harmondsworth: Penguin, 1990), but neither applies it to the revisions.

19.   Horne, *James and Revision*, ch.3.

20.   Anthony J. Mazella, 'James's Revisions', in *A Companion to Henry James Studies* (ed. Daniel Mark Fogel; Westport, CT: Greenwood Press, 1993), pp. 312-14.

21.   See Mark Anderson's consideration of these issues in relation to pedagogy and interpretation in 'Anorexia and Modernism, or How I Learned to Diet in All Directions', *Discourse* 11. 1 (1988), pp. 28-41.

22.   *The Art of the Novel: Critical Prefaces by Henry James* (New York: Scribner's, 1934), pp. 339-40.

23.   *Art of the Novel*, p. 135.

24.   *Art of the Novel*, p. 310.

25.   *Art of the Novel*, p. 230.

26.   *Art of the Novel*, pp. 233, 266.

27.   *Art of the Novel*, p. 154.

28.   *Art of the Novel*, p. 196.

29.   *Art of the Novel*, p. 201.

30.   *Art of the Novel*, p. 10.

31.   *Art of the Novel*, pp. 84-86.

32.   See 'The New Novel', in *Henry James, Selected Literary Criticism* (ed. Roger Gard; Harmondsworth: Penguin, 1987), pp. 595-614.

33.   F.R. Leavis, *The Common Pursuit* (Harmondsworth: Penguin, 1976), p. 228. One could compare Arnold Bennett writing of his 'fastidiousness', his probably never having had a pint of beer, the 'thinness' of his stories, and his essays 'packed close with vitamines'. 'A Candid Opinion on Henry James', *Evening Standard*, 27 January 1927.

34.   *Henry James Letters*, IV. *1896-1916* (ed. Leon Edel; Cambridge, MA: Belknap Press, 1984), p. 415.

35.   *Letters*, IV, pp. 494-95.

36.   Dorothy Richardson, 'About Punctuation', in Scott (ed.), *The Gender of Modernism*, p. 416. First published in *Adelphi* 1/11 (April 1924).

37.   Paglia, *Sexual Personae*, pp. 616-17. Paglia describes James's late style as 'a miasma, a new version of the female swamp of generation' (p. 621).

38.   Thomas M. Leitch, 'The Prefaces', in Fogel (ed.), *Companion*, p. 65.

39.   Quoted by Edel from Case 97 of Mackenzie's *Angina Pectoris* (1923), *Letters*, IV, p. 518.

40.   *Letters*, IV, pp. 299-301.

41.   *The Letters of Henry James* (ed. Percy Lubbock; 2 vols.; New York: Scribner's, 1920), II, pp. 96, 104.

42.   *Letters*, IV, pp. 483, 394.

43.   *Art of the Novel*, pp. 337-39.

44.   *Art of the Novel*, pp. 344-45.

45   Gilbert Seldes, 'The Mind of an Artist', *The Dial*, July 1920, p. 88.

46.   *Art of the Novel*, p. 17.

47.   Mark Seltzer, *Bodies and Machines* (New York: Routledge, 1992), pp. 49-90.

48.   Seltzer, *Bodies and Machines*, p. 3 *et passim*.

49.   William James approved of Fletcherism (without seeing it as a universal cure): see comments made in 1904 in *William James: Selected Unpublished Correspondence 1885-1910* (ed. Frederick J. Down Scott; Colombus: Ohio State University Press, 1986), pp. 329, 351.

50.   Green, *Fit for America*, pp. 242-57.

51.   'The Place of Affectional Facts' (1905), *The Writings of William James: A Comprehensive Edition* (ed. John J. McDermott; Chicago: University of Chicago Press, 1977), pp. 272, 277.

52.   See 'The Experience of Activity' (1905), in McDermott (ed.), *Writings of William James*, pp. 277-91.

53.   Leon Edel, 'The Architecture of Henry James's New York Edition', *New England Quarterly* 24 (1951), pp. 169-78; Millicent Bell, *Edith Wharton and Henry James: The Story of a Friendship* (New York: Braziller, 1965), p. 167. On the New York Edition as a marketing strategy, see the final chapters of Michael Anesko, *'Friction with the Market', Henry James and the Profession of Authorship* (New York: Oxford University Press, 1986), and Anne T. Margolis, *Henry James and the Problem of Audience* (Ann Arbor, MI: UMI Research Press, 1985).

54.   *Letters*, IV, p. 250.

55.   Mazzella, 'James's Revisions', p. 314.

56.   *Art of the Novel*, p. 347.

57.   *Letters*, IV, p. 498.

58.   Schwartz, *Never Satisfied*, p. 81.

59.   Stuart Ewen, *All Consuming Images: The Politics of Style in Contemporary Culture* (New York: Basic Books, 1988), ch. 8 (p. 179 cited).

60.   Cited in Irving Norton Fisher, *My Father Irving Fisher* (New York: Comet Press, 1956), pp. 183-84.

61.   Elaine Showalter, *Sexual Anarchy: Gender and Culture at the Fin de Siècle* (London: Bloomsbury, 1981), p. 16.

62.   *Letters*, IV, pp. 380, 415.

63.   Anesko, *'Friction with the Market'*, p. 151.

64.   Wollen, *Raiding the Icebox*, p. 20. This is, as he suggests, part of the paradigm shift in Modernism, away from artifice and display (coded as feminine) towards functionality and the machine-æsthetics of 'efficiency' (coded as masculine).

65.   *The Selected Letters of Henry James* (ed. Leon Edel; New York: Farrar, Straus and Cudahy, 1955), p. 159.

66.   See for example Daniel Bell, *The Cultural Contradictions of Capitalism* (New York: Basic Books, 1966); Ewen, *All Consuming Images*; and (for a literary version) David Trotter, 'Too Much of a Good Thing: Fiction and the "Economy of Abundance"', *Critical Quarterly* 34/4 (1992), pp. 27-41. Seltzer rightly points out (*Bodies and Machines*, p. 60) that this story of a Fall into 'consumerism' has been positioned by different writers at very different points in the history of Capitalism; nevertheless large-scale shifts in patterns of production took place in the period, and perhaps more importantly, these shifts were noticed by contemporary social commentators.

67.   On Patten, see Daniel M. Fox, *The Discovery of Abundance: Simon N. Patten and the Transformation of Social Theory* (Ithaca: Johns Hopkins University Press, 1967); on earlier economists and consumption, see Trotter, 'Too Much', p. 29.

68.   See Lawrence Birkin, *Consuming Desire: Sexual Science and the Emergence of a Culture of Abundance, 1871-1914* (Ithaca: Johns Hopkins University Press, 1988), pp. 12-13.

69.   Fletcher, 'What Sense?', Part II of *Glutton or Epicure*, p. 5.

70.   See Anson Rabinbach, 'Neurasthenia and Modernity', *Incorporations* (ed. Jonathan Crary and Stanford Kwinter; New York: Urzone, 1992), pp. 178-89.

71.   *Art of the Novel*, p. 340.

72.   *Art of the Novel*, pp. 304-305.

73.   *Art of the Novel*, p. 341.

74.   On this issue, see Anesko, Margolis (n. 53 above), and Jonathan Freedman, *Professions of Taste: Henry James, British Æstheticism, and Commodity Culture* (Stanford: Stanford University Press, 1990).

75.   On James, advertising, and consumption, see Jennifer Wicke, *Advertising Fictions: Literature, Advertisement and Social Reading* (New York: Colombia University Press, 1988), ch.3.

76.   Ezra Pound, 'Henry James', *Instigations* (New York: Boni & Liveright, 1920), p. 160. Appositely, Pound introduced his essay as 'a dull grind' in its digestion of James's whole corpus (p. 106).

77.   *Ivory Tower*, p. 296.

78.   *Ivory Tower*, p. 329. See Seltzer's Foucaultian account of surveillance in *Henry James and the Art of Power* (Ithaca: Cornell University Press, 1984); and John Goode's analysis of

character as self-possession in 'Character and Henry James', *New Left Review* 40 (1966), pp. 55-75.

79.   *Ivory Tower*, pp. 270, 338.

80.   *Ivory Tower*, p. 330.

81   Seltzer, *Bodies and Machines*, p. 57.

82.   *Ivory Tower*, p. 227.

83.   *Ivory Tower*, p. 333.

84.   *Ivory Tower*, p. 259.

85.   See Gillian Brown, 'The Empire of Agoraphobia', *Representations* 20 (1987), pp. 134-57.

86.   Henry James, 'The Art of Fiction', *Literary Criticism: Essays on Literature, American Writers, English Writers* (ed. Leon Edel; New York: Library of America, 1984), p. 44.

87.   Dana J. Ringuette, 'The Self-Forming Subject: Henry James's Pragmatic Revision', *Mosaic* 23 (1990), pp. 115-30 (p. 119 cited).

88.   William C. Spengemann, *A Mirror for Americanists: Reflections on the Idea of American Literature* (Hanover: University Press of New England, 1989), p. 109.

89.   *Ivory Tower*, p. 72.

Film

Lee Grieveson

KNOWABLE MAN:
DRIVE FOR LIFE

The Drive for a Life is a one-reel film made in 1909 by the director D.W. Griffith for
the American Mutoscope and Biograph Company. It tells the story of a young man
abandoning his mistress in order to marry a respectable girl. The young man, named
Harry Walker by the bulletin which accompanied the film, visits the Widow Lebrun
and announces his forthcoming marriage to Mignon.[1] Lebrun pleads with Walker to
stay but he leaves and visits Mignon at her family home. He produces a ring, they
kiss, and as he leaves she is surrounded by her family who admire the ring. Lebrun
then goes out on an errand as Walker is showing off his motor car to Mignon and
the two routes intersect, so that Lebrun follows Walker and Mignon whilst they
remain unaware of her presence. Lebrun returns home and proceeds to forge Walker's
signature on a note to Mignon accompanied by a box of poisoned candy. There is an
insert shot of Lebrun injecting the candy with poison, followed by an intertitle which
reads: 'Forging his handwriting, the poisoned candy is sent on its terrible mission'.
Walker arrives at Lebrun's house to return some letters and discovers the attempt to
poison Mignon and sets off in a race-to-the-rescue, arriving just at the moment
Mignon and her family were about to eat the candy. The film ends as they kiss.

The 'cinema' between 1895 and 1907—more accurately, the not yet cinema—differs
from a later classical cinema above all in the conception of the relations between film
and viewer, inasmuch as these relations can be inferred from developing histories of
exhibition practices and from analyses of textual modes of address. Understood as a
distinct mode of representation, this 'cinema' embodies a different logic of the relation between viewer and film, a different thinking about the status of the image in
film, and a different conception of space and narrative from a later industrial logic of
film production. Within the film texts, the autonomy of the single shot without
scene dissection produces a logic of spatial coherence which overrides that of
temporality or causality. The image manifests what Noel Burch terms a 'topological
complexity', demanding from the spectator an active 'reading' of differing subject
positions, setting up then a fundamentally different logic of vision and knowledge
which functions for Burch to maintain 'the externality of the spectator subject'.[2] In
Tom Gunning's influential formulation, this is a 'cinema' of 'exhibitionistic confrontation rather than diegetic absorption':[3] a logic of representation which eschews
the 'suturing' of classical point of view structures and the temporal solicitation of an

incorporeal subject for a structure of spatial coherence and a solicitation of a resolutely social subject.[4]

A number of film scholars have discerned a series of shifts in this logic which coalesce around 1907-1909, a shift that then functions as something like the stuttering emergence of a new discourse, finally formalized from around 1917. Certainly this periodisation is part of an analytical method and does not reflect clear divisions across film production and form, but there are a series of definable shifts within the industrial configuration of the (becoming) cinema within these years which reflect—and effect—the 'cinema's' turn to narrative as its main form of textual and ideological support. There are two strands to this temporal scheme: one, the development and hegemony of narrative—a shift to an articulation of temporality alongside the solicitation and suturing of an incorporeal spectator-subject—and two, the construction of cinema as a particular form of commodity within the context of industrial shifts and shifts in exhibition practices. This itself necessitates, in Lea Jacobs' words, 'a conception of the industry as a site of a discursive logic',[5] a logic whose genealogy might be traced via the wholesale reorganization of the industry in 1909 with the formation of the monopolistic Motion Pictures Patents Company and the 1909 establishment of a National Board of Censorship.[6]

The specifically filmic articulation of narrative is then predicated on develop-ments in analytical editing (scene dissection via the stitching together of various shots) which dramatizes space and time differently, in the process producing images as, in Elsaesser's words, 'motivated views (implying an act of showing) and semiotic acts (elements of a discourse)'.[7] The formal organization of time and space becomes progressively organized in view of the production of certain effects for a spectator, so that a specific narrative logic is set in play which is also a logic of the subject and the spectator, now positioned 'at the imaginary apex of a textual geometry'.[8] Here is where the shifting hierarchies of knowledge in *The Drive for a Life* would be sited: the complex moving shot of Lebrun following Walker and Mignon and the rendering of the race-to-the-rescue via parallel editing—a series of shots showing Walker's race and Mignon endlessly about to eat the candy—is predicated on a hier-archy of knowledge subsuming spectator and characters and is productive of what Tom Gunning calls a 'sense of the hand of the storyteller as he moves us from place to place, weaving a new continuity of narrative logic'.[9] This kind of parallel editing is then positioned by Tom Gunning as a 'narrativizing of the possibilities of filmic discourse'.[10]

This logic of signification and subjectivity involves both theoretical and histori-cal questions. That is, the 'suturing' of a transcendent and unified spectator has long been established as the central moment of films engagement with ideology, yet this suturing also has a historical narrative. As Miriam Hansen points out, the very word 'spectator' was only introduced around 1910; prior to that the film viewer was still referred to by the plural term 'audience'.[11] This increasing subjectification of cine-matic discourse must be placed within various configurations of power—ranging across the film industry, a disciplining of an unruly exhibition context, and a broader 'political technology' of subjectification. My emphasis here is then twofold (though these aims are, as I shall suggest, linked in various ways): firstly, *The Drive for a Life* and its narrative organization must be positioned within the context of the historical

and theoretical issues broached above; secondly, following Michel Foucault's definition of a genealogical aim 'to maintain passing events in their proper dispersion',[12]
I want to site the text in various matrices of dispersion around masculinity, sexuality
and its relation to the social body. It is worth noting here though at the outset that
the representation of gender within cinema does have its own discursive logic, so that
the specificity of cinema—as a mode of representation, as a certain configuration of
viewer and text, and as an industry devoted to the production and circulation of a
certain commodity—must also be taken into consideration in this relationship across
film texts and discourses which circulate outside them.

     This genealogy of narrative function and cinematic discourse will be pursued
here in relation to a series of contemporaneous discourses and knowledges which
aspire to order the domain of the sexual in relation to the social, and which constitute
the body and its sexuality as social processes (medical, anthropological, eugenic, social
hygiene discourses and so on). In Foucault's work on sexuality and what he terms
'governmentality', sexuality—and, arguably, gender—is understood as a set of truth
effects of a political technology, so that what we call sexuality is 'the set of effects
produced in bodies, behaviours and social relations' by the deployment of a 'complex
political technology'.[13] This is approached under the term 'bio-power', a dispersed
matrice of power concerned with the bringing of 'life and its mechanisms into the
realm of explicit calculation'. This drive for life—for in one sense that is what is
involved in this configuration—is undertaken firstly via a focus on the 'body as a
machine: its disciplining, the optimization of its capabilities, the parallel increase of
its usefulness and its docility' and, secondly, via a focus 'on the species body, the body
imbued with the mechanisms of life and serving as the basis of the biological
processes: propagation, births and mortality, the level of health'.[14] These two levels of
an anatomo-politics of the body and a bio-politics of the population are 'linked
together in a whole series of relations' which are effectively read by Foucault as the
development of a 'new kind of relationship between the social entity and the
individual'.[15] In this respect, the subject is positioned by Foucault as a product of an
epistemological configuration, being inextricably emmeshed in political strategies
and involved with the power–knowledge effects applied by discourse. Subjection—
in a moral and physical sense—is carried out by means of a dual functioning of
discourse which socializes bodies by making them amenable to the definition and
organization of the restraints and coercions to be applied. This is a category of power
which 'categorizes the individual, marks him by his own individuality, attaches him
to his own identity, imposes a law of truth on him which he must recognize' and
which then 'makes individuals subjects'.[16] These broader questions around
subjectification, around the sexual and the social body are approached here then both
as part of a broader project of a genealogy of 'cinema' and as part of a (partial)
genealogy of 'masculinity'.

The Drive for a Life begins with an intertitle which reads: 'The young man determines
to put away an unworthy past for a higher future'.[17] Walker's 'unworthy past' is his
'improper' relationship with the Widow Lebrun. He has decided to change: this is a
narrative of transformation (and a transitional narrative) that is both a transformation

of sexuality (in the sense of its repositioning into a marital relationship) and of masculinity. The intertitle stresses 'young man', suggesting a move into maturity. The narrative is established on an explicit temporal schema which, however, precedes the text, so that Walker's transformation of knowledge has in fact already taken place. Instead of the epistemological drive or hermeneutic structuration of classical narrative—where the problem of knowledge is so insistently that of woman—just the playing out of a shift in knowledge which raises the question (unanswered in the text) of Walker's motivation. It is possibly here though where Walker's 'determination' enters—'the young man *determines* to put away an unworthy past'—a word that seems to me curiously out of place, invoking at its edges a form of dissatisfaction, or of the determined subjective realignment of Walker with a set of moral norms, a system of moral 'worth'. This 'determination' becomes then a representation—and a narrative beginning—of a subjective assimilation to a system of morality in relation to sexuality, this process in which, in Foucault's formulation, 'the individual delimits that part of himself that will form the object of his moral practice, defines his position relative to the precept he will follow, and decides on a certain mode of being that will serve as his moral goal. And this requires him to act upon himself, to monitor, test, improve, and *transform* himself.'[18]

Walker's transformation—and the movement of narrative—is from a position of asocial sexuality to a manifestation of a sexuality in accord with the social formation. This transformation seems to me to parallel a series of debates and campaigns around 'masculinity' as some form of 'danger', debates and campaigns which coalesce within a social hygiene discourse (and which I want to analyse in more detail below). 'Masculinity' enters discourse—becomes an object of knowledge—as both problem of knowledge and governance; that is to say, what is produced as 'masculinity' brings with it, as part of its production, the demand for a discursive policing, so that masculinity is produced as, in Judith Butler's words, 'a regulatory fiction'.[19] Far from a disembodied masculine 'knower', what emerges across this discursive configuration is a concern precisely over 'knowable man'—and this insistently around knowledge of the sexual body in relation to the social body—so that 'masculinity' itself is imbricated in various formations of power and is complexly fragmented in relation to power.[20] A series of discourses then insistently suggest that masculinity must transform its 'unworthy' instincts to produce a 'higher future'.

This generalized concern around the sexual and social body can also be traced out in the stuttering emergence of filmic narrative, itself so insistently centred around threats to a family structure and around a narrativization of the formation of the heterosexual couple (this regime of narrative might itself be read as a major enforcer of what Butler terms 'the epistemic regime of presumptive heterosexuality').[21] This concern can be seen in the brief genealogy of the narrational function of cinema given above. There is a proliferation of films prior to 1907 which exhibit a sort of exhibitionistic pleasure in displaying the unfaithfulness of husbands (and, very occasionally, wives), a series of 'shrewish' wives, and a series of films depicting men's unwillingness to get married. For example: *The Divorce* (1903) shows a husband who, upon leaving his house, accidentally drops a letter which his wife finds and reads and later, with a detective, finds him in a hotel with another woman. *A Search for Evidence*

(1903) tells a similar story and *The Story that Biograph Told* (1903) shows a man flirting with his secretary whilst an office junior surreptitiously films them and later exhibits the film at the nickelodeon the man and his wife attend. *The Henpecked Husband* (1905) shows how, according to the bulletin, 'a henpecked husband is jawed to a finish by a nagging wife'.[22] Both *No Weddings Bells for Him: The Attractions of Married Life do not Appeal to this Bachelor* (1906) and *Trial Marriages: Experiences of a Bachelor in the Modern Matrimonial Game* (1907) present married life as undesirable for the single male. Post 1907—and that clearly stands as a somewhat arbitrary delineation—there seems to emerge a greater stress on the constitution of the heterosexual couple, of the family, of the sanctity of the family structure, and then on a series of re-mappings of what constitutes 'legitimate' masculinity and femininity (and here is where one would position *The Drive for a Life*). This shift must be positioned both within the context of the film industry making efforts to appeal to a middle class audience and to produce cinema as 'respectable', a production that necessitates the construction of a set of film texts—these films that Adolph Zukor had associated with a 'slum tradition'—as 'other' to that construction. This is a moment in the construction of cinema as what Elsaesser terms 'a species of discourse'.[23]

To return to *The Drive for a Life* from this perspective is to position this text as a sort of dramatization of this shift, so that the 'putting away' of Walker's 'unworthy past'—his affair with Lebrun—and the 'higher future' of marriage to Mignon dramatizes both an assimilation of the sexual to the social body and a shift then from a narrative of overt sexuality to one of morality. In the specific context of the sexual male body, this process of assimilation to the social is undertaken via a dichotomization of that body: the splitting of Walker into (and across) unworthy past–youth–sexuality and higher future–maturity–marriage. This is a structure which can be discerned across a wider body of texts, although most commonly there is a splitting across a hero and villain figure (and this usually around an innocent and morally 'pure' heroine). Deviancy is here coded across various icons of difference, in relation to class, ethnicity and race (in fact, the villain will often be in a position of superiority over the heroine—he will be her supervisor at work, her guardian, even her father, though here the threat is less direct and more often in the way the father will encourage unwanted advances generally for his own social advancement).[24] It is also clear that the oscillation across this space marked out as 'masculinity' insistently takes place in relation to sexuality, so that the villain becomes a figure of sexuality out of control and his eventual defeat and punishment marks a repositioning of that sexuality.

The splitting of diegetic material is discernable in a splitting of the formal procedures of the text. Writing specifically about Griffith, Tom Gunning has suggested that the narratives of this period of his work are almost always based on an initial splitting of the narrative core which produces several narrative threads which are then gradually woven together. This dividing of the pursuer and pursued—or, more commonly, attacker–victim–rescuer—creates a formal-dynamic patterning, emotional suspense and a quite different conception of diegetic space (dispersed but linked by temporal simultaneity via 'the hand of the storyteller').[25] A diegetic splitting of masculinity across the hero and villain clearly leads to this fragmentary narrative core, though it must also be noted that *The Drive for a Life* does not follow this external splitting but instead renders it internally, replaying it on a temporal schema so that the 'young man' was sexuality out of control but now this is in the 'unworthy past'. Masculinity is here divided against itself.[26] The continuity across the two structures is in relation to sexuality, so that masculinity is produced as problematic within the film texts and broader discursive structures because of these seemingly irrational and powerful sexual drives which cut across the body, linking high and low, and which then produce masculinity as an unstable nexus of conflictual desires and demands. The further point here is that the splitting of the narrative core is at the same time a splitting of sexuality across some form of anti-social sexuality (which is associated both with 'deviant' masculinity and femininity) and a sexuality assimilated to the social. There is then a conjunction of textual containment—linked in the text with a play around *driving*—and containment of a produced deviancy in relation to sexuality.

Alongside the internalization of a split masculinity in *The Drive for a Life* there is an externalization of a doubled femininity, a structure that then produces the text as a curious mirror image to those films which feature a hero and villain fighting over an innocent heroine. The split across Lebrun and Mignon is produced by the text as a split across sexually active–available woman and asexual–pure woman; again, this is a split across the positioning of sexuality in relation to sociality, producing Lebrun in the process as a 'being thoroughly saturated with sexuality'.[27] The *mise en scène* associated with the two women presents a clear contrast: Mignon is insistently positioned in the centre of the frame, surrounded by her family, all dressed in white, whereas Lebrun's home is darker, less grand, more cluttered. Lebrun lives alone and, according to the bulletin, is a widow, a positioning that places her within a tradition of early film texts representing sexually active widows, often in conjunction with their lack of maternal attentiveness. This is a set of texts which clearly evince a concern with the moral 'problem' of undomesticated feminine sexuality.[28] Lebrun's threat to domesticity is also present in the text in her entrance into the public space of the text unchaperoned, a move that sets in play her attempt to poison the constitution of the heterosexual couple.

Lebrun's threat to Walker and Mignon's marriage, her status as widow, her entrance into the public space of the text, the implied opposition to Mignon, all seem to position her as a coded representation of the prostitute, a figure widely constructed within social-hygiene discourse as a manifestation of 'the social evil'. There is a conjunction of the characterization—such as it is—of Lebrun and the characterization of the prostitute, and this primarily around a representation of un-domesticated–asocial sexuality, a presence in public space (the prostitute as street-walker[29]) and, more central here, around the representation of prostitution and associated venereal diseases as a 'poisoning' of the family. This representation is central to the constitution of a social-hygiene discourse, closely linked to a theory of congenital venereal disease—propagated through the years 1885-1910—which produces venereal disease, and the prostitute who is seen to transmit it, as a threat of degeneration via a 'poisoning' of the family and the social. Venereal diseases in this period were commonly referred to as 'family poison':[30] it is here where the poisoned candy of Lebrun must be placed, so that the candy—itself an image of innocence— masks a devastating ability to literally poison Mignon, her family, and the 'higher future' of

Mignon and Walker's marriage, a poisoning quite clearly linked to 'unworthy' sexuality.[31]

As has become all too apparent, venereal disease can stand as a sort of stress point in the delineation of the relation of the individual to the social, being produced insistently as a literalization of a decaying social order. Around the turn of the nineteenth and twentieth century there was quite clearly a flurry of activity around these questions, which both animated a social purity movement and a developing discourse of social-hygiene.[32] For example: Prince Morrow, a leading figure in the American social-hygiene movement—founder in 1905 of the Society of Sanitary and Moral Prophylaxis and author of the influential 1904 *Social Diseases and Marriage*— asserted that venereal diseases 'in their essential nature… are not merely diseases of the human body, but diseases of the social organism'.[33] The body and the social collide here over 'unworthy' sexuality. The further point pursued by Morrow (and others) is the dissolution of the family structure inherent in the transmission of these diseases: 'No other disease is so susceptible of hereditary transmission, and so fatal to the offspring'—being part of 'that relentless law of Nature which visits the sins of the fathers upon the children'—and which becomes 'an actual cause of the degeneration of the race'.[34] The whole question of eugenics and of variations on what Foucault terms 'state directed racism' enters here: as Morrow suggested in an article entitle 'Eugenics and Venereal Disease', 'the effect of venereal disease is to produce a race of inferior beings, by *poisoning* the sources of life, and sapping the vitality and health of the offspring' becoming then 'directly antagonistic to the eugenic ideal'.[35]

For Morrow and others working within various configurations of reform discourse it was precisely the 'sins of the fathers' that was at issue. Venereal disease was seen as entering the family structure via the straying of the father so that there was 'more venereal infection among virtuous wives than among professional prostitutes'.[36] As Morrow pointed out, venereal diseases 'link the debased harlot and the virtuous wife in the kinship of a common disease'.[37] To reposition this discourse in relation to *The Drive for a Life* is instructive: the narrative function of the candy is to link Lebrun (as 'debased harlot') and Mignon ('virtuous wife' to be), a structure that is then predicated both on their (ideological and spatial) separation and the threat of the dissolution of this separation, a threat of a boundary breakdown across 'debased harlot' and 'virtuous wife'. The structure of parallel editing (and its acceleration) puts in place an ideological separation that is threatened but ultimately upheld (in *The Drive for a Life* this is both the threat of eating the poisoned candy but also, it seems, the threat that opens the text of Walker's choice of partners: in one sense, the drama of the penetration of the poisoned candy must replay an earlier, though unrepresented, drama of Walker's temptation by 'unworthy' sexuality). What is interesting about this structure of parallel editing and the erection of a distinction between Lebrun and Mignon is precisely the flimsy nature of that distinction, the overt possibility of a boundary breakdown between them which in the text is linked to some form of 'boundary breakdown' within Walker. That is, the opposition of Lebrun and Walker is tenuous precisely because of Walker, because of his oscillation across the two figures and the two positions in relation to sexuality. It is, after all, via his handwriting that the candy is accepted by Mignon, so that the 'family poison' is authored, at one remove, by Walker: it is both him, and not him. And in many ways the buttressing of Walker's position on one side of that handwriting—the distinction of fake from real—constitutes the narrative trajectory of the text.

Morrow and the broader configuration of social purity and social-hygiene discourse insistently produced the problem of 'family poisoning' as a problem of male sexuality, of what Morrow termed 'male unchastity'. 'The male factor', Morrow asserted, 'is the chief malefactor'.[38] Morrow called on sex education—and the stress should be on education, on the dissemination of knowledge—to 'include as a cardinal feature a correction of the false impression instilled in the minds of *young men* that sexual intercourse is essential to the health and that chastity is incompatible with full vigour'.[39] It is here then where *The Drive for a Life*—and a number of other film texts—can be positioned, as a text similar then to a series of advice manuals, to those texts that, in Foucault's words, serve as 'functional devices that would enable individuals to question their own conduct, to watch over and give shape to it, and to shape themselves as ethical subjects'.[40] The text then, and it stands here as metaphoric for a moment in the constitution of cinematic discourse, offers a mode of address as advice, constructing spectators in a particular way as moral subjects.

There are a number of issues which emerge out of this interface between reform discourse and a developing cinematic discourse. Firstly, the referential subject of these texts—this set of concerns around the body and the social—is interlinked with a shift in the strategies of filmic narrative. Secondly, an external discursive construction of the cinema—as either capable of 'uplift' or as excrescence on the social body— interweaves with an internal construction, so that what emerges as 'cinema' is intimately connected to a series of discursive struggles over what is not yet 'cinema'. Like Foucault's approach to a history of sexuality—a history that 'must be written from the viewpoint of a history of discourses'[41]—the 'cinema' itself can be approached via discourses about the cinema. Thirdly, and closely linked to this, a genealogy as an attempt 'to maintain passing events in their proper dispersion' must pay attention to a whole series of discourses around the reform of the cinema and the reform of the social. These social-reform discourses are, Lynda Nead suggests, 'one of the centres in the nineteenth century which produced definitions of sexuality' and are also, as I have suggested, imbricated in the production of definitions of cinema, which itself becomes, in Teresa De Lauretis's formulation, 'a technology of gender'.[42] There are important questions of discursive productivity, interchange and transformation here.

Within the context of a political technology of gender and sexuality my interest here is in the entrance of masculinity into various configurations of knowledge. This phrase 'knowable man' that I have appropriated for the title of this paper is used by Foucault in *Discipline and Punish*, where, in a discussion of the inscription of power– knowledge onto the (genderless) subject, Foucault refers to 'knowable man' and places after it, in parentheses, 'soul, individuality, consciousness, conduct, whatever it is called'.[43] The epistemological configuration of subjectivity—which is both a question of an inscription of knowledge onto the subject and a self-inscription—is linked to a range of techniques for controlling and making manageable new multiplicities of individuals associated with nineteenth-century modernity. This production of what

Foucault also terms 'the docile body' required 'the involvement of definite relations of power; it called for a technique of overlapping subjectification and objectification; it brought with it new procedures of individualization'.[44] The production of 'knowable man' via an overlapping of subjectification and objectification is re-specified here: the question is precisely over knowledge and masculinity, of masculinity being produced within knowledge and power. This is not to deny the positioning of femininity within discourse as a problem of knowledge, merely to draw attention to a concomitant imbrication of masculinity within power.

These 'new procedures of individualization' might also be read back into the brief sketch of recent development in film history which opened this paper. That is to say, the related development of character psychology, motivation, narrativization, the 'invention' of spectatorship—in effect, a widespread reconfiguration of the relations between an observing subject and modes of representation—might be approached via Foucault's genealogy of subject-effect.[45] For now this is moving too far ahead. Perhaps though such an analysis might begin with an image of the 'arrival' of a 'new' knowledge of the subject in America in 1909, an image which also— though in a slightly different way than that related here—invokes an image of infection: Freud arriving at Ellis Island, turning to Jung and (according to Lacan) saying, 'they don't realize we are bringing them the plague'.

With many thanks to Steve Neale, Elizabeth Cowie, Peter Kramer, Tom Gunning, Vanessa Martin, Sue Wiseman, Thomas Austin and Howard Booth.

Notes

1.   The American Mutoscope and Biograph Company produced one page bulletins to advertise films to exhibitors, who would themselves often place the bulletins within the space of the nickelodeon. There is also evidence of bulletins being used by film lecturers who described and explained the action of the film as it was happening to the audience. The bulletin for *The Drive for a Life*, no. 233, is collected in *Biograph Bulletins* (ed. Kemp R. River; Los Angeles: Locare Research Group, 1971). There is some ambiguity here between the film text and the bulletin as to the precise relationship between Lebrun and Walker. The bulletin suggests that Lebrun 'had mistaken his platonic attentions for love' though this is I think clearly contradicted by the text, which suggests that there was some form of non-platonic relationship between them in a number of ways. Firstly, an intertitle refers to Walker 'putting away an unworthy past for a higher future', constructing then his relationship with Lebrun as in some way 'unworthy'; secondly, Walker returns some letters to Lebrun which are then constructed as love letters; thirdly, this reading provides a motivation for Lebrun's subsequent actions. The further issue would then be this disparity across the bulletin and the film text, so that the bulletin denies the (suggested) salacious opening of the film—which sets in play what I am reading here as a narrative trajectory of a transformation of masculinity—in an attempt to reaffirm a morality which the text itself reaffirms at the close. This different logic of image and text is indicative of a discursive struggle over constructions of 'cinema' as a moral discourse, an issue I shall pursue throughout this paper.
2.   Noel Burch, *Life to Those Shadows* (London: BFI, 1990), p. 150.

3.   Tom Gunning, 'The Cinema of Attractions: Early Film, Its Spectator and the Avant-Garde', in Thomas Elsaesser, *Early Cinema: Space Frame Narrative* (ed. T. Elsaesser; London: BFI, 1990), p. 59 (this essay was first published in *Wide Angle*. 8, 3/4 [Fall 1986]).

4.   The term 'suture' as used within film theory refers to the discursive 'join' between the textual system of a film and the spectator it solicits such that within the configuration of classical narrative cinema the spectator is seen to be bound into a circumscribed 'position' of subjectivity. For an elaboration of this theory see Stephen Heath's *Questions of Cinema* (Bloomington, IN: Indiana University Press, 1981) and Kaja Silverman's *The Subject of Semiotics* (Oxford: Oxford University Press, 1983). Miriam Hansen's argument is that the collective address of early cinema is radically different from the suturing of an individual spectator-subject and that this suturing must then be read as a historically specific imposition of power, as a production and policing of an audience which threatened disorder in terms of class and gender relations. Miriam Hansen, *Babel and Babylon: Spectatorship in American Silent Cinema* (Cambridge, MA: Harvard University Press, 1991).

5.   Lea Jacobs, 'Industry, Self Regulation and the Problem of Textual Determination', *The Velvet Light Trap* 2 (Spring 1989), p. 4.

6.   See especially Tom Gunning's work on the interpenetration of textual and industrial logic in 'Weaving a Narrative: Style and Economic Background in Griffith's Biograph Films' in *Early Cinema* (this essay was first published in *Quarterly Review of Film Studies* [Winter 1981]) and in *D.W. Griffith and the Origins of the American Narrative Film* (Chicago: University of Illinois Press, 1991). The National Board of Censorship is a crucial element in the production of a cinematic discourse, of the construction and delimitation of understandings of cinema, its social function and the uses to which it might be put. On its formation see: Gunning, 'The Cinema of Attractions'; Eileen Bowser, *The Transformation of Cinema, 1907-1915* (Berkeley: University of California Press, 1990); Larry May, *Screening Out the Past: The Birth of Mass Culture and the Motion Picture Industry* (Oxford: Oxford University Press, 1980); Daniel Czitrom, 'The Redemption of Leisure: The National Board of Censorship and the Rise of Motion Pictures in New York City, 1900-1920', *Studies in Visual Communication* 10, 4 (Fall 1984); and Czitrom, 'The Politics of Performance: From Theatre Licensing to Movie Censorship in Turn-of-the-Century New York', *American Quarterly* 44, 4 (December 1992).

7.   *Early Cinema*, p. 15.

8.   *Early Cinema*, p. 304.

9.   Gunning, 'Weaving a Narrative: Style', *Early Cinema*, p. 340. The shot of Lebrun following Walker and Mignon creates several distinct spaces within the diegesis, setting in play a hierarchy of knowledge which positions the spectators alongside Lebrun, providing then a perspective on her motivation—the shot is followed simply by an intertitle proclaiming 'Jealousy'—which is effectively a brief moment of identification with her. This structure clearly also builds up narrative suspense. See Ben Brewster's discussion in 'A Scene at the Movies', in Elsaesser (ed.), *Early Cinema*, p. 322; first published in *Screen* 23. 2 (July 1982); Elsaesser's discussion in *Early Cinema*, p. 315; and Tom Gunning's reading in *D.W. Griffith*, pp. 210-11.

10.   Gunning, *D.W. Griffith*, p. 190.

11.   *Babel and Babylon*, p. 84.

12.   Michel Foucault, 'Nietzsche, Genealogy, History', in *Language, Counter-Memory, Practice: Selected Essays and Interviews* (ed. Donald F. Bouchard; trans. Donald Bouchard and Sherry Simon; Ithaca: Cornell University Press, 1977), p. 143.

13.   Foucault, *The History of Sexuality: An Introduction* (trans. Robert Hurley; Harmondsworth: Penguin, 1979), p. 127. The relation of gender to Foucault's history of sexuality has been much discussed. In an insightful reading, Teresa de Lauretis has suggested

that Foucault's 'critical understanding of the technology of sex did not take into account its differential solicitation of male and female subjects, and by ignoring the conflicting investments of men and women in the discourses and practices of sexuality, Foucault's theory, in fact, excludes, though it does not preclude, the consideration of gender'. *Technologies of Gender: Essays on Theory, Film, and Fiction* (Indianapolis: Indiana University Press, 1987), p. 3. De Lauretis's attempt to reinscribe gender back into Foucault's schema is pursued here.

14.   Foucault, *History of Sexuality*, p. 139.

15.   Foucault, 'The Political Technology of Individuals', in *Technologies of the Self: A Seminar with Michel Foucault* (ed. Luther Martin, Huck Gutman and Patrick Hutton.; London: Tavistock Publications, 1988), p. 153. Foucault suggests that the reconfiguration of power structures attendant upon modernity produced the family as 'the privileged instrument for the government of the population', positioning it then as a 'linking role between general objects regarding the good health of the social body and individuals' desire or need for care'. Foucault, 'Governmentality' in *The Foucault Effect* (ed. Graham Burchell, Colin Gordon and Peter Miller; London: Harvester Wheatsheaf, 1991), p. 100, and Foucault, 'The Politics of Health in the Eighteenth Century', in *Power/Knowledge* (ed. Colin Gordon; New York: Pantheon Books, 1980), p. 174. There arises here the question of the validity of Foucault's analysis in the specific context of the US. Alisa Klaus's admirable *Every Child a Lion: The Origins of Maternal and Infant Health Policy in the United States and France, 1890-1920* (London: Cornell University Press, 1993) approaches this question and argues convincingly for a significant continuity across a discursive policing of the family in both France and the US.

16.   Foucault, 'The Subject and Power' in Hubert Dreyfus and Paul Rabinow, *Michel Foucault: Beyond Structuralism and Hermeneutics* (Chicago: University of Chicago Press, 1983), p. 212.

17.   This is the opening intertitle of the copy of the film available for viewing at the National Film Archive in London though it is not present in the copy available for viewing in the Library of Congress in Washington. I am indebted to Tom Gunning for pointing this out to me. As the intertitle closely resembles all the other intertitles within the film it seems to me to be original. This could perhaps mean one of two things: either the intertitle was lost in the remaining American print, or that the British version was originally sent out with different intertitles.

18.   Foucault, *The Use of Pleasure: The History of Sexuality, Vol. 2* (trans. Robert Hurley; New York: Pantheon Books, 1986), p. 28.

19.   Judith Butler, 'Gender Trouble, Feminist Theory, and Psychoanalytic Discourse', in *Feminism/Postmodernism* (ed. Linda J. Nicholson; London: Routledge, 1990), p. 337.

20.   This is not to deny the sexualization of the female body as an object of knowledge that proliferates in the discourses of medical science, religion, art, literature, popular culture and so on. Indeed, as a number of feminist scholars have suggested, femininity is insistently produced within this configuration as an epistemological quandary: if masculinity can ultimately be 'knowable', femininity remained the 'dark continent'. See especially Mary Ann Doane, *Femmes Fatales: Feminism, Film Theory, Psychoanalysis* (London: Routledge, 1991) for a sustained consideration of discourses around knowledge and femininity. For a reading of this logic in relation to masculinity, see my review article in *Screen* 35.4 (Winter 1994).

21.   Judith Butler, *Gender Trouble: Feminism and the Subversion of Identity* (London: Routledge, 1990), p. viii.

22.   The bulletin for this film, and for others mentioned here, is collected in River, *Biograph Bulletins*.

23.   *Early Cinema*, p. 303. Adolph Zukor talked of his aim 'to kill the slum tradition in the movies', and Griffith himself talked of an ambition to 'translate a manufacturing industry

into an art and meet the ideals of cultivated audiences' (both quoted by Miriam Hansen, *Babel and Babylon*, p. 64). There was clearly a widespread association of early film with 'low morals' and a widespread attempt to reform this constitutes a significant moment in the constitution of 'cinema'.

24.   Films that I have seen here would include *The Mill Girl* (1907), *Falsely Accused* (1907), *A Beast at Bay* (1912), and *Alma's Champion* (1912). Ben Brewster suggests that the structure of a supervisor villain–worker hero fighting over an innocent heroine—a structure that Brewster reads into *The Paymaster* (1907) and *The Tunnel Workers* (1906)—might be linked to the class address of these films, an address which begins to shift for Brewster from around 1910. Brewster, 'A Scene at the Movies', in *Early Cinema*, p. 324.

25.   Gunning, 'Weaving a Narrative', pp. 336-48.

26.   This internal division can be related to the increasing 'psychologisation' of characters within film texts. Kristin Thompson has suggested that 'character psychology forms the basis of numerous changes that distinguish the classical cinema from the primitive cinema. It serves both to structure the causal chain in a new fashion and to make the narration integral to that chain'. Thompson in David Bordwell, Kristin Thompson and Janet Staiger, *The Classical Hollywood Cinema: Film Style and Mode of Production to 1960* (London: Routledge, 1985), p. 177. Thompson quotes from a screenplay manual written in 1921 which asserted that 'A story is the record of a struggle…man's inner conflict of the 'good nature' against the 'bad nature' —of conscience against evil inclination…' (pp. 180-81). Clearly *The Drive for a Life*, produced earlier than the manual, articulates a movement towards the dramatization of this 'inner conflict'.

27.   Foucault, *History of Sexuality*, p. 104.

28.   For example, *The Widow* (1903) shows a widow crying over her deceased husband until she receives 'a caller, a young man'. The bulletin points out that 'the change of emotions is exceedingly effective' (River, *Biograph Bulletins*, p. 104). In *You Will Send Me to Bed, Eh ?* (1905) a young boy is taken to bed because his mother, a widow, is expecting a call from a suitor. The boy sneaks in and pulls off his mothers wig as the suitor is proposing. *The Boy Under the Table* (1905) tells a similar tale and *Mother's Angel Child* (1905) is again similar though here the child is a daughter and the film ends with the suitor leaving the house in disgust. An interesting series develops here, clearly constructing widows as a problematic manifestation of sexuality which is, at the same time, presented as dangerous to the family structure. This is truly a cinematic policing of the family.

29.   As Mary Ann Doane suggests, an increased fascination with the figure of the prostitute in the late nineteenth century 'was emblematic of the new woman's relation to urban space. The conjunction of the woman and the city suggests the potential of an intolerable and dangerous sexuality, a sexuality which is out of bounds precisely as a result of the woman's revised relation to space, her new ability to "wander"'. Doane, *Femmes Fatales*, p. 263. See also Christine Buci-Glucksmann, 'Catastrophic Utopia: The Feminine as Allegory of the Modern', *Representations* 14 (Spring 1986) for the development of a similar perspective. It is perhaps significant that in *The Drive for a Life*—at least in its bulletin—it is the male character who is literally named 'Walker'.

30.   As Allan M. Brandt points out in *No Magic Bullet: A Social History of Venereal Disease in the United States Since 1880* (Oxford: Oxford University Press, 1985), p. 9. Alain Corbin, in *Women for Hire: Prostitution and Sexuality in France After 1850* further suggests that 'the obsessive figure of hereditary syphilis imposed the stigmata of degeneracy' (trans. Alan Sheridan; Cambridge, MA: Harvard University Press, 1990), p. 250.

31.   The further point here is around the impact of censorship and this widespread attempt to construct cinema as a moral discourse on film form and style. That is to say, it is clear that

beginning from around this period film texts become insistently suggestive of a sexuality which is both there and not there, as Lea Jacobs suggests in 'Industry Self-Regulation and the Problem of Textual Determination'.

32.   See Paul Boyer, *Urban Masses and Moral Order in America, 1820-1920* (Cambridge, MA: Harvard University Press, 1978), Mark Connelly, *The Response to Prostitution in the Progressive Era* (Chapel Hill: The University of North California Press, 1980); David J. Pivar, *Purity Crusade, Sexual Morality and Social Control, 1868-1900* (London: Greenwood Press, 1973); John D'Emilio and Estelle B. Freedman, *Intimate Matters: A History of Sexuality in America* (New York: Harper and Row, 1988); and Ruth Rosen, *The Lost Sisterhood: Prostitution in America, 1900-1918* (Baltimore: Johns Hopkins University Press, 1982).

33.   Prince Morrow, 'A Plea for the Organization of a Society of Sanitary and Moral Prophylaxis', in *Transactions of the American Society of Sanitary and Moral Prophylaxis* I (1906), quoted in D'Emilio and Freedman, *Intimate Matters*, p. 206. The society later became the American Social Hygiene Association.

34.   Prince Morrow, *Social Diseases and Marriage* (New York, 1904), p. 78; Morrow, 'Blindness of the Newborn', *Transactions of the American Society for Sanitary and Moral Prophylaxis* (April 1908), quoted in Brandt, *No Magic Bullet*, p. 14; Morrow, *Social Diseases and Marriage*, p. 79.

35.   Morrow, 'Eugenics and Venereal Disease', *Proceedings of the Child Conference for Research and Welfare* 2 (1910), quoted in Brandt, *No Magic Bullet*, p. 19.

36.   Morrow, *Social Diseases and Marriage*, p. 14. The further problem here for Morrow and others is then in the possibility that women can become infertile as a result of venereal diseases. For example, Dr. Abraham Wolbarst asserted that 'The flower of our land, our young women, the mothers of our future citizenship are being mutilated and unsexed by surgical life-saving measures because of these diseases'. Wolbarst, 'The Venereal Diseases: A Menace to the National Welfare' in *New York State Journal of Medicine*, June 1913, quoted in Brandt, *No Magic Bullet*, p. 15.

37.   Morrow, 'Eugenics and Venereal Diseases', quoted in Brandt, *No Magic Bullet*, p. 32.

38.   Morrow, *Social Diseases and Marriage*, p. 340.

39.   Morrow, *Social Diseases and Marriage*, p. 355. My emphasis. There was a whole series of texts advising 'young men' on how to achieve 'masculinity' proliferating within this period. For example, in a 1914 text entitled *Ten Sex Talks for Boys* Irving David Steinhardt asserted that sexual intercourse 'should never be indulged in before marriage...The sexual relation is absolutely unnecessary to you or to any other man'. Quoted in D'Emilio and Freedman, *Intimate Matters*, p. 206.

40.   Foucault, *Use of Pleasure*, p. 13.

41.   Foucault, *History of Sexuality*, p. 69.

42.   Lynda Nead, *Myths of Sexuality: Representations of Women in Victorian Britain* (Oxford: Basil Blackwell, 1988), p. 150; de Lauretis, *Technologies of Gender*, p. 13.

43.   Foucault, *Discipline and Punish: The Birth of the Prison* (trans. Alan Sheridan; New York: Vintage Books, 1979), p. 305.

44.   Foucault, *Discipline and Punish*, p. 305.

45.   Jonathan Crary's brilliant *Techniques of the Observer: On Vision and Modernity in the Nineteenth Century* undertakes such a reading in relation to broader shifts in the configuration of vision, linking them back to 'the construction of a new kind of subject or individual in the nineteenth century' (Cambridge, Massachusetts: MIT Press, 1992), p. 14.

Brian Caldwell

MUSCLING IN ON THE MOVIES:
EXCESS AND THE REPRESENTATION OF THE MALE BODY
IN FILMS OF THE 1980s AND 1990s

In *Camera Obscura*, May 1988, Constance Penley and Sharon Willis assert that the title of the issue 'Male Trouble' refers not so much to men in trouble, but to the 'idea of masculinity itself (which) is both theoretically and historically troubled'. They argue that,

> Under the pressure of feminism and gay politics, and as a result of the demands of advanced capitalism for new kinds of workers, men are being asked to respond as men in new and different ways.[1]

Popular media and literature, they suggest, have served up 'a bewildering variety of images of contemporary masculinity' often 'overtly contradictory images'. It is not difficult to provide examples of such a variety of images. Films such as *Big* (1988) which focus on boys in men's bodies, present an image of a physically adult male released from the demands of maturity; effectively a licence to indulge in boyish irresponsibility. In an article entitled 'The Last Real Man in America' David Leverenz notes the following description of Sean Connery as depicted on the cover of *Gentlemen's Quarterly*, July 1989:

> Dressed in a creamy ivory tuxedo, standing with arms folded against a beige background, visible only to the waist, he embodied elegance, sensuality and virility.[2]

Not only is the last real man in America not an American, he apparently does not exist below the waist either. Leverenz's consideration of the film *Batman* (1989) indicates the potential span of images of masculinity. The quasi-aristocratic Bruce Wayne (played by Michael Keaton) becomes half-beast and descends into 'a world that seems hell-bent on robbing every man of a father and virility'.[3] In the face of such opposition Batman asserts a recuperated masculinity, rising above, or below, the boy-like Bruce Wayne.

This spectrum of available images has a number of potential consequences. Penley and Willis are prompted to consider masculinity 'as it is crucially inflected by class, race, and ethnicity'. There is thus a perceived need both to pluralize and to contextualize masculinity. The multiplicity of images also potentially exposes the ways in which masculinities are either constructed, reconstructed or both since, if more than one image exists, by implication the constituent elements and structures are different and can be contrasted. An example of a literally constructed masculinity is served up in *Aliens* (1986). As the crew emerge from their sleeping pods and begin exercising, Vasquez, played by Jenette Goldstein, raises herself on an exercise bar and displays her muscled body. A male member of the crew asks, 'Hey, Vasquez—have you ever been mistaken for a man?' Vasquez replies, 'No, have you?' Exercise develops the building blocks of a muscular, instantly recognizable and apparently uncomplicated masculinity. However, the anxiety implicit in the first question is reflected or inflected in the second, and underlined by the significant absence of an answer. If masculinity, or to be precise an image of masculinity, can be developed by Vasquez the status of the masculinity displayed by the male members of the crew becomes problematic. Which, for example, is negative, and which is print?

The intention in this paper is to concentrate on representations of excessive masculinity, on both the methodology of that representation and its ideological underpinnings. Examples include films featuring the excessively muscled bodies of Arnold Schwarzenegger and Sylvester Stallone. Schwarzenegger's body has for example been described by one critic as 'a condom stuffed with walnuts', whereas Stallone, particularly in the *Rambo* films, has been referred to as Fenimore Cooper's 'leatherstocking on steroids'.[4] More significantly in terms of filmic representation, Gaylyn Studlar and David Desser refer to Stallone's 'glistening hypermasculinity' as John Rambo and note how this is 'emphasized in the kind of languid camera movements and fetishizing close-up usually reserved for "female flashdancers"'.[5]

Rambo III (1988) places the eponymous hero in self-exile in Thailand, supporting himself by engaging in martial arts contests. The contests allow Stallone's half-naked body to be presented as a spectacle to be looked at by the spectator. The camera admiringly circles the body, utilizing close-up shots to display first the muscled back then the heavily muscled front torso. In each case Stallone adopts conventional body-building poses to display his physique. The body is posed for the receptive camera, which obligingly closes in at appropriate moments, that is when the optimally flexed muscles are at their most prominent. The specific code of masculinity employed is registered initially if problematically as an image on and of the body, available for the consumption of the spectator.[6] The excess of masculinity, represented in the overwrought body of the actor, is underlined by the loud music and loud voices, the crowded and animated *mise-en-scène*, and the rapid editing. All serve to orchestrate the male body as spectacle, as an object to be looked at, much in the manner in which traditionally the female body has been presented in mainstream film.

The male body has thus muscled in on the site previously occupied by the object of the male voyeuristic gaze, and in so doing prompts a range of questions. Pam Cook, for example, asks simply, 'What are the consequences of placing the male body at the centre of visual display?'[7] Miriam Hansen asks more specifically, 'If a man is made to occupy the place of erotic object, how does this affect the organization of vision?'[8] One response from the male spectator might well be discomfort due to the eroticism, actual or potential, which derives from the visual display of the male body. In addition the male spectator, forced to gaze narcissistically at an image of himself, may well experience additional discomfort since the exaggerated proportions of the body image on screen point to his own inadequacies. As a consequence there is an incentive either to mask the cause of the discomfort, or more feasibly, to distract attention from it. Thus for example the violence which seems inseparable from such displays of excessive masculinity (whether in the *Rambo* sequence, *The Terminator* [1984] and *Terminator II* [1991] or in a significant number of films about the war in Vietnam) may reinforce the masculine image or may seek to distract from it. The body, actively enmeshed in a *mise-en-scène* of violence will no longer hold the fixed gaze of the spectator, and since violent acts usually imply consequences, a further reassurance will be the promise of a return to narrative. The body posed momentarily as the object of the male gaze, either voyeuristic or narcissistic, or both, reasserts itself as subject in a cause and effect sequence of events.

Yvonne Tasker notes similar ambiguities when she suggests that the 'over-developed and over-determined body' of the muscular male hero could be either 'a triumphal assertion of traditional masculinity' or 'an hysterical image'.[9] Stallone–Rambo evokes the stature of the classic warrior and recalls images of the gladiator of epic film and thus could be said to represent the body triumphant. However in conventional terms, Rambo–Stallone may equally represent a failed masculinity. Thus his reluctance to speak and the manner in which the camera concentrates on his hair, eyes and pectoral muscles could equally suggest a masculinity in crisis. The play of the camera and its implicit feminization of the hero, in filmic terms at least, underlines this interpretation.

The constructions of masculinity are also on view. The bodies of Stallone and Schwarzenegger are clearly structured or restructured. In one sense they are literally self-made men, but, as Margaret Walters notes, 'paradoxically, body building is the most purely narcissistic and, in that sense, most feminine of pastimes'.[10] This self conscious aspect of body building is perhaps what prompts Barbara Creed to observe that such actors are performing the masculine. In a literal sense as actors they obviously are, but the excessive nature of the masculinity on view denotes a constructed performance, one verging on the caricature.[11] Tasker indeed links the notion of performance of the masculine to questions of masquerade and parody, and asserts:

> In terms of the muscular hero, it is possible to argue that these male
> figures offer a parodic performance of masculinity, which both enacts and
> calls into question the qualities they embody.[12]

The manner in which masculinity is both exaggerated and foregrounded and yet implicitly exposed as artifice or construct points up the paradox of the performance. The process of simultaneous assertion and denial may act as a defence designed to deflect anxiety about the idea of masculinity itself, but may equally draw attention to that anxiety. Thus the representations of the heavily muscled body in films featuring Stallone and Schwarzenegger present ambiguities of masculinity if not masculinity in crisis. It is quite possible to argue that the link between narcissism and the feminine is more tenuous than Margaret Walters assumes. However the hyperbole of the masculine image demands attention from the spectator who is thus encouraged to question not only why such excess is presented, but how it is constructed. The image of masculinity on view thus draws attention to its own artifice, prompting questions about what constitutes an appropriate masculinity, not least because the excess on view is clearly not obtainable by the majority, if any, of the male spectators.

Such ambiguities in part develop because it is the body which is used as a register of gender. The way in which body-building in general and the play of the camera in particular tends to feminize the image of the male body has already been noted. However, the cultural categories of masculinity and feminity, the histories and values associated with them, cannot be defined and contained within the image of the body. Tasker for example coins the term 'musculinity'[13] to indicate the way in which developed musculature transgresses the binary gender divide. Tasker refers to the muscled bodies of Sigourney Weaver in the *Alien* trilogy and Linda Hamilton in *Terminator II* to illustrate her point. The question addressed to Vasquez in *Aliens* (1986), 'Have you ever been mistaken for a man?', centres on her muscled body and implies that masculinity can be acquired or built by the female. However such conventional marks of the masculine could be read as foisting a masculine code on the female. Antony Easthope argues that contemporary popular culture imposes on a man 'the burden of having to be one sex all the way through' with the result that 'his struggle to be masculine is the struggle to cope with his own femininity'.[14] One aspect of this struggle, assuming that it exists, may be that popular culture will seek to empower the feminine but only if she is coded as masculine. Masculine power is legitimised albeit vicariously. Thus the muscled bodies of for example Weaver and Hamilton, armed with phallic weaponry, encapsulate their own ambiguities.

The representations of masculinity(ies) in both the Weaver–Hamilton and the Stallone–Schwarzenegger examples involve an excess of muscle and consequently an excess of masculinity. Such cinematic excess can be defined as referring to 'heightened material elements in a film that surpass the requirements of narrative progression and frequently even undermine or contradict the narrative',[15] or as 'those aspects of the work which are not contained by its unifying forces' (where film is considered as a struggle of opposing forces in which some forces 'strive to unify a work').[16] Literally then excess is that which is more than is required, used or consumed. Images of excessive musculature are often accompanied by excessive sound, rapid camera movement or rapid editing, or all three, contributing to and emphasizing the excess of the image. Such excesses of masculinity(ies) draw attention to the representational hyperbole, but also exposes the processes of film. The spectator is aware of both the construction of a masculinity and the construction of a film sequence.

In *Terminator II* (1991), for example, the spectator watches the physically constructed body of the actor act the role of cyborg. In the early sequences of the film, as he enters a café in search of clothes, the point of view repeatedly shifts so that instead of looking at the cyborg the spectator looks with him. The *mise-en-scène* is presented at first directly, then as if through the Terminator's computer screen. The graphics on the screen, the colour red which suffuses the image and the distorted soundtrack all signal that the muscled cyborg is a construction. The visual and aural excesses underline that his masculinity is an artifice. Yet ironically it is the constructed non-human cyborg who violently overthrows the brute excess of masculinity represented by the bikers. Such an indulgence of excess carries consequences for the narrative, for the construction of meaning and, perhaps most significantly, for the spectator. Each will be addressed with specific reference to excesses evident in the representation of masculinity.

Both definitions of excess cited earlier foreground the effect of excess on the narrative. For Thompson excess works against the structures which seek to unify the film whereas for Springer excess threatens to surpass, undermine or contradict the narrative. In short, excess disrupts narrative progression. It is as if the narrative is freeze-framed, so that the spectator is released from its demands and allowed to feast on the spectacle of excess. In the genre of the musical the relationship between excess (specifically the song and dance routines) and the narrative is easier to explain. The song and dance might amplify, develop or reflect on the narrative; that is tell us more of what we already know, tell us more of what we want to know, or allow the cast to step outside of the narrative and talk or sing about what is happening. It is less easy to explain the relationship between such muscular excesses as have been noted earlier and the narrative within which they are contained. Such spectacles of masculinity seem to exist in their own right and could be placed almost anywhere on the plot line. In some ways such images are akin to that of the separate head and shoulders shot of the cowboy which was offered to exhibitors and which could be projected at the beginning or at the end of Edwin S. Porter's *The Great Train Robbery* (1903), particularly because they draw attention to themselves as distinct freestanding images rather than as one part of a cause and effect sequence.

Excess draws attention to the process of film-making. If it is accepted that generally Hollywood film seeks to construct a seamless narrative, that is it seeks to mask its own devices, then in films where excess occurs it might be expected that an extra effort will be made to disguise such breaks in smooth narrative progression. In fact excess can both cause the break and serve to disguise either the resultant or existing narrative fractures or both. Hollywood films of the Vietnam war provide an apposite example since they often experience significant problems in the construction of a fluently progressive narrative, not least because they often insist on utilising the World War II combat movie genre—a genre designed to demonstrate success in war—to represent a war that was lost. One attempted solution to such difficulties is the use of the voice-over narration, to guide the spectator across the fractures which narrative alone fails to negotiate. Another potential solution is to commandeer excesses of masculinity, violence or both.

This process can be traced through a consideration of the consequences of excess for meaning in film. For Susan Jeffords, combat films are 'about the construction of the masculine subject'.[17] In an obvious material way the male body is under threat from the enemy who in Vietnam war films are often characterized as feminine. The threat, that is the potential deconstruction of masculinity, is masked by an excess of violence, in dialogue and action. In *Full Metal Jacket* (1987), for example, Animal Mother's reaction to the threat posed by the sniper who has already wounded two of the American soldiers is a display of excessive heroism. Spitting almost as many expletives as bullets, he charges at the enemy (in fact a 16 year old Vietnamese girl). The spectacle of filmic excess in this case provides a cultural corollary to military imperialism; the spectacle depends upon the excess of American firepower and indeed implicitly economic power since the excessive discharge from the M.60 could be (and was) afforded. This display of extreme masculine heroism is ironically juxtaposed with the evident risking of that masculinity's destruction. The excess compensates for the de-stabilizing of the masculine position, and, since Animal Mother has disobeyed orders to make the charge, for the destabilizing of masculine authority.

For Jeffords the excess of combat films is 'produced by and relieves moments of crisis in the construction of the masculine subject'. Thus in *Platoon* (1986) Chris Taylor (played by Charlie Sheen) is increasingly under threat, not least because he is caught between the 'good' Sergeant Elias and the 'evil' Sergeant Barnes. He finally reemerges as the self-acknowledged 'child born of two fathers'. The excesses associated with the variously muscled hard bodies on display and the combat violence have effectively sought to disguise three factors: firstly the inevitable destabilization of masculinity which occurs during combat; secondly the exchange of power from the two fathers to the son; and thirdly the reproduction or reconstruction of gender, that is the hero reborn as a stable masculine subject.[18] It could be noted that the transfer of power is within an exclusively male world where the mother is redundant. However the black American soldiers and the Vietnamese are also excluded from the equation so that white Anglo-Saxon Protestant masculinity is the exclusive site of power.

It could also be argued that whilst excess seeks to mark the unstable transfer and reconstruction of male power, it also has a tendency to over-compensate. Not only are the implicit threats to stable definitions of masculinity brought into focus but the attractions of instability and the threat to authority are revealed. The gap (symbolic wound?) which is opened in the patriarchal structure at the point of transference of power may well be exaggerated by the excessive attempt to disguise it. Thus in *Platoon* Chris Taylor is presented with a variety of temptations which seek to lead him away from accepting the conventional responsibilities of the male soldier. He is, for example, temporarily drawn into an underworld of drink, drugs and rock n' roll, lured away from authority and responsibility by the excesses of contemporary siren voices. The spectator is also distracted, in this case from the demands of the narrative, in order to be entertained by the seductive images and sounds of sensual pleasure. The central character and the spectator share a point of view and are equally vulnerable to the spectacle of excess, which in turn seeks to distract the attention of both, but partic-ularly the spectator, from the destabilizing of traditional male authority.

Mulvey's argument on the masculinization of the spectator position is pertinent here,[19] but there are other consequences for the spectator whether male or female. The spectator of filmic excess, according to Claudia Springer, is not only treated to an arresting spectacle, but also to heightened visual and auditory stimuli which in turn encourage feelings of intensity and exhilaration.[20] The spectator is effectively distanced from the visual image not sutured by conventional patterns; for example the shot-reverse-shot sequence in which the spectator apparently shares the point of view of the major, usually male, characters sequentially and is thus drawn in or stitched into the narrative. Instead, the spectator looks at rather than with the major characters. Specific subjective engagements are diffused and a visual and subjective distance is created as the spectator momentarily steps out of the narrative binds.

However, the spectator may not entirely escape, but remain caught between attraction and repulsion, pleasure and unpleasure. In films of the Vietnam War the attraction may be to the hero's restraint and (usually) his guaranteed survival, whereas unpleasure may be experienced at the excess of violence or carnage and the threat of sharing the hero's apparently imminent death. As if to emphasize this ambiguity, loosely a pattern of sadistic and masochistic pleasures–unpleasures, the punishment and suffering meted out to the bodies of the central character are characteristically dwelt upon. Thus in the *Deerhunter* (1978) the unpleasure experienced because of the sadistic treatment of the American soldiers held captive by the Viet Cong (or by the North Vietnamese Army since the two are rarely rendered distinct in American films of the Vietnam War) is tempered by the knowledge that Michael, played by Robert De Niro, will almost certainly remedy the situation and exact a suitable vengeance. However the physical and psychological suffering experienced by the soldiers is dwelt upon in lingering close-ups of their anguished faces; the spectator experiences unpleasure but also pleasure at their stoic, masochistic endurance.

Excess can thus serve not only to disguise but also to draw attention to the disrupted, fractured narrative. Either way the spectator is encouraged to sit back and watch the spectacle unfold. The spectator is freed, however transiently, from the constraints brought about both by identification with the central characters' point(s) of view and also from the need to solve or resolve the enigma of the plot. Thus the spectator is left 'dangerously' liberated to read the text in a variety of ways, to bypass the dominant or preferred readings, and is allowed to negotiate his or her own path within the ambiguities and fractures created by cinematic excess.

The problematic position of masculinity in contemporary popular culture has it seems spawned in turn examples of compensatory masculinities. The excesses of musculature and violence in the films examined construct a spectacular masculinity which appears to dominate both the narrative and the gaze of the spectator. Inscribed within this excessive masculinity are, however, the seeds of its own anxiety. The over-compensation exposes ambiguities in the representation of the male body not least because it has muscled in on the territory previously occupied by the female body. The camera's fetishizing gaze, still geared to the representation of the 'other', tends to amplify such feminization of the male body to the point of parody. The encoded ambiguities and anxieties are reinforced because the process of building the masculine image is exposed; the spectator, male or female, is made aware of masculinity as construct. The spectator is liberated and permitted to muscle in on the building sites of meanings and masculinities. Cinematic excess in general and the display of musculature in particular thus ironically fail to produce a definitive masculinity.

Notes

1.   C. Penley and S. Willis, *Camera Obscura: A Journal of Feminism and Film Theory* 17 (May 1988), pp. 4-5.
2.   D. Leverenz, 'The Last Real Man in America: From Natty Bumppo to Batman', *American Literary History* 3, 4 (Winter 1991), p. 753.
3.   Leverenz, 'The Last Real Man', p. 769.
4.   H. Schechter and J.F. Semeiks, 'Leatherstocking in Nam: Rambo, Platoon and the

American Frontier Myth', *Journal of Popular Culture* 24, 4 (Spring 1991), p. 23.
5.   G. Studlar and D. Desser, 'Never Having to Say You're Sorry: Rambo's rewriting of the Vietnam War', *Film Quarterly* XLII, 1 (Fall 1988), p. 15.
6.   A. Easthope asserts that, 'gender can be defined in three ways: as the body; as our social roles of male and female; as the way we internalise and live out these roles'. See Easthope, *What a Man's Gotta Do: The Masculine Myth in Popular Culture* (London: Paladin, 1986), pp. 2-3.
7.   P. Cook, 'Masculinity in Crisis', *Screen* 23, 3-4 (1982), p. 40.
8.   M. Hansen, 'Pleasure, Ambivalence, Identification: Valentino and Female Spectatorship', *Cinema Journal* 25, 4 (Summer 1986), p. 10.
9.   Y. Tasker, *Spectacular Bodies: Gender, Genre and the Action Cinema* (London: Routledge, 1993), p. 109.
10.   M. Walters, cited in S. Cohan, 'Masquerading as the American Male in the Fifties: Picnic, William Holden and the Spectacle of Masculinity in Hollywood Film', *Camera Obscura: A Journal of Feminism and Film Theory* 25-26 (January-May 1991), p. 61.
11.   B. Creed cited in Tasker, *Spectacular Bodies*, p. 111.
12.   Tasker, *Spectacular Bodies*, pp. 110-11. See also J. Riviere, 'Womanliness as Masquerade', in *Formations of Fantasy* (ed. J. Burgin, J. Donald, and C. Kaplan; London: Methuen, 1986)
13.   Tasker, *Spectacular Bodies*, p. 3.
14.   Easthope, *What a Man's Gotta Do*. The argument, that popular culture will seek to empower the female, but only if she accepts the codes of the masculine, could be applied to for example *Thelma and Louise* (1991). In this film however the female protagonists are not burdened with the marks of the masculine, but do inhabit the terrain of a traditionally male narrative structure, colloquially referred to as the 'buddy movie'.
15.   C. Springer, 'Anti-War Film as Spectacle: Contradictions of the Combat Sequence', *Genre* XXI, 4 (Winter 1988), pp. 480-81.
16.   K. Thompson, 'The Concept of Cinematic Excess', in *Narrative, Apparatus, Ideology: A Film Theory Reader* (ed. P. Rosen; New York: Columbia University Press, 1986), p. 130.
17.   S. Jeffords, 'Masculinity as Excess in Vietnam Films: The Father/Son Dynamic', *Genre* XXI, 4 (Winter 1988), p. 489.
18.   G. Zavitzianos has argued that clothes which are associated with paternal authority, such as military uniforms, are used to stabilize the body image. See G. Zavitzianos, 'The Object in Fetishism, Homeovestism and Transvestism', *International Journal of Psychoanalysis* 58 (1977), pp. 487-95.
19.   L. Mulvey, *Visual and Other Pleasures* (Basingstoke: Macmillan, 1991), pp. 14-26. For the purposes of this paper I have ignored the current debates about gendered spectatorship.
20.   Springer, 'Anti-War Film as Spectacle', pp. 479-82.

Filmography

Aliens	(20th Century-Fox/Brandywine,1986, dir. James Cameron, 137 mins.)
Batman	(Guber-Peters/Warner, 1989, dir. Tim Burton, 126 mins.)
Big	(20th Century-Fox, 1988, dir. Penny Marshall, 102 mins.)
Deerhunter	(Universal/EMI, dir. Michael Cimino, 183 mins.)
Full Metal Jacket	Warner, 1987, dir. Stanley Kubrick, 116 mins.)
Platoon	(Hemdale, 1986, dir. Oliver Stone, 120 mins.)
Rambo III	(Carolco, 1988, dir. Peter Macdonald, 101 mins.)
The Terminator	(Hemdale, 1984, dir. James Cameron, 108 mins.)
Terminator II	(Carolco, 1991, dir. James Cameron, 135 mins.)
Thelma and Louise	(Pathe/Main, 1991, dir. Ridley Scott, 128 mins.)

Contemporary Fiction

James Annesley

COMMODIFICATION, VIOLENCE AND THE BODY:
A READING OF SOME RECENT AMERICAN FICTIONS

Contemporary American narrative's preoccupation with bodily violence is apparent
to the most casual of observers. These concerns have been brought to the fore by,
among other things, the recent emergence of Quentin Tarantino as one of America's
leading screen-writers and directors and the debate generated by the brutal tone of
his films *Reservoir Dogs*, *True Romance* and *Pulp Fiction*. Tarantino's notoriety has been
matched in the literary world by the controversy that accompanied the publication
of Bret Easton Ellis's novel *American Psycho*. The interesting thing about these pieces
is, however, that their portrayals of extreme violence are neither unusual nor unprecedented. The gruesome scenes and brutal images presented by Ellis and Tarantino are
not shocking deviations from the mainstream, but elements that are characteristic of
it. This widespread emphasis on representations of corporeal violence can be seen in,
for example, the films of Abel Ferrara, Jonathon Demme's *Silence of the Lambs*, the
Raymond Carver stories 'So much water so close to home' and 'Tell the women
we're going', Ray Shell's and Jess Mowry's tales of urban deprivation and drug-
addiction, the Vietnam novels of Bobbie Ann Mason and Jayne Anne Phillips and the
revisions of Western mythology offered by Clint Eastwood in *Unforgiven* and Cormac
McCarthy in *Blood Meridian*. The prevalence of this kind of imagery in recent
American film and fiction demands interpretation and this paper intends to contribute to that project by reflecting on the deployment of representations of corporeal
violence in one particular strand of modern American writing, the strand that has
come to be known as blank fiction.

Blank fiction is a new tendency in American writing. This fiction, which has
been described as the work of a 'Generation X' and labelled in alternative terms as
'the fiction of insurgency', 'blank generation fiction' and 'Brat Pack fiction', can be
identified by its characteristic use of flat, stunned prose styles and the employment of
authorial perspectives that seem cold, distanced and voyeuristic.[1] Jay McInerney,
Donna Tartt and Tama Janowitz are writers who have established themselves working
within this form and affinities exist between their work and the less familiar fiction
of authors like Darryl Pinckney, Lynne Tillman and Joel Rose. The tonal and stylistic
similarities shared by these novelists are paralleled by a common set of thematic
preoccupations. Their narratives are predominantly urban in focus and intimately
concerned with the dynamics of popular culture. More significantly, blank fiction
displays a willingness to engage with the kind of experimental subject matter that

obsessed Bataille, Burroughs and De Sade. Blank novels are about 'sex, death and subversion' and this thematic continuity means that these novels return repeatedly to images of the violated human body.[2] Blank fiction's concern for images of brutality finds specific articulation in Dennis Cooper's novel *Frisk* and Brian D'Amato's *Beauty* and it is upon these texts that this paper will concentrate.[3] The intention is to link a discussion of the way the body is represented in these two novels with a reading of wider social and economic forces by suggesting that the brutal and objectified images used by Cooper and D'Amato reflect an environment that is, in a different way, being brutalized and objectified. Their fictional descriptions of bodily carve-ups and aggressive penetrations register the economic forces carving up, penetrating and brutalizing the social body of modern America.

An analysis of the role played by the concept of beauty in these narratives offers a useful way of establishing the problem and developing the arguments needed to read the portrayal of bodily violence from a materialist perspective. These texts focus on beauty and the body's æsthetic and establish, through these *foci*, a sense of the forces that link the individual human body with the economic body. In both *Frisk* and *Beauty*, the body's visual æsthetic is the mechanism through which capitalism gets to grips with the personal. *Beauty* is both a received judgment on the body's appearance and a means of putting an economic valuation on that appearance. The complex functioning of the idea of beauty thus engages the body in the exchange system and provides the means through which the body is transformed into a commodity.

D'Amato's *Beauty* is a novel about plastic surgery, about the purchasing of beauty. It describes the activities of a New York sculptor who leaves the world of art and becomes an illicit cosmetic surgeon, using new and untested techniques to radically alter the faces of his female customers. These slickly performed but ghoulish procedures represent brutalization: they attack the flesh, penetrate and mould it into new shapes. Despite the controlled violence of these processes, D'Amato emphasizes the quality of the results achieved. His artist–surgeon does not perform minor alterations, he completely restructures faces. The crude cosmetic surgery of silicon and liposuction is replaced by a fantasy surgery that totally transforms the body.

This narrative introduces a number of crucial ideas, the most important of which is the understanding that cosmetic surgery provides a means of marketing and commercializing the body's appearance. Beauty, something previously considered to be 'free' and 'natural' is, as a result of cosmetic surgery, made available to those with money. The central feature of D'Amato's representation of cosmetic surgery is that he puts beauty up for sale in absolute terms. The fantasy operations he imagines are freed from the constraints imposed on real cosmetic surgery by factors like age and bone structure. The only thing *Beauty*'s surgical procedures need is money. D'Amato's text thus describes a situation in which beauty is totally commodified. The novel's central character complains that 'It's horrible the way some people try to convince you that you can't buy beauty.'[4]

At this point it is essential to acknowledge that the connection between money and beauty is not unique to a world in which the kind of fantastic transformations described by D'Amato are possible. Cosmetic surgery is nothing new. The histories of foot-binding and infibulation, for example, give an sense of the extent and antiquity of practices intended to refine the body's appearance. More importantly, the cultural norms that define the beautiful face must be read in terms that appreciate the role played by the taste of dominant and wealthy power groups in their construction. However, the practices described in *Beauty* establish links between economics and the body that are of unprecedented strength and directness. The situation D'Amato imagines is one in which the body, and specifically the female body, is being completely fetishized. This fetishism holds clears echoes of Marx's sense of the dehumanizing consequences of commodity fetishism. Marx writes:

> The mysterious character of the commodity form consists therefore simply in the fact that the commodity reflects the social characteristics of men's own labour as objective characteristics of the products of labour themselves, as the socio-natural properties of things.[5]

Marx's position finds a specific resonance when read alongside D'Amato's text and prompts a recognition of the way his novel represents cosmetic surgery as a process of dehumanization that is both abstract and physical. The objectification of labour described by Marx is an objectification that takes place on the level of social psychology. In D'Amato's text this abstract process is translated into real corporeal event. The body is operated upon and, as a result, enters the exchange system. The dehumanizing consequences of commodification are thus exactly paralleled by the dehumanizing consequences of creating the commodity through the surgical brutalization of the body. All the dehumanizing effects of commodification identified by Marx are present in this system. The difference is, however, that this economic relation involves an extra level of dehumanization that takes place in a way unforeseen in Marx's original discussion. *Beauty* thus represents a situation in which commodification has an impact on human experience that is more intense and more extreme than that originally envisaged by Marx.

This sense of a heightened level of commodification can be linked to the theoretical interpretation of late capitalism advanced by Ernst Mandel. Mandel's concern is to outline the specific character of late twentieth century capitalism and to contrast contemporary economic relations with those of earlier periods. He writes:

> The age of late capitalism, with its accelerated technological development and the…massive extension of intellectually qualified labour, drives the contradictions of the capitalist mode of production to its highest pitch.[6]

Mandel's thesis differentiates late capitalism from preceding modes of production by identifying the increased intensity of capitalist activity in this period. Late capitalism is capitalism at it 'highest pitch', an 'accelerated' capitalism where the increased intensity of economic activity creates conditions in which capital's contradictions become more severe. This interpretation of the intensification of capital is developed into a more specific reflection on commodification by Frederic Jameson who argues 'late, multinational, or consumer capitalism…constitutes… the purest form of capital yet to have emerged', and suggests that this period is characterized by a 'prodigious expansion of capital into hitherto uncommodified areas'.[7] The links between Jameson's position and the arguments offered by Mandel are clear. However, there are differences and it is important to recognize the way Jameson refines Mandel's argument and connects it more directly to reification: where Mandel sees increased contradictions in late capitalism, Jameson sees increased commodification. In Marx's view commodi-fication precipitates particular kinds of contradictions. Jameson's position outlines a specific arena and context for these contradictions, contradictions which develop as a result of what Mandel identifies as the general intensification of the capitalist mode of production. Jameson's ideas thus provide a precise way of reading the commer-cialization of the body presented by D'Amato. *Beauty*'s somatic preoccupations reflect Jameson's suggestion that late capitalism involves an expansion of capital's sphere of influence into 'hitherto uncommodified areas'. Clear parallels exist between the lan-guage and ideas associated with economic invasion and penetration and this dis-cussion of the invasion and penetration of the human body by, simultaneously, the operations of cosmetic surgery and the commodification that attends those operations.

The relationships between this economic model and D'Amato's text can be strengthened by considering the central role played by æsthetics in the promotion of products. This function is illustrated in *Beauty*'s portrayal of the artist–surgeon's search for an image of the supposedly perfect face. His energy is concentrated on an attempt to construct a composite image of different faces using the already commodified images of fashion models and film stars. He uses these airbrushed, idealised images of beauty as the templates for his own creations and transforms them into new com-modities. This triumph of commodification means that the advertising devices become products in their own right; D'Amato's artist surgeon turns advertising into reality in the faces he constructs. A perfectly commodified system results with the product and the promotion melding into one. Capital, in D'Amato's world, instead of selling through advertising, now sells advertising itself. The circle closes completely when the women who have been transformed using images from fashion and the cinema become themselves fashion models and film stars. One scene in the novel captures this play on levels in particularly clear terms. D'Amato describes his surgeon visiting a department store and discovering that the mannequins in the shop have been modelled on one of his surgically transformed women:

> One day I went shopping in Barney's…there was a whole gang of her there, unmoving, five garishly swimsuited, variously wigged clones, staring down at me with lifeless eyes through the window. Apparently a mannequin company had made a head design based on her; kind of an interesting reverse switch, I guess, but I sort of lost interest in shopping that day.[8]

Life is not imitating art, it is imitating advertising, with that imitation then becoming advertising itself.

The centrality of the concept of beauty to the processes of product promotion has been explored by W.F. Haug, and the applicability of his *Critique of Commodity Æsthetics* to this reading of Beauty is striking. Haug identifies the æsthetic illusion, the beautiful appearance, as a key element in the marketing process. Haug argues that 'within the commodity system of buying and selling, the æsthetic illusion—the commodity's promise of use value—enters the arena as an independent function of its selling'.[9] In D'Amato's novel it is clear that the women who have had their faces transformed are not just the products and the customers, they are the advertising as well. In a curious way their beauty has become an 'independent function' of the process of selling cosmetic surgery. A cosmetic surgeon's clients are living advertisements for that surgeon's skills and D'Amato capitalizes on this fact and brings these commodifying and recommodifying forces into focus. In Haug's view this cycle of images, and the power that accompanies those images, is an inevitable part of the æsthetics of marketing. He suggests that 'Æsthetic innovation, as the functionary for regenerating demand, is thus transformed into a moment of direct anthropological power and influence'.[10] The implication is that beauty, as superficial appearance, takes on an authority that is at odds with its superficiality. Marketing's need for æsthetic innovation, and the power those innovations yield, create complicated sets of relationships between the commodity and the consumer. Rachel Bowlby offers a similar kind of interpretation when she argues

> The commodity makes the person and the person is, if not for sale, then an object whose value or status can be read off with accuracy in terms of the things he has and the behavioural codes he adopts.[11]

The commodity's transformative potential is, in Bowlby's terms, associated with the æsthetic illusions supplied with the commodity. This transformative potential is literalized in D'Amato's text which represents the anthropological power of the advertising image in a way that sees those images being themselves anthropomorphized. Bowlby's understanding of the commodity's power to 'make' the person, finds vivid reflection in *Beauty*'s portrayal of a world in which the authority of the æsthetic illusion is unparalleled.

The interrelationships that D'Amato constructs between the commodity, the commodity's image, the consumer and the body thus offers a means of shedding light on Mandel's view of late capitalism's heightened contradictions and Jameson's sense of the intensification of commodification in the late capitalist period. D'Amato's text creates an environment in which the body takes on a number of contradictory roles and becomes the site in which conflicting forces meet. It is the consumer and the consumed, the selling point and the product. The fact that the dehumanizing consequences that attend the body's commodification take effect in a way that allows the objectified body to become, in its own way, an æsthetic illusion and thus complicit in its own objectification is one of the most striking twists in D'Amato's narrative. This reading of *Beauty* is thus organized in terms that re-examine the forces that Jameson and Mandel identify as characteristic of late capitalism. The fact that brutalization, dehumanization and exploitation are dominant themes in D'Amato's text makes this association even more interesting as it offers the possibility of establishing an interrogative perspective on this mode of production. Late capitalism is shown breaking into new markets and effecting human experience in a specific and disturbing ways as it penetrates the limits of the body and commodifies the physical core of experience and subjectivity.

The problem with this reading is, however, that it relies on assumptions that figure the body in ways that contradict more established critical positions. The suggestion here is that the penetration of the body represents a diminishment of human experience. Corporeal limits are signalled as precious and the breakdown of those limits is marked in negative terms. This contradicts the orthodox postmodern line which places the piercing of the body's limits in a positive light by arguing that such denaturalizations disrupt the imaginary unity of the body and undermine positions that draw their strength from biologically determined reasoning. Recent criticism has made a great deal of, for example, the significance of the female cyborg, interpreting her as a figure that articulates the artificiality of the construct of the body.[12] A cyborg's prosthetic organs are read as an expression of her ability to define herself and her own body rather than having her body defined for her. Judith Butler's *Bodies that Matter* considers these issues on a theoretical level by asking the question 'are bodies purely discursive?' and interrogating the relationship between materiality and bodily identity.[13] These interpretations do not, however, work well when linked to the denaturalizing processes of cosmetic surgery which enforce dominance rather than deconstruct it. In the kind of cosmetic surgery described in *Beauty*, the penetration and transformation of the body is a process that works to reproduce cultural norms. The women created are not cyborgs, they are mannequins. Rather than breaking up culturally constructed ideas about the female body, cosmetic surgery carves those constructions deeper into the skin.

Beauty's representation of cosmetic surgery provides a clear opportunity for interpreting its brutal treatment of the body in economic terms. The potential for reading the depiction of bodily violence in Cooper's *Frisk* in this way is, however, less obvious. *Frisk* revolves around the lives of a group of young gay men. The novel describes them sleeping with their friends, acting in porn films, prostituting themselves and taking drugs. The central character, Dennis, is haunted by the recollection of being shown, while still an adolescent, the pornographic image of an apparently dead boy. The teenage memory of this 'snuff' picture plays on Dennis's mind and provides the background for his adult obsessions with masochism and murder. At the end of the novel he moves from Los Angeles to Amsterdam. The penultimate section of the book is in the form of a long letter written by Dennis to a former lover that describes a series of brutal sexual murders that he has apparently committed, with the help of two accomplices, while he's been in Holland. Dennis's accounts of these murders represent the human body in terms that are completely objectified and dehumanized. The letter explains how

> We cut him apart for a few hours and studied everything inside the body, not saying much to one another, just the occasional, Look at this, or swear word, until there was nothing around but a big, off-white shell in the middle of the worst mess in the world. God human bodies are such garbage bags.[14]

There is no sense here that the corpse is in any way connected with humanity. It is a thing to be mutilated. It is the 'worst mess in the world'. This inhuman atmosphere is heightened by the lack of communication between Dennis and the other murderers, just grunting at each other, swearing and making phatic observations.

The potential for establishing an interpretative response to this piece in economic terms is not immediately apparent. Traces of the economic sphere can, however, be observed in this section's complete objectification of the body. The language of transforming living matter into dead echoes Marx's interpretation of commodity fetishism as a kind of metaphorical death. It is possible to strengthen this position by considering the way *Frisk* makes connections between the murders and coprophilia. The letter describes, for example, a section that includes the following dialogue between Dennis and the punk kid he is murdering. Cooper writes:

> I'd never wanted to eat someone's shit before, but I was starved for the punk's. I asked him if it had been eaten before. He mumbled, No, let me go. I asked him if he'd like me to eat it. He said, Are you really going to kill me? I said no very casually. Then I repeated my question. He said he didn't know what I meant. I said if he'd shit in my mouth we'd let him go. He said okay.[15]

This piece establishes links between commodification, excrement and murder, links that can be interpreted by considering Norman O. Brown's discussion of 'filthy lucre' in *Life Against Death*. Brown states that 'Money is inorganic dead matter which has been made alien by inheriting the magic power which infantile narcissism attributes to the excremental product.'[16] The relationship established here between excrement and money is a relationship that is reflected in *Frisk*'s description of Dennis's bargain with the punk. Dennis, employing a system of exchange that uses excrement instead of money, encourages the punk to try and buy his freedom with his 'filthy lucre'. This commercial proposition commodifies the punk's body and simultaneously devalues it by pricing it in excremental terms. The important point is that this devaluation takes place on both metaphorical and literal levels as the body is simultaneously subjected to the abstract mortifications of the reifying process and the real mortifications of violent death. The casual brutality described in *Frisk* is thus linked to this dehumanizing transaction, a transaction that generates 'dead matter' in economic terms (the commodity), in psychological terms (excrement) and in real terms (murder).

It is possible to strengthen this sense of the relevance of Brown's ideas by considering the way his argument develops into a reflection on what he identifies as the fundamental human need to produce objects that are both 'alien' and 'dead'. Brown writes:

> Excrement is the dead life of the body, and as long as humanity prefers a dead life to living, so long is humanity committed to treating as excrement, not only its own body, but the surrounding world of objects, reducing all to dead matter and inorganic magnitudes.[17]

Brown's understanding of humanity's commitment to treat 'as excrement...the surrounding world of objects' gestures towards a connection between his position and Marx's interpretation of commodification's objectifying impact. The problem with this relationship is that Brown's work is resolutely ahistorical. His argument reads the

human tendency to reduce everything to 'dead life' along essentialist lines and suggests that there is 'something in the structure of the human animal which compels
him to produce superfluously'.[18] The ahistoricism of Brown's stance can, however, be
broken down by putting a historical slant on his attempt to locate history's meaning
in individual psychology. Brown's suggestion that surplus is produced in response to
a fundamental human impulse is thus projected onto a historical axis and reinterpreted
as a manifestation of the intrinsically overproductive character of capitalism. The his-
toricization of this thesis creates an opportunity to develop these ideas on death, excrement and the body into a wider reflection on the dehumanizing and objectifying
forces of commodification. This approach enables *Frisk*'s representation of coprophilia
and the violence to be viewed in a way that illuminates the increasingly dehumanizing conditions generated by the intensified levels of commodification in late capitalism.
The parallels between Brown's argument and the imagistic scheme employed by
Cooper prompt a recognition of the economic dimension in *Frisk* and thus provide
a framework for interpreting the text's repeated emphasis on scenes that involve the
transformation of living matter into dead. Look, for example, at the following section
in which one of Cooper's characters visits a doctor's office.

> The most interesting thing inside the office were charts showing human
> anatomy, one male, one female. Covering most of the wall, they showed
> life-size, young-looking people whose flesh had been peeled off at
> various points. The purplish stuff inside the wounds made Joe think of a
> pair of pyjamas he'd worn when he was seven or eight.[19]

The important thing here is the way the reflections on the colour of the inside of the
human body turn into a recollection of an object. The pyjamas are indistinguishable
from the image of human tissue and the whole structure of the character's response
to the body involves a kind of reification.

The opportunities for reading *Frisk*'s treatment of the body in these economic
terms can be extended by examining the text in a more straightforward way and
looking at its content. The commercial focus in *Beauty*'s descriptions of cosmetic
surgery is mirrored in *Frisk*'s representation of pornography and prostitution. In *Frisk*,
as in *Beauty*, the æsthetic illusion of the commercialised body is both the economic
value of that body and an actual corporeal attribute. Once again evaluations of the
body's physical appearance and assessments of its beauty are seen to lock the human
frame into commercial relationships. In porn acting the beauty of the body determines the value of the performer. In a similar way, the æsthetics of the body
determine the value of the prostitute. Porn and prostitution are not, of course, new
types of commercialisation and it is difficult to argue that they, in themselves, represent the intensification of capital identified by Jameson and Mandel. What is
important in *Frisk* is, however, the way these professions dominate. Everybody sells
their body in this accelerated flesh-market.

This reading of the violent imagery in *Frisk* must be tempered by an appreciation
of the fact that the murders described are in fact nothing more than the product of
Dennis's fantasies. The letter is a fiction and nobody really gets hurt. Even the 'snuff'

photograph that has such a significant effect on Dennis's imagination is shown to be a fake. In this respect *Frisk* appears to be a novel that gestures towards familiar post-modern concerns about the ontological status of fiction. The material perspective of this paper seems to be at odds with a text that is apparently so intent on interrogating the whole problem of materiality and representation. This is the line Elizabeth Young takes in her essay 'Death in Disneyland: the work of Dennis Cooper'. Young suggests:

> Cooper's central concern is something that has obsessed postmodern theorists. Faced with a seamlessly hyperreal society, apparently in-vulnerable to negation or political change, theorists have struggled to articulate a 'real' that escapes representation.[20]

Young's Baudrillardian reading locates Cooper's work within the æsthetic flux of postmodern writing and implicitly rejects interpretations grounded on material concerns. The fundamental problem with Young's approach is, however, that it is unable to step outside the boundaries of postmodern thought and remains caught up in exactly the kind of hyperreality she describes. Cooper is condemned to replicate Baudrillard in a way that leaves Baudrillard's postmodern pronouncements un-challenged and traps *Frisk* in a cyclical logic in which fiction can only reflect on a 'seamlessly hyperreal' world. A materialist reading of these fantasies, on the other hand, breaks down this sense of the hyperreal and allows *Frisk* to be engaged in terms that interpret the social significance of its fantasies. It is possible to strengthen this position by considering the way Cooper's text, in its combination of the brutal and the banal, seems to invite reflection on the meaning of those relationships. The glossy character of *Frisk*'s style, a style that enables Cooper to move so smoothly between the horrific and the mundane, appears to articulate a range of specific anxieties about the meaning of violence and the status of the body. The text's superficial and blank response to corporeality compels the reader to reflect on these conditions and encourages a search for elements that have been displace in the narrative's attempt to appear empty. The effort to trivialize and debase the human body becomes, when viewed in this way, an approach that almost insists *Frisk* be interpreted in terms that reject those trivializing processes. Cooper's method loads the body with significance and legitimates perspectives that read the body as a site in which the impact of wider forces, and particularly wider material forces, are registered.

This reading of *Frisk*'s representations of bodily violence is thus located within a framework of ideas derived from the analysis of commodification in late capitalism. *Frisk*, like *Beauty*, employs its images of the brutalized body to reflect on wider forces of dehumanization. The reading proposed here translates the mundane violence of Cooper's and D'Amato's texts onto an axis that measures these descriptions against an interpretation of the casual cruelties of the everyday economy. This assessment of the gratuitous blood-letting portrayed in *Beauty* and *Frisk* is an assessment that gestures towards the possibility of establishing a wider understanding of modern American narrative's general preoccupation with brutality, an understanding that sees in this preoccupation a reflection of the complex relationships that have developed between commodification, violence and the body.

Notes

1.   These definitions are taken from Douglas Coupland, *Generation X* (London: Abacus, 1992); Robert Siegle, *Suburban Ambush: Downtown Writing and the Fiction of Insurgency* (Baltimore: Johns Hopkins University Press, 1989); and Elizabeth Young and Graeme Caveney, *Shopping in Space: Essays on American 'Blank Generation' Fiction* (London: Serpent's Tail, 1992), pp. v–vi.

2.   *High Risk 2, Writings on Sex, Death and Subversion* (ed. Amy Scholder and Ira Silverberg; London: Serpent's Tail, 1994).

3.   Dennis Cooper, *Frisk* (London: Serpent's Tail, 1991); Brian D'Amato, *Beauty* (London: Grafton, 1993).

4.   *Beauty*, p. 307.

5.   Karl Marx, *Capital* (trans. Ben Fowkes; London: Penguin Books, 1976), I, p. 164.

6.   Ernst Mandel, *Late Capitalism* (trans. Joris de Bres; London: Verso, 1978), p. 267.

7.   Fredric Jameson, *Postmodernism, or, The Cultural Logic of Late Capitalism* (London: Verso, 1991), p. 36.

8.   *Beauty*, p. 279.

9.   W.F. Haug, *Critique of Commodity Æsthetics: Appearance, Sexuality and Advertising in Capitalist Society* (trans. Robert Bock; London: Polity Press, 1973), p. 17.

10.   *Critique of Commodity Æsthetics*, p. 44.

11.   Rachel Bowlby, *Just Looking: Consumer Culture in Dreiser, Gissing and Zola* (London: Methuen, 1985), p. 26.

12.   Donna Haraway, 'A Cyborg Manifesto: Science, Technology and Socialist Feminism in the Late Twentieth Century', in *Simians, Cyborgs and Women: the Reinvention of Nature* (ed. Donna Haraway; London: Free Association Books, 1991). This paper was first published as 'A Cyborg Manifesto: Science, Technology and Socialist Feminism in the 1980s', *Socialist Review* 80 (1985).

13.   Judith Butler, *Bodies that Matter: On the Discursive Limits of 'Sex'* (London: Routledge, 1993), p. 67.

14.   *Frisk*, p. 106.

15.   *Frisk*, p. 99.

16.   Norman O. Brown, *Life Against Death* (2nd edn; Middletown, CT: Wesleyan University Press, 1985), p. 279.

17.   *Life Against Death*, p. 295.

18.   *Life Against Death*, p. 256.

19.   *Frisk*, p. 51.

20.   Elizabeth Young, 'Death in Disneyland: the Work of Dennis Cooper', in Young and Caveney, *Shopping in Space*, p. 260.

Richard Canning

TALES OF THE BODY?:
PROBLEMS IN MAUPIN'S PERFORMATIVE UTOPIA

This essay is more about the search for a body, or bodies, in the first three volumes of Armistead Maupin's *Tales of the City* series than a rumination on the status of the body within the text.[1] Much of it comprises an attempt to establish why I think readers of Maupin should be looking for textual bodies in the first place; bodies which, in the end, largely do not materialize. I engage with a number of theoretical positions, some of which (those concerning gender, sexuality and identity) seem transparently to impact upon notions of the 'body'; others of which—theories of reader-response and narratology—may only do so indirectly, or by analogy. If I risk marginalizing—until the last few pages—those same bodies I seek to draw attention to, it is because I am more interested in bringing together three apparently distinct matters: the way(s) in which Maupin's *Tales* seek to be read; the constitution—imagined and actual—of their readership; and the presentation of identity in and beyond the body within these volumes.

There is a further logic at work here, however circuitous, for it is precisely the absence of a sense of bodiliness in Maupin's characterizations which interests me—a striking absence given, as I shall argue, that protagonists in the *Tales* behave performatively, rather than according to fixed or essential notions of identity. This performativity would surely remain conditional upon a performing *body*; yet Maupin's characters repeatedly fail to perform in ways which might indicate an identity. I am thinking here especially of sexual identities and performances, and in particular of the remarkable sexual unperformativeness of the chief gay character, Michael.

I have concentrated on *Tales, More Tales* and *Further Tales* as Maupin's later volumes respond and correspond to very different circumstances. Werner J. Einstadter and Karen P. Sinclair have noted the tonal difference between the first trilogy and the second—*Babycakes, Significant Others* and *Sure of You*, describing it as the replacement of the 'whimsicality of the seventies' by the 'severity of the eighties'.[2] Maupin himself has acknowledged the significance of abandoning his initial farcical plot structure for *Babycakes* in the light of the emerging epidemic.[3] In part, my arguments rest on Maupin's engagement with his readership as the *Tales* were serialized daily in the *San Francisco Chronicle*. This relationship was destabilized by the political partisanship he felt was a necessary response to AIDS; indeed, the last volume, *Sure of You*, was not serialized at all.[4] Plots slacken, subplots wither, and the characteristic tone of levity proves increasingly hard to sustain.

Adam Mars-Jones has associated the abruptness of this rupture with the undermining of both the *Tales'* formal and ideological foundations by AIDS:

> AIDS attacked the central principle of soap opera, the democracy of problems, the approximate interchangeability of crises. What could conceivably act as a counterweight to a virus that was not only fatal in its operations, but apparently discriminatory in its targets?[5]

Maupin's *Tales* had indeed established such a kind of pluralist democracy, in the inter-actions of the members of Mrs. Madrigal's household in Barbary Lane, with their assortment of genders and sexualities. Elsewhere, Mars-Jones has compared the effect of the syndrome on fiction to that on lives: in both, 'a story [is] interrupted by a foot-note that grows to book length, the text never resuming'.[6] This comment captures the trajectory of the later *Tales*: after the planned comic plot of *Babycakes* is discarded, the series is quickly dominated by a darker tone. Likewise, the pluralist ethos of the earlier *Tales* cannot survive the sharper political division between conservative and liberal creeds in eighties America—over gay and other issues. For from the outset, Maupin's deference to his readership, manifest in the *Tales'* serialization in mainstream newspapers, involved not simply a reflection of their individual situations, but equally a fiction, a dream, a political project: to illustrate that gay and straight, male, female, and transsexual, white and black characters could get along.

This is an act of authorial performance. Indeed, the serialization of the *Tales* justifies comparison to the nineteenth century serial novel, which, according to Katherine Tillotson, restored 'the original context of performance' to storytelling.[7] Maupin has confessed to a love of public readings, where he 'feels like an entertainer'.[8] Likewise, he has attributed the accidental discovery of his prose style to him being 'extremely conscious of trying to hold [the reader's] attention, and that meant suspense and humor—laughs—all done in a very terse way'; to Maupin, 'the cardinal sin of writing is to alienate the reader'.[9]

The requirement not to alienate any part of the daily audience of his first fiction had tangible consequences. The sustained model of liberal pluralist values—Barbary Lane—resulted from Maupin's awareness of the social diversity of his readers: 'the strength of *Tales of the City* was, from the very beginning…that it included everyone in this large canvas, so that all of us, gay and straight, could see our lives reflected in some way' (Maupin: 1993). Yet this statement simultaneously reveals just how Maupin broke his universal readership down into two constituencies from the start: 'gay' and 'straight'; labels to which we might usefully append, respectively, 'marginal–subcultural' and 'dominant–mainstream'. The *Tales* distinguish themselves immediately from novels like Andrew Holleran's *Dancer from the Dance* or Larry Kramer's *Faggots*: peer works directed not only at a gay readership, but at knowing readers from a particular gay subculture.[10] Maupin's account of gay life is comparably authentic, but its presentation is complicated by his envisaged audience.

Seen historically, the attempt at offering a pluralistic 'reflect[ion]' draws on a novelistic tradition of incorporating homosexual characters in mixed communities which predates gay emancipatory thinking: James Baldwin's *Another Country*; Iris

Murdoch's *The Bell*, for example.[11] Yet it differs from such works in two ways. First, Maupin's depiction of gay characters operates within the context of a wider gay sub-culture, however problematically this hinterland is presented. The *Tales* are set in San Francisco, not in Cleveland (Mary Ann's hometown). It is Maupin's straight characters who suffer isolation, struggle to form friendships and build a sense of belonging, of community. The boot of cultural norms is on the other foot: Mary Ann admits to finding the number of gay men 'terribly depressing',[12] Brian fails to convince a girl at the mixed baths that he isn't gay,[13] and Mona despairs of ever finding an attractive straight man in the city.[14] Venetia, a character in Philip Lloyd-Bostock's *The Centre of the Labyrinth*, similarly asks herself on arriving in San Francisco: 'Had she really come to live in a city where heterosexuals wore badges saying, "Hi! I'm straight"?'[15] Gay characters, far from being marginal, troubled, or deviant, occupy a privileged, centre-stage position. As Einstadter and Sinclair put it, 'while he clearly accepts sexual diversity, Maupin nevertheless situates gayness on the higher moral ground. Such basic qualities as loyalty, trust, friendship and humility are all practised in nobler fashion by the gay protagonists'.[16]

Nevertheless—and this is the second contrast—it is not so much that gay is being played off against straight, as that the overtly liberal ethos of Barbary Lane is being contrasted with conservative, religious or small-town elements of mainstream American culture and society—which Maupin has elsewhere described as 'still held tight in the grip of our Calvinist roots…[W]e're a fundamentalist nation'.[17] Mars-Jones has said that

> To gay readers these books offered an extraordinary experience, of having their difference neither denied nor insisted on, but dissolved for the duration—far less of an existential branding in this jaunty utopia than, say, coming from Cleveland.[18]

Maupin's *Tales* begin by addressing 'all of us', then, but according to a dual, both–and model of who 'we' Americans are: principally, both gay and straight. Though Mrs. Madrigal's radical libertarianism might purport to encompass other sexual identities— 'Dear…I have no objection to anything', she says ambiguously of Mary Ann's enquiry about living with pets—and Maupin introduces the pædophile Norman in *Tales* (though promptly kills him off), the protagonists who endure divide cleanly according to their sexualities. Mary Ann and Brian pair off as straights; Michael and Jon (later, Thack) as gay men. Bisexuality is consigned to a marginal comment by Michael on 'switch hitters' and to the figure of Beauchamp Day, whose duplicity seems insep-arable from his sexuality (and vice-versa), and who is killed off in *More Tales*.[19] One further caution is necessary when thinking of Maupin's utopia as poly-sexual: arguably, he signals his reluctance to incorporate a lesbian sensibility or experience within Barbary Lane by consigning Mona's relationship with a woman to the *Tales*' prehistory (having tried it, she declares herself 'a lousy dyke'[20]). She then decamps, bound for an unconsummated convenience marriage and life among the English nobility. The DeDe–D'Orothea relationship does develop through the series—but, significantly, outside the parameters of Barbary Lane. Women come to occupy a less-explored, and increasingly less sympathetically drawn, corner of heterosexuality.

Maupin's conditioning of narrative in accordance with his conception of a dual readership relates well to recent comments on narrativity by Wayne Booth and Wolfgang Iser Booth, asserting the influence of authorial ideals of readership upon fiction, quotes Saul Bellow:

> The writer cannot be sure that his million [readers] will view the matter as he does. He therefore tries to define an audience. By assuming what it is that all men ought to be able to understand and agree upon, he creates a kind of humanity.[21]

Booth concluded that, in writing, an author necessarily has in mind an 'implied reader', against which (s)he puts forward an 'implied author': 'one that his most intelligent and perceptive readers can admire'.[22] Consequently, 'the most successful reading is one in which the created selves, author and reader, can find complete agreement'.[23] Maupin's problem, by analogy, in portraying the mixed community of Barbary Lane, lies in persuading the decidedly less integrated gay and straight readerships of the *Tales* not merely of its credibility, but of their placing in relation to it: what consent may be inferred from their reading?

It becomes more useful to invoke Wolfgang Iser's modification of Booth's over-rigid model. To Iser, readers do not straightforwardly adopt a role 'implied' in the structure of fictional texts. Rather, a tension is set up between text and reader; between 'the role offered by the text and the reader's own disposition'.[24] Reading and writing are not simple collaborative acts; they form an 'asymmetr[ical]' or uneven exchange.[25] The reader's role—filling in 'the blanks and negations arising out of the text'[26]—remains of a different order to that of writing. As J.V.M. Lotman puts it, 'the tendency to complicate the characters is the author's; the contrastive black-white structure is the reader's'.[27] Still, Maupin's creation of a fictional world predicates the *range* of interpretative choices, rather as sociologist Pierre Bourdieu's paradigm of the 'habitus' does of an individual's range of behavioral choice.[28] From this range a reader produces one—or several—undefinitive reading(s).

The linkage of reading- and writing-strategies assumes a correlation not only between these acts or performances, but equally between an author's construction of character and his or her conceptualization of (a) readership(s). Readers engage with and project themselves into the fictional world in such a way that W. J. Harvey's comments on characters apply just as much to readers:

> The character moves in the full depth of his conditional freedom; he is what he is but he might have been otherwise. Indeed the novel does not merely allow for this liberty of speculation; sometimes it encourages it to the extent that our sense of conditional freedom…becomes one of the ordering structural principles of the entire work.[29]

The reader's own habitus—manifest in his or her deportment; what Bourdieu terms the 'hexis', 'embodied, turned into a permanent disposition…of *feeling* and *thinking*'[30]—is brought to bear on a reading of characters themselves sited in a distinct, if fictional, habitus. Iser improves on Booth's simple model by pointing out the difficulty of extricating starting positions—what we might, for argument's sake, consider essences—in this symbiotic exchange. He emphasizes instead the 'game going on between author and reader': 'I am not sure to what extent one could separate the image of an implied author from the part that each plays in the game'.[31] This 'game' coerces the reader into pleasurable self-questioning, as:

> For the duration of the performance we are both ourselves and someone else. Staging oneself as someone else is a source of æsthetic pleasure…The need for such a staging arises out of man's decentred position: we are, but do not have ourselves…Wanting to have what we are, that is, to step outside of ourselves in order to grasp our own identity, would entail having final assurances as to our origins, but as these underline what we are, we cannot 'have' them…[L]iterature is not an explanation of origins; it is a staging of the constant deferral of explanation, which makes the origin explode in its multifariousness.[32]

'Staging oneself' by reading fiction then compares to wider manifestations of desiring, of '[w]anting to have what we are'. In his or her subsequent performative behaviour, the reader risks losing sight of his or her origins, so opening up the possibility—and risk—of change. As Wallace Martin has glossed Iser's theory: 'the self that begins reading a book may not be quite the same as the one that finishes it…[T]he reader is a transcendental possibility, not yet realized, that exists and changes only in the process of reading'.[33] It is here that the didactic element in authorship becomes apparent. Every questioning of a text affords, equally, readerly self-questioning: a process precipitated by the suspension of one's real self for an 'implied' self-as-reader, by agreeing to enter into the 'game' of fiction. Maupin, for example, allows for the inclusion of a reader carrying with him or herself the same 'Calvinist' baggage of a conservative family upbringing as Mary Ann, by opening up the world of Barbary Lane through her arrival in it; equally, though, her readjusting perspective as the *Tales* progress dares that same reader to follow suit, or else lose the security of his or her place within their fictional order.

This potential for identity transformation through the game of reading mirrors that inherent in other acts of performance, as Judith Butler argues in her influential book on identity constructions, *Gender Trouble*.[34] This implies that any given identity felt by the reader—of politics, gender, sexuality—to be essential, or fixed, may prove performative, or mutable, 'constituting the identity it is purported to be'[35] rather than reflective of essence. Maupin's *Tales* make play with identity on the same presumption: that such essences are regulatory 'fabrications' which invariably support the Judeo-Christian cultural norm of the family; and—again in Butler's words:

> [R]eality is fabricated as an interior essence…[A]cts and gestures, articulated and enacted desires, create the illusion of an interior and organizing gender core, an illusion discursively maintained for the purposes of the regulation of sexuality within the obligatory frame of reproductive heterosexuality.[36]

Butler argues that sexuality too is constructed and constrained through the 'phantasmatic' paradigm of an essentialized gender, required to sustain 'compulsory heterosexuality'.[37] Undermining this illusion may be possible, not by the adoption of further, apparently oppositional identities, but through gender parody—the parody not of 'original[s]', but 'of the very notion of an original'.[38] Maupin seems to offer just such a parody of gender in transsexual Anna Madrigal, whose hermaphroditic omni-science stems from the fact that she both 'is' woman and 'was' man.

The exposure of all ontologies of identity as fabricated is Butler and Maupin's common purpose. Where the revelation of Madrigal's gender switch undermines the illusion of gender fixity, Brian's experience at the baths undermines the consolations of sexual 'essence'. He is unable to prove the immanence of his heterosexuality to the girl he would seduce; it is not tangible, so she refuses to believe in it.[39] Brian learns that his sexuality can only be proven by being acted out: performed—the very performance, ironically, the girl teasingly refuses him.

Throughout the *Tales*, behaviour offers a surer guide to what people 'are' than the names they adopt for themselves. Maupin asks how one can 'be' anything, if it is not evident in behaviour; in performance. The alternative family of Barbary Lane can be taken as parodic: subverting the claim to naturalness and precedence of the biological family. Maupin's theft of conventional familial rhetoric constitutes an assault on the hegemony of heterosexual values inherent in, and sustained by, the social paradigm of the family. In what sense, the *Tales* ask, do Michael's parents amount to family, when their behaviour contradicts familial ties of loyalty? How could one object to the description of Madrigal's household as family when it *performs* as one?

Butler argues that radical, libertarian politics requires not the proclaiming of identity, but its deconstruction through parody:

> [T]he task here is not to celebrate each and every possibility *qua* possibility, but to redescribe those possibilities that *already* exist, but which exist within cultural domains designated as culturally unintelligible and impossible…Cultural configurations of sex and gender might then proliferate or, rather, their present proliferation might then become articulable within the discourses that establish intelligible cultural life, confounding the very binarism of sex, and exposing its fundamental unnaturalness.[40]

To her, this might more obviously suggest the subversive potential of drag, or butch–femme lesbian roleplaying. Maupin, however, realizes the same project through the introduction of gay characters—and a transsexual—outside of what be a 'culturally intelligible' context: the gay subculture depicted and addressed by gay authors like Kramer and Holleran. Butler might argue that these latter's portrayal of separate, differently-ordered gay lifestyles—in Holleran's case particularly, so consciously contrasted to the familial order of his gay protagonists' origins—was a fruitless 'celebrat[ion]' of this newly-possible hedonism. Maupin, contrastingly, brings *his* gay character Michael well out of the Castro ghetto—and back into a behaviourally recognizable but essentially different family, thus rendering his sexuality 'articulable' to mainstream readers. Madrigal's household works to reveal how fabricated the more commonplace unit of the family is. In Butler's words:

> The replication of heterosexual constructs in non-heterosexual frames brings into relief the utterly constructed status of the so-called hetero-sexual original. Thus, gay is to straight not as copy is to original, but, rather, as copy is to copy. The parodic repetition of 'the original'…reveals the original to be nothing other than a parody of the idea of the natural and the original.[41]

Maupin deploys one particular narrative device to effect precisely the sense of 'gay [being]…as copy is to copy'. Plot twists around and back on itself, the experiences of gay and straight characters anticipating and echoing each other, with the result that the reader is hard pressed to identify which event is 'original', and which 'cop[ies]'. The 'marriages' of Michael to Jon and Brian to Mary Ann offer a good example. Michael finds Jon just after Brian finds Mary Ann. The gay couple make their pledge after Michael's apparently psychosomatic illness—an attack of Guillain-Barre—follows the stress of coming out to his mother.[42] Yet on the opening of *Further Tales* the gay coupling is already over, rewritten as doomed from the beginning. Whereas *More Tales* stressed the continuity and similarity between hetero- and homosexual relationships, *Further Tales*, it seems, will mark Michael's return to gay hedonistic individualism. His time with Jon, he emphasizes, could not be compared to a straight marriage, with its 'nasty heterosexual role-playing'.[43] He tells gay fellow traveller Ned that he had had '[l]ots of buddy nights at the baths. I can't even count the number of times I rolled over in bed and told some hot stranger: "You'd like my lover".'[44] This contradicts his euphoric dismissal of the importance of sex when 'married': 'All his adult life he had searched for someone to do nothing with in bed. And now he had found him, this bright, generous person, whose love was so strong that sex was in perspective again'.[45] Yet no sooner has Michael indulged sexually than he regrets it—renouncing the word 'gay', defending only 'being homosexual', and seeking 'another way to be queer'.[46] Ned quips that Michael is 'gayed out' and 'could become a lesbian';[47] Michael counters that lesbians 'date, for Christ's sake. They write each other bad poetry'.[48]

The stage is now set for the reconciliation of Michael and Jon, the narrative's—and Michael's—account of gay relationships having come full circle. Michael hints at the spiral structure within which his life—and the *Tales*—is structured: 'I run in cycles, I guess…As soon as the moon changes, I want to be married again. I want to sit in a bathrobe and watch *Masterpiece Theatre* with my boyfriend.'[49] Rejecting the sexual objectification which had trapped both himself and straight Brian in *Tales*, Michael now swings toward a desire for domestic contentment which is figured as feminine: it is the natural province of women-loving women; Michael's 'cycles', subject to the moon, invoke menstruation.

Further Tales ends with a recapitulation of the entire plot. Jon returns, reproving Michael for his dedicated, performative sexual indulgence: 'You're not having a life, Michael—you're fucking the Village People, one at a time'.[50] Brian defends Michael against gaybashers and is hospitalized. From his hospital bed, he proclaims his love for Mary Ann and they plan to marry, just as Jon and Michael did at the end of *More Tales*. The symmetry is double-edged, stressing both the mutability of such pledges, and the open chance of a second try, should things fall apart. Mary Ann then urges Michael and Jon to remarry. The final triumph of the artificial family of Barbary Lane over biology—and, arguably, its highpoint over the six novels—occurs, somewhat fantastically, when even Mary Ann declines to invite her own mother to her wedding, preferring 'just family...I mean...my family here'.[51]

Maupin's fiction dares to suggest that the performance of reading itself allows for—reveals, perhaps, to the reader—the possibility that his or her own set of identities or values may have become naturalized by repetition—petrified, perhaps—but are by no means as natural or essential as they appear. The reader's desire for escape-in-fiction implies a preparedness to be decentred, moved from the prescriptiveness of origins (in the terms of the book, where the reader 'is' before opening it). This desire mirrors that which initially draws Maupin's protagonists to San Francisco: I shall now look at how Maupin uses this city as ideal site for his performative utopia.

Maupin's San Francisco, like his novels, is nobody's origin: 'Nobody's *from* here', as Brian informs Mary Ann.[52] Barbary Lane not only facilitates but imposes performative self-examination upon its inhabitants. A Calvinist set of values is contrasted to Madrigal's own liberal pluralism, and then thrown into jeopardy. Maupin challenges the reader's complicity in—or at least identification with—this mainstream culture by analogy with the three characters—Brian, Michael and, most obviously, Mary Ann—who will themselves away from familial origin, and in so doing, initiate the construction of the Barbary Lane utopia. Peter Brooks' theorization of the mechanics of plot can usefully be invoked here. In *Reading for the Plot*, Brooks notes the importance of characters' desire to plot development, terming Balzac's protagonists 'desiring machines', whose 'presence in the text creates and sustains narrative movement through the forward march of desire, projecting the self onto the world through scenarios of desire imagined and then acted upon'.[53] Brooks sees this desire as a necessary deviation from the normative standards of any origin, for:

> Deviance is the very condition for life to be 'narratable': the state of normality is devoid of interest, energy, and the possibility for narration. In between a beginning prior to plot and an end beyond plot, the middle—the plotted text—has been in a state of error: wandering and misinterpretation.[54]

Maupin has similarly admitted to a 'rose-tinted' view of San Francisco as 'a place that lets people find themselves more closely and get in touch with their dreams' (quoted Ellicott). It is through the *Tales*' opening scene, in which Mary Ann wilfully rejects her origins in favour of wandering, deviating, dreaming of another life, that they are rendered narratable—and that the reader is allowed his or her own escape into fictionality. The *Tales* close on Mary Ann's departure—a symmetry Maupin has noted.[55]

His characters sustain plot only insofar as they choose to deviate from conservative familial values. These values seemingly overlap with traditional career aspirations: at the outset, Mary Ann tells her mother she won't be returning to her regular job in Cleveland;[56] her final despatch to New York is precipitated by a reactivated lust for career success (hence, we must qualify Brooks' concept of 'desiring' characters as engines for plot: only certain desires are thus sanctioned in the *Tales*). Mona's biological mother, Betty, 'Made a Living in real estate' and had 'joined the Reagan campaign in Minneapolis', leading Mona to conclude that her real mother must be Anna Madrigal, 'a woman so in tune with creation that even her marijuana plants had names';[57] with typical perversity, Madrigal turns out to 'be' or 'have been' Mona's father. The misery of the career-driven Halcyons in the early *Tales* contrasts with the utopia of Barbary Lane; Maupin has admitted that his real-life heroes all 'have a willingness to put their personal fulfillment on the top of their priorities, above career'.[58]

Mary Ann's rejection of Cleveland—even the name suggests the divisiveness of smalltown values—is inseparable from the assertion of her desire: the need to 'start making my own life' (similar sentiments are found in Michael's coming-out letter).[59] Warned that San Francisco will seduce her out of her own essential self—or, rather, her presumption of herself as essential—Mary Ann symbolically accepts her new performative mobility, in a clear signposting to readers of the demands made on them by the fiction they are entering:

> Her mother began to cry. 'You won't come back. I just know it.'
> 'Mom... please...I will. I promise.'
> 'But you won't be the same!'
> 'No! I hope not.'[60]

San Francisco, nobody's origin, becomes a playground of experimental self-evasion; what Frances FitzGerald in her book of travel journalism *Cities on a Hill* has called 'a kind of laboratory for experimentation with alternate ways to live... This was play; it was at the same time a meditation on the arbitrary nature of gender roles and costumes.'[61] FitzGerald was describing the gay Castro exclusively, however. Herein lies a problem with Maupin's use of San Francisco. It is complicated by the division between his two 'implied' readerships. He is forced to confront the ambiguous status of a city commonly seen not merely as liberal and pluralist—and so gay-friendly— but, equally, as simply gay: as in FitzGerald's article. Maupin's universalism requires that he deny the shift in perception whereby liberal values would become those solely of gay culture: to believe in them, you would (have to) be gay. Accordingly, Barbary Lane includes a gay character, but is not a gay household. It is sited far from the Castro, the nearest thing among America's gay urban enclaves to a gay 'community', according to sociologist Stephen O. Murray;[62] 'a city separated from the outside world' to FitzGerald;[63] 'the gay Mecca' to one gay journalist.[64] Brian, by remaining loyal to West Coast liberalism, prevents this latter's collapse into a gay politics in the later *Tales*; Michael, equally pivotally, and earlier, 'badmouth[s] the ghetto ten times a day',[65] so illustrating that gay life exists beyond and outside Castro separatism.

Like the narrative, however, Michael oscillates—somewhat inconsistently— between asserting the importance of gay identification and renouncing a gay lifestyle which seeks to elevate this difference to a geographically, constituently separate world. In the letter to his parents, Michael emphasizes how the city opened up a liberal, pluralist community beyond gayness: 'Being gay...has shown me the limitless possibilities of living'; 'San Francisco is full of men and women, both straight and gay, who don't consider sexuality in measuring the worth of another human being'.[66] Murray similarly terms the city a 'haven of tolerance'.[67] Still, the heavy stress on its pluralism only underlines the danger of the city's reputation slipping into nothing but homosexual. Brian is told that his search for a straight sexual encounter must mean he is furtively gay.[68] Although Mary Ann's mother associates San Francisco vaguely with 'hippies and mass murderers', her daughter paraphrases this as meaning 'Sodom and Gomorrah'.[69] Similarly, when Philip Lloyd-Bostock's character Venezia calls San Francisco 'the most sexually liberated city in the world', her antagonist Sibylla laments its reputation as 'Babylon by the Bay'.[70] FitzGerald refers to the common belief that the city is built on poor moral as well as geological foundations: '[t]he beginnings of the AIDS crisis had felt like the first tremors of an earthquake'.[71]

The assertion that '[n]obody's *from* here' has a literal and figurative truth, again inseparable from the city's status as a repository for large-scale migration of gay men. This phenomenon dates at the latest from the forties, according to Murray: of a sample of gay men living in the Bay Area, only 4% had been born nearby.[72] Visiting the city has become cultural shorthand for declaring one's gayness, as when David in Gary Glickman's novel *Years from Now* finds himself confronting 'the trick question, the San Francisco test'.[73] An interlocutor asks if David has been to the city as a means of identifying whether he is gay.

Figuratively, San Francisco offers a clear counterpoint to familial ethics; what David Bergman, in his *Gaiety Transfigured*, calls 'the straight myth':

> the belief that homage to the family can only be shown through duplication...in the heterosexual world, the failure to reproduce the family is an attack on the family. Homosexual sex is an act that goes to the etymological root of iconoclasm.[74]

'Nobody's *from* here': San Franciscan pluralism threatens to identify the city not as protecting the values of both mainstream culture and others, but merely as a resting point for these (gay) others; a site outside and beyond the familial order of the rest of America. It becomes a place which, like the gay subculture it supports, cannot bring forth progeny and so has to recruit from outside. The phobic mythologization of gay men as involved in a process of perpetual induction—seduction, even—to ensure the continuation of the subculture is transposed onto the entire city. This prejudice is confronted when Michael refutes his mother's charge that he was 'recruited' into homosexuality in San Francisco.[75]

Patently, unlike ethnic subcultures, gay society cannot achieve stability by replicating the dominant social unit of the family; only *despite* and *away from* it.[76] The importance of Barbary Lane is that it stands as a surrogate family, built on incremental loyalties, not on ties of blood—yet one which nevertheless can accommodate different sexualities and genders. Yet its status as parody is strengthened by its

pluralism, too. This paradigm of the alternative family stands in contrast to the uni-
formity and masculinity of the Castro, 'a world in which there were apparently neither
women nor children', according to Lloyd-Bostock's Jerome.[77]

Maupin is well aware of the danger of slippage in the early *Tales*' inclusion of
gay themes evidently of great interest to him. This, and the context of serialization
in which they appear, explains Michael's almost schizophrenic existence on the edge
of two commonly distinct worlds. It also accounts for the descriptive conservatism of
the novels. For if (homo)sexual identity is performative, it follows that a key manifestation of it must be in its performance and bodily locus: the act of gay sex.
Logically, one would expect to find this performance related in the *Tales*—but this is
something serialization doesn't allow Maupin to do. His singular position—as gay
recounter of gay experience to a gay and straight readership—is thus problematized.
However defining his protagonists' sexuality to their identity; however, critical their
sexual experience, Maupin cannot detail the intricacies of gay sexual difference.

His solution is to revert to a portrayal of gay sexuality as social given—more
essence than performance. Such a portrayal might be glossed as founded in liberal
heterosexuality; based on the 'liberal hope' long identified by Dennis Altman in his
Homosexual: Oppression and Liberation: 'that homosexuals will come to merge
imperceptibly into society as we now know it'.[78] The following two excerpts, from
very different sources, illustrate the parameters within which such representation
invariably operates:

> *Don't dwell too much on the sexual aspects of homosexuality.* Don't peer too
> closely into the bedroom of a Gay son or daughter—you wouldn't with
> a straight child, would you?...If, however, the Gay child insists on
> drawing you unwillingly into personal sexual discussion, you have every
> right to protest: 'Spare me the details—and did you remember to send
> your grandfather a birthday card?'[79]

> 'I'm a healthy, strapping boy again, and Jon and I can...well, never mind
> that part. Plus—oh, miracle of miracles!—my mother sent me a pound
> cake yesterday.'[80]

The first comes from a book of advice to the parents of gays and lesbians; the second,
from the characteristically over-sweet closing episode of *More Tales*. Both offer
portraits of gay men and women conspicuously framed within the family. Both consciously address a heterosexual audience—in the second case, the gay Michael Tolliver,
speaks to the straight and straight-minded reader through her or his fictional substitute,
Mary Ann Singleton. In both cases, the spectre of gay sexual performance is raised—
only to be exorcized, curtailed within the readership's presumed adherence to 'family
values': effectively, to heterosexuality. Gay desire is suspended; reconstituted as a
problematic given.

Nor is this a rare or distant phenomenon. Marlon Riggs, discussing the eroticism
of his film *Tongues Untied* criticized a similar conservative tendency in gay-produced
cinema—to avoid the 'threatening' nature of 'the physicality of our identity', thus
'mak[ing the] work easy for straights to consume by erasing our sexuality as physical

people engaged in physical intimacy'.[81] In this respect, Maupin retreats from a performative characterization of sexual identity. Michael's gayness is accepted—for convenience—as essential or natural.

Michael himself adopts the same tactic—a strategic reversion to essence—in coming out to his mother. His sexuality was 'something I knew, even as a child, was as basic to my nature as the color of my eyes'.[82] The fundamentalist model of heterosexuality as predetermined or inherited and of homosexuality as acquired or learnt is reversed: Michael's journey west allows him to discover the person he always was, and escape an acculturated—so, acquired—set of heterosexual values purporting to comprise essence.

The comparison with Riggs may seem misplaced; the making and watching of gay films have been subject to different conditions to the writing and reading of gay fiction. But the mixed readership of the syndicated *Tales* places Maupin closer to the constraints on—and consequent restraint of—both gay film-makers and pre-emancipatory gay writers than to peer gay novelists. Equally, though, the *Tales* anticipate a retreat from all-gay environments to the context of the family which has characterized much post-AIDS gay literature: novels which 'don't ever talk about sex', in Edmund White's words;[83] plays like Larry Kramer's *The Destiny of Me*, described by the author as 'part AIDS agit-prop, part family drama'.[84] David Bergman considers this to belong to a much more long-standing tendency, arguing that, from the Violet Quill group on, gay novels have failed to offer a new myth of gay living which escapes the 'received heterosexual conception of gay man's fate' as tragic.[85] Bergman feels such a myth might reconcile the two polar contexts of gay fiction— 'the sexual world and the familial world'—and save the gay novel from being (as he believes it now is) 'fractured, divided against itself, without a satisfactory resolution'.

Maupin's *Tales* seemingly support such a reading. His positive rendering of gay characters occurs only within the context of the surrogate Barbary Lane family—as, conversely, the solipsistic lives of Andrew Holleran's protagonists suffuse them with a tragic heroism. Similarly Edmund White has noted that, of the three gay protagonists in Maupin's last novel *Maybe the Moon*, 'the sympathetic gay character is absorbed into a circle of straight friends'.[86] By definition, Maupin's 'family', like the orthodox domesticity these other novels contrast with gay urbanity, restricts Maupin's narrator's ability to examine gay sexuality. He knows that (a part of) his readership would prefer not to consider the detail of gay coupling, just as Michael reads the same disinclination into Mary Ann.

Maupin's alternative family might provide the best chance of Bergman's two worlds being brought together—just as he might have hoped of his two readerships. Though Barbary Lane can be seen as radically performative, subversive along the lines advocated by Butler, Maupin's universalism can just as easily be read as effectively neutering his gay characters. The representation of gay sexuality seems sanitized compared even to morally conservative yet descriptively graphic works such as Larry Kramer's *Faggots* or Fierstein's *Torch Song Trilogy* (though Fierstein's fantastic, conservative construction of a gay family eclipses the sexual daring of early scenes).[87] Maupin's gay characters have states of desire and satiety, separated by strategic chapter endings or '***'s. To some degree, the same evasive closure characterizes heterosexual encounters too. Mary Ann's night of passion with Simon ends before the act, with her 'cup[ping] her hands against the small marble mounds of his ass'.[88] Still, in the morning scene which follows, she 'gave his cock a friendly yank'[89]—a detail unthinkable in Michael's sexual encounters, and one which presages the (hetero)sexual explicitness of the unserialized *Maybe the Moon*.

Torch Song Trilogy offers the most useful contrast, in its evident presumption of a mixed (theatrical and later cinematic) audience. Nicholas de Jongh saw Fierstein's 'aspiration' as assimilationist, to 'emphasise gay affinities with heterosexuals rather than differences'.[90] He projects gay lifestyles within a familiar, familial order as Maupin does: ultimately, his protagonist Arnold 'wishes to homosexualize the heterosexual marriage'.[91] Yet, though Fierstein locates Arnold 'safely' this side of the urban hedonism of his foil character, the absent Murray—just as Maupin does, playing Michael off against Ned—the easy accommodation of a mainstream audience implied by this 'highly conservative theory of gay identity'[92] is at least complicated by the immediate, upfront portrayal of backroom bar culture (even de Jongh admits the piece has 'other, less conservative aspirations'[93]). Arnold penetrates the secrets of the backroom—and is himself penetrated, the shock of which he recounts at length in monologue.[94] On stage the theatricality of the moment is underlined by a gesture toward the play's artificial privileging of its audience: much of the humour rests on Arnold's panic at not being able to see what or who he is doing; the visual humour for the audience residing in the manifestation of this panic in Arnold's well-lit features.

The elision of gay sexual performance in the *Tales* is accompanied by a subtler transposition of gay identity into a succession of iconic material images, kept just as distant from Michael as he strains to keep his parents away from the Castro. When gay icons do figure, they are rendered comically unthreatening, as when the roller-skating gay 'nuns' appear.[95] Overall, the minimizing of gay sexual expression elides Michael's character. It also inevitably accentuates his sexual need in the beforeness of each sexual encounter, and the reason he is drawn to the ghetto in the first place: 'there was a lot to be said for sheer numbers when you were looking for company'.[96] Unlike Holleran or Kramer, Maupin alludes to the farther shores of gay sexuality only nominally—and then to discount their representativeness. Typical is the joke that Michael and Jon had 'an S & M relationship…Streisand and Midler…It was pure, unadulterated hell…We fought all the time'.[97]

Repeatedly any hint of a less pristine subculture is lanced through a comic deflation which invariably also re-feminizes gay desire—as if to reassure the main-stream reader that the newer assertiveness and fashionable masculinity among gays is merely superficial. '[M]urky legends' of homicidal sadists tempt Michael to 'sick with Mary Tyler Moore'.[98] The orgy room 'empties during Mary Hartman'.[99] A trick of Michael's only owns a set of handcuffs because he is a policeman.[100] Michael tells of his disappointment when going home with 'some…male-type…A nice mustache, Levi's, a starched army shirt…strong', only to find his true femininity manifest in the bathroom: 'Face creams and shampoos for days. And on top of the toilet tank they've always got one of those goddamn little pedestals full of colored soap balls!'[101] Ned, personification of the masculinized Castro, knows how to 'stand in a corner at Badlands'—but he can still sew.[102]

Michael himself shrugs off the trappings of gay urban subculture while still occupying its centre. Though he dislikes poppers, he has used them.[103] He prefers country and western to the 'mystic tribal rite' of disco, but the latter 'had simultaneously delighted and intimidated' him.[104] He is euphoric when separated from San Franciscan gay subculture, watching Nevadan '[q]ueers doing cowboy dancing'—men unlike his peers, 'content to shriek for Judy at Carnegie Hall'.[105] Asked to slow dance by an Arizonan, he is astonished to find himself following in the woman's role; 'doing things backwards' in the cause of 'romance'—a quality sacrificed in the physicality of disco.[106]

Michael's delight at being removed from the polarities of '[t]wo prevailing cultures—one very straight, one very gay...[which] had successively denied him this simple pleasure'[107] conceals the fact that Maupin's narrative effectively reappropriates gay desire as feminine, and gay desirability as masculine: a highly conservative construct, and kin to the tragic tales of thwarted gay love in pre-emancipatory novels like *The City and the Pillar*.[108] Though Michael's straight-acting partner is clearly homosexual, his social transgressiveness—in that his masculinity is more than skin-deep, more than playacting or performance—is one to which the San Franciscan gay subculture Michael is doomed to return to can never aspire.

In contrast to the conservative rendering of gay sexuality throughout the *Tales*, Maupin insisted on explicitness in describing the (heterosexual) encounters of his heroine Cadence Roth in *Maybe the Moon*—defending it as (in interviewer Patrick Gale's paraphrase) 'essential if [my] readers were to confront their ignorance and prejudice' towards the undersized.[109] Serialization contextualizes this difference, but it hardly explains the disparity between this later connecting of Cadence's desires with her identity, Maupin 'relish[ing]...the little flickers of distaste' people register on hearing the sex scenes between short and tall protagonists (Gale), and the sexless characterizations of Jeff in the same novel, and of Michael in the *Tales*. Maupin seeks to satisfy both readerships in the latter by encoding gayness according to an æsthetic precedent as old as Wilde: homosexuality as a matter of taste.

How, then, can Maupin's reversion to essence in circumventing gay sexuality, be squared with the presentation of Barbary Lane as a performative family? Perhaps it is only by accepting Bergman's view of gay and familial worlds as oppositional—indeed, narratologically incompatible. The radicalism of Maupin's liberal theft of family rhetoric in describing his performative family involves, simultaneously, a descriptive conservatism in relation to sex and the body. It is sobering in this context to remember that American public service television, widely believed to have scrapped plans for further *Tales* adaptations following complaints by the Right about a single gay kiss, does not see it that way.[110]

Notes

1.   Armistead Maupin, *Tales of the City* (New York: Harper & Row, 1978); *More Tales of the City* (New York: Harper & Row, 1980); *Further Tales of the City* (New York: Harper & Row, 1982); collected in *Tales of the City: Omnibus I* (London: Chatto & Windus, 1989).

Citations from these volumes will refer to page numbers from the Omnibus edition.

2.   Werner J. Einstadter and Karen P. Sinclair, 'Lives on the Boundary: Maupin's Complete *Tales of the City*', *Journal of the History of Sexuality* I, 4 (1991), pp. 682-89; here, p. 686.

3.   Armistead Maupin, 'Introduction' to *Tales of the City: Omnibus II* (London: Chatto & Windus, 1990), pages unnumbered.

4.   *Tales, More Tales, Further Tales* and *Babycakes* were serialized in the *San Francisco Chronicle; Significant Others* in the *San Francisco Examiner*.

5.   Adam Mars-Jones, 'Tweak My Nipple', *London Review of Books*, 25 March 1993, p. 21.

6.   Adam Mars-Jones, 'Introduction' to *Monopolies of Loss* (London: Faber & Faber, 1992), pp. 1-8; here, p. 2.

7.   Katherine Tillotson, *Novels of the Eighteen-Forties* (London: Oxford University Press, 1956), p. 36.

8.   Armistead Maupin, quoted by Susan Ellicott, 'A Life in the Day of', *Sunday Times Magazine,* 7 March 1993, p. 62.

9.   Armistead Maupin, speaking at a public reading, Northgate Hall Lesbian and Gay Centre, Oxford, 4 March 1993.

10.   Andrew Holleran, *Dancer from the Dance* (New York: Morrow, 1978); Larry Kramer, *Faggots* (New York: Random House, 1978).

11.   James Baldwin, *Another Country* (New York: Dell, 1963); Iris Murdoch, *The Bell* (London: Chatto & Windus, 1958).

12.   *Tales*, p. 42.

13.   *Tales*, pp. 97-98.

14.   *Tales*, pp. 76-77.

15.   Philip Lloyd-Bostock, *The Centre of the Labyrinth* (London: Quartet, 1993), p. 140.

16.   Einstadter and Sinclair, 'Lives on the Boundary', p. 685.

17.   Armistead Maupin, quoted by Tina Ogle, 'Frisco Inferno', *Time Out*, 8-15 September. 1993, pp. 16-17; here, p. 16.

18.   Mars-Jones, 'Tweak My Nipple', p. 21.

19.   *Tales*, p. 19, 58.

20.   *Tales*, p. 180.

21.   Saul Bellow, quoted without attribution by Wayne Booth, *The Rhetoric of Fiction* (Chicago: University of Chicago Press, 1961), p. 118.

22.   Booth, *Rhetoric*, p. 395.

23.   Booth, *Rhetoric*, p. 138.

24.   Wolfgang Iser, *The Act of Reading: A Theory of Æsthetic Response* (Baltimore: Johns Hopkins University Press, 1978 [1976]), p. 37.

25.   Iser, *Act of Reading*, p. 169.

26.   Iser, *Act of Reading*, pp. 169-70.

27.   J.V.M. Lotman, *Die Struktur. literarischer Texte* (trans. Rolf-Dietrich Keil; Munich: W Fink, 1972), p. 418; quoted Iser, *Act of Reading*, p. 125.

28.   For Pierre Bourdieu's definition of the 'habitus', see his *Outline of a Theory of Practice* (trans. Richard Nice; Cambridge: Cambridge University Press, 1977 [1972]), p. 72; and *The Logic of Practice* (trans. Richard Nice; Cambridge: Polity, 1990 [1980]), p. 64. On the habitus, see Richard Jenkins, *Pierre Bourdieu* (London: Routledge, 1992), ch. 4: 'Practice, Habitus and Field', pp. 66-102; esp. pp. 74-84.

29.   W. J. Harvey, *Character and the Novel* (London: Chatto & Windus, 1965), p. 147.

30.   Bourdieu, *Outline*, p. 93.

31.   Wolfgang Iser, *Prospecting: From Reader Response to Literary Anthropology* (Baltimore: Johns Hopkins University Press, 1989), p. 63.

32. Iser, *Act of Reading*, pp. 244-45.

33. Wallace Martin, *Recent Theories of Narrative* (Ithaca: Cornell University Press, 1986), p. 162.

34. Judith Butler, *Gender Trouble: Feminism and the Subversion of Identity* (London: Routledge, 1990).

35. Butler, *Gender Trouble*, p. 25.

36. Butler, *Gender Trouble*, p. 136.

35. Butler, *Gender Trouble*, pp. 30, 148.

38. Butler, *Gender Trouble*, p. 138.

39. *Tales*, pp. 97-98.

40. Butler, *Gender Trouble*, pp. 148-49.

41. Butler, *Gender Trouble*, p. 31.

42. *More Tales*, p. 424.

43. *Further Tales*, p. 523.

44. *Further Tales*, p. 523.

45. *More Tales*, pp. 453-54.

46. *Further Tales*, p. 596.

47. *Further Tales*, pp. 597, 596.

48. *Further Tales*, p. 596.

49. *Further Tales*, p. 665.

50. *Further Tales*, p. 726.

51. *Further Tales*, p. 747.

52. *Tales*, p. 46.

53. Peter Brooks, *Reading for the Plot: Design and Intention in Narrative* (Oxford: Clarendon Press, 1984), pp. 39-40.

54. Brooks, *Reading for the Plot*, p. 139.

55. In an interview by Anthony Quinn, 'An Elf-Hero with a Case of the Mauves', *The Independent*, 6 March 1993, p. 31.

56. *Tales*, p. 10.

57. *Tales*, pp. 84, 85.

58. Quoted by James Cary Parkes, 'Moon Talking', *Pink Paper*, 14 March 1993.

59. *Tales*, p. 10.

60. *Tales*, p. 10.

61. Frances FitzGerald, *Cities on a Hill: A Journey through Contemporary American Cultures* (London: Picador, 1987 [New York: Simon & Schuster, 1986]), p. 12.

62. Stephen O. Murray, 'Components of a Gay Community in San Francisco', in *Gay Culture in America* (ed. Gilbert Herdt; Boston: Beacon Press, 1992), pp. 107-46.

63. FitzGerald, *Cities on a Hill*, p. 87.

64. Frank Browning, *The Culture of Desire: Paradox and Perversity in Gay Lives Today* (New York: Crown, 1993), p. 2.

65. *Tales*, p. 85.

66. *More Tales*, pp. 415, 414.

67. Murray, 'Components', p. 128.

68. *Tales*, pp. 97-98.

69. *Tales*, pp. 10-11.

70. Lloyd-Bostock, *Centre of the Labyrinth*, pp. 148, 145.

71. FitzGerald, *Cities on a Hill*, p. 97.

72. Murray, 'Components', p. 125.

73. Gary Glickman, *Years from Now* (London: Heinemann, 1988 [New York: Knopf, 1987]), p. 138.

74.   David Bergman, *Gaiety Transfigured: Gay Self-Representation in American Literature* (Madison–London: University of Wisconsin, 1991), p. 208.

75.   *More Tales*, p. 414.

76.   Browning, *Culture of Desire*, pp. 4–10.

77.   Lloyd-Bostock, *Centre of the Labyrinth*, p. 215.

78.   Dennis Altman, *Homosexual: Oppression and Liberation* (London: Angus & Robertson, 1972 [New York, 1971]), p. 219.

79.   Gloria Guss Back, *Are you Still my Mother? Are you Still my Family?* (New York: Warner Books, 1985), p. 230.

80.   *More Tales*, p. 494.

81.   Quoted by Andrea R. Vaucher, *Muses of Chaos and Ash: AIDS, Artists and Art* (New York: Grove Press, 1993), p. 135.

82.   *More Tales*, p. 414.

83.   Vaucher, *Muses of Chaos and Ash*, p. 125.

84.   Interviewed on 'Arena: Larry Kramer' (BBC2, 5 February 1993).

85.   The Violet Quill was a group of American gay writers including Edmund White and Andrew Holleran which met in the 1970s to discuss ongoing projects. See David Bergman, *The Violet Quill: A Reader* (New York, 1994), p. 196.

86.   Edmund White, 'Larger than life', *Times Literary Supplement* (5 February 1993), p. 19.

87.   Harvey Fierstein, *Torch Song Trilogy* (London: Methuen, 1984 [New York: Gay Presses of New York, 1981]).

88.   Armistead Maupin, *Babycakes* (New York, 1984); references here to *Tales of the City: Omnibus II* (London, 1990); here, p. 194.

89.   *Babycakes*, p. 207.

90.   Nicholas de Jongh, *Not in front of the Audience: Homosexuality on Stage* (London: Routledge, 1992), pp. 171–72.

91.   De Jongh, *Not in front of the Audience*, p. 163.

92.   De Jongh, *Not in front of the Audience*, p. 171.

93.   De Jongh, *Not in front of the Audience*, p. 163.

94.   Fierstein, *Torch Song Trilogy*, pp. 14–16.

95.   *Tales*, p. 187.

96.   *Tales*, p. 85.

97.   *Further Tales*, p. 522.

98.   *Tales*, p. 85.

99.   *Tales*, p. 220.

100.   *Further Tales*, pp. 903–904.

101.   *Tales*, pp. 155–56.

102.   *Further Tales*, p. 597.

103.   *Further Tales*, pp. 643–44.

104.   *Further Tales*, p. 645.

105.   *Further Tales*, p. 644.

106.   *Further Tales*, p. 645.

107.   *Further Tales*, p. 645.

108.   Gore Vidal, *The City and the Pillar* (New York: E.P. Dutton, 1948).

109.   Patrick Gale, 'Writing himself out of the Gold-Plated Cage', *Daily Telegraph Review*, 1 September 1992, p.xii.

110.   The television adaptation of the first *Tales of the City* was directed by Alastair Reid for Channel Four Television (1993); co-funding for this and future series was sought from the American television network PBS.

Science Fiction

Amanda Boulter

Polymorphous Futures:
Octavia E. Butler's *Xenogenesis* Trilogy

Octavia Butler's writing identifies her as a distinctive voice within science fiction. She works within and against the conventions of the genre, drawing upon familiar themes (such as alien contacts, telepathy or immortality) to expose and reconfigure the implicitly sexist and racist assumptions that, until the 1960s, characterized science fiction. Her narratives evoke African legend and African-American history as well as contemporary black (and) feminist politics. From the mid-1970s Butler's novels have consistently featured black women as their protagonists, an assertion of black female identity that has not only challenged the unthinking racism and sexism of the science fiction pulps, but has also highlighted the repetition of a white hegemony within the emerging sub-genre of feminist science fiction.

Throughout the 1970s and 1980s, Butler was the only recognized African-American woman writing in the genre, and her texts resonate with this oppositional perspective. She characterizes herself as a 'black feminist science fiction writer from Southern California', locating her writing within her particular social and historical experience as a black woman in the United States.[1] However, as Adele Newson also observes, Butler generates a 'characteristic ambivalence towards her message' that disturbs didactic or partisan readings of her texts.[2]

Butler's science fiction creates powerful images of black women in a genre in which and from which they have traditionally been marginalized and excluded. Amber, the heroine of Butler's first published novel, *Patternmaster* (1976),[3] is in many ways, as Dorothy Allison points out, prototypical of all of Butler's heroines.[4] She is a powerfully independent woman who has survived abuse because she can not only heal but also kill when necessary. The Patternist series continues to feature such strong, black heroines: Mary in *Mind of My Mind* (1977); Alanna in *Survivor* (1978); and Anyanwu in *Wild Seed* (1980).[5]

Frances Smith Foster argues that the heroines in Butler's Patternist series represent 'a new kind of female character in both science fiction and Afro-American literature'.[6] That Butler's heroines are complex and powerful, however, does not suggest a break with black writing in America, so much as demonstrate the connections between Butler's science fiction and other black, especially women's, writing. Foster's characterization of Butler's protagonists as 'combinations not only of Eve and Madonna, but also of God and Satan' might equally describe Toni Morrison's Sula or Pilate as Butler's Mary or Alanna.[7] Butler has suggested that her characters reflect her experience of radical Black politics in the 1960s which made her wary of absolutist assumptions about the heroism or complicity of previous generations. She argues that the representation of African-American history must acknowledge more complex models of resistance. Describing the experiences of her mother and grandmother who were both 'treated like a non-person; something beneath notice' in white society, she remembers both their absorption of these judgments and their strength in defying them.[8] Butler's texts represent strong and powerful women, but her heroines also show the heroism of expedience and the victory of survival.

Sandra Govan has identified 'difference, adaptability, change and survival' as the thematic threads which weave together Butler's writing in the 1970s, 'as tightly as the first pattern...linked the Patternists'.[9] The concept of change is, for Butler, a defining characteristic of science fiction, and she argues that representing change is 'one of the biggest challenges' she faces as a writer.[10] The novels she published in the 1980s are thematically comparable to the earlier Patternist series in their emphasis upon the exploration of change, but in these later texts the focus is less upon the external transformation of a community or environment than upon the internal trans-formation of the body. Clay's Ark (1984) and the Xenogenesis trilogy (Dawn [1987], Adulthood Rites [1988] and Imago [1989]) all envisage human evolution in terms of a biological transformation mapped out upon and within the body. Only in the l990s, in Parable of the Sower (1993), does Butler's emphasis once again return to the explo-ration of primarily ideological changes in religion, power and social organization.

In Butler's fiction during the 1980s human biology was represented as the catalyst for, rather than the impediment to, social change, a reconceptualization of the body that coincided with the contemporary speculations of popular science. The 1980s witnessed a cultural and scientific optimism about the role of biotechnology in treating 'anti-social' behaviour. Daniel Koshland, the editor of Science magazine, stated in 1989 that the massive project to identify the three billion nucleotides of the human genome promised to reveal the causes of those diseases 'that are at the root of many current societal problems'.[12] As Evelyn Fox Keller notes, such rhetoric identifies alcoholism, manic-depression, schizophrenia, and even homelessness as examples of genetically determined conditions, and these (largely unfounded) statements generate corresponding changes in the general terms of the nature-nurture debate.[13]

For the new genetics 'nature' rather than 'nurture' is the harbinger of change. Human biology promises greater mutability than the depressed and resistant environments of the contemporary West. In the 1970s feminists argued, contra Freud, that biology did not equal destiny, because society and technology could overcome nature. In the 1980s and 1990s, however, scientists are reinstating the primacy of that biological equation to insist that biology is destiny, but that the social and not the natural world is its ultimate programmer.

In Clay's Ark and the Xenogenesis trilogy Butler draws upon cultural speculations about biotechnology to redefine the alien-contact motif. In these texts the encounter between the human and the alien is represented as a genetic symbiosis that disturbs the relationship between 'self' and 'other'. The aliens penetrate the humans' flesh and reconstruct the microscopic codifications of the human genome, altering the pattern of genes which, according to some biotechnologists, define the essence of humanity.[14] In *Clay's Ark* an extra-terrestrial virus invades human cells, mutating them as the alien and human DNAs merge. Infected humans are more alert, faster and stronger than they were before, but the urge to infect others is compulsive as the virus, like the 'selfish gene', seeks its own replication.[15]

The *Xenogenesis* trilogy is a post-holocaust narrative in which the survivors of nuclear World War are rescued or captured by an alien species, the Oankali. The humans are stored in suspended animation for two hundred and fifty years while the Oankali repair and replenish the devastated Earth. When they are 'awakened' they learn that the Oankali are drawn to humans because they are compelled to perform an inter-species gene trade. The Oankali are natural genetic engineers who achieve health, knowledge and sexual pleasure through their manipulation of DNA. They share their skills with humanity, genetically improving human memory, strength and longevity. This generosity however is subtended by a ruthlessness of purpose. They also alter reproductive cells, effecting an involuntary sterilization among humans, to ensure that all future human children will be the product of human-Oankali matings.

For the Oankali, the fusion of biologies and cultures represents a utopian evolution, but for the humans it represents a devastating loss of identity. The humans must adapt to survive, but the nature of their survival transcends their identity as *homo sapiens*. Butler draws out the complexities of power and identification within this alien contact through the character of Lilith, the black heroine of *Dawn*, who, as one of the first to be 'awakened' by the Oankali, learns to live among and love her adoptive Oankali family. The Oankali have three sexes, male, female and Ooloi who form three-parent families. The females gestate children within their bodies, but the embryo is created within the body of the Ooloi who extracts reproductive material from its mates and manipulates it within a special organ called a yashi. When Lilith has adjusted to the Oankali's alienness (they are humanoid but covered in worm like tentacles) she is used by the Oankali to awaken other humans and accustom them to this alien contact. Lilith forms a sustaining and permanent relationship with a young Oankali Ooloi, Nikanj, and yet in spite of her love for it she encourages human resistance and never abandons her desire for escape. She aligns herself with the Oankali, in response to aggressive human behaviour, but these associations remain complex, guilty and always incomplete.

Marketing The Face of Humanity

The third person narrative of *Dawn* is focused upon Lilith's perceptions, so that the reader must identify with her as both the protagonist and the ambassador of humanity. Butler has said in interview that her readership is mainly white, and I would add that her publication by mainstream science fiction presses, such as Warner in the United States, and VGSF in Britain, suggests that this readership is also predominantly male.[16] In other words, Butler's publishing history indicates that her audience approximates the demographic proportions of the general science fiction readership. In interview she attributes her popularity as a writer to her commitment to story-telling and her refusal to be 'too pedagogical or too polemical' in her fiction.[17] Unlike Joanna Russ or Samuel Delany, Butler does not experiment with narrative structures or expectations to continually estrange or challenge the reader. Neither does she write for a specific audience: she divides her readers into three distinct, but inevitably overlapping, categories, 'feminists, science fiction fans, and black readers'.[18] In *Xenogenesis*, Butler uses the comfortable conventions of third person and first person narratives to draw the reader into a series of empathetic relationships with progressively more 'alien' identities. Our perceptions are directed by a black woman in *Dawn*, a black 'construct' male in *Adulthood Rites* and finally a polymorphous, newly gendered (Ooloi) 'construct' in *Imago*.

Butler also explicitly contrasts her fiction to other science fiction narratives which homogenize humanity as a singular identity. Criticizing those science fiction writers who identify the universal (WASP) Man as the essence of humanity, she suggests that:

> many of the same science fiction writers who started us thinking about the possibility of extraterrestrial life did nothing to make us think about here-at-home human variation—women, blacks, Indians, Asians, Hispanics, etc. In science fiction of not too many years ago, such people either did not exist, existed only occasionally as oddities, or existed as stereotypes.[19]

The human characters in the *Xenogenesis* trilogy have been rescued mainly from the Southern Hemisphere, recreating a human community in which the white Euro-American peoples are no longer dominant. Butler's male and female human protagonists are black, Chinese, Hispanic and white.

Butler's explicit critique of white-only science fiction, and her own commitment to representing human diversity is not, however, reflected in the marketing of her texts. The artwork for *Dawn*, especially, indicates the resistance science fiction publishers have had to signifying humanity as black and female. The British VGSF edition portrays a racially ambiguous female face emerging from a ring of tentacles. More remarkably, the jacket illustration for the Warner edition in the US pictures Lilith as, in Donna Haraway's words, 'an ivory white brunette mediating the awakening of an ivory white blond woman'. Haraway adds that this misrepresentation allowed several (presumably white) readers to read *Dawn* 'without noticing either the textual cues indicating that Lilith is black or the multi-racialism pervading *Xenogenesis*'.[20] This refusal to 'see' Lilith as a black woman suggests that these readers worked to produce a narrative that supported their expectations of science fiction as a white genre. Stephanie Smith adds that the representational 'violence' of the artwork for *Dawn* was repeated by Warner's cover for *Imago* (1989) which presented 'the polyphonic, polymorphous Jodahs' (a human Oankali Ooloi) as 'a half-naked Caucasian woman with weird tentacles'.[21]

These marketing strategies echo the editorial advice that Butler was given which suggested that she should avoid including black characters in her texts because 'they change the character of the story'. She reports anecdotally, 'he [the editor] went on to say that well, perhaps you could use an alien instead and get rid of all this messiness and all those people that we don't want to deal with'.[22] The suggested inter-changeability of black people and aliens confounds the problems of identification in *Dawn*. For this (white male) reader–editor, Lilith, as both black and female, might appear to be effectively more estranging and generically unfamiliar than the Oankali. For a black woman reader, however, the complexities of the relationship between Lilith and the aliens might suggest the ways in which black women have themselves been made to figure 'the other of the other' in Western patriarchy.[23] The attempted erasure of the characters' racial identity (and by extension Butler's racial identity) through these editorial and marketing decisions allows white readers to (mis)interpret her texts to reinforce a racialized hegemony that whitifies the genre.

The Body as Text: Defining the Human

Butler records that the stimulus for her trilogy came from Ronald Reagan whose Republican policy of 'limited' or even 'winnable' nuclear war inspired the holocaust that immediately pre-dates the narrative of *Dawn*. She adds that he also focused her conception that humanity was genetically flawed.[24] In *Xenogenesis* the Oankali define this fatal flaw as the 'Human Contradiction' or 'Human Conflict'. Humans are (self-) destructive because their bodies have a 'mismatched pair of genetic characteristics':[25] intelligence and hierarchical behaviour. This dangerous combination is both 'fright-ening and seductive…deadly and compelling'[26] to the Oankali whose desire for diver-sity and difference makes humanity's alienness irresistible, both sexually and scientifically (these impulses are not differentiated by the Oankali as they are by the humans).

   Butler, however, has been criticized for representing 'human nature' in such biologist terms. Hoda Zaki asserts that:

> Butler's unmediated connections between biology and behaviour have an
> implicit corollary: that abandoning the human body is a necessary
> prerequisite for real human alteration. This represents an essentially
> retrogressive view of politics (*i.e.* collective human action), which she
> never sees as offering the solution to social or political problems.[27]

Zaki rightly identifies such biologism as a potential *cul-de-sac* for radical politics. But she demonstrates the dangers of such biological reductivism by means of a similar textual ·reductivism. The narrative essentialism, which draws from biologism and naturalism, is neither consistent nor monolithic, but always ambivalent. As Diana Fuss argues, the representation of essentialism within a text must not in turn be 'essentialized' by critics, but must be read in terms of its narrative motivation.

   The Oankali claim to understand the nature of humanity through their intimate knowledge of living human flesh, but they nevertheless repeatedly misinterpret or wrongly predict human behaviour. Their biological certainty does not 'solve' the mystery of 'human nature' (as indeed some contemporary geneticists claim for their own mapping of human DNA) but rather focuses the problems of definition onto the body, which is positioned as the primary signifier of human identity. The human characters also define their humanity in terms of a genetic integrity, but for them the body does not in and of itself denote humanity. They position the body as the lesser term within a mind–body split, which demands that bodily impulses be regulated by social values. In *Dawn*, the newly awakened humans draw upon the redundant ideologies of twentieth-century America to reconstruct themselves as human in the face of the alien. The Oankali, however, do not recognize such Cartesian dualism. In *Xenogenesis*, the body remains a contested signifier: it represents both a genetic and a cultural 'text' that resists monological interpretations.[29] As living texts the humans are not only 'read' by the Oankali, they are also re-written.

The assertion in *Xenogenesis* that human identity is genetically determined may flirt with a dangerous reductivism, but it also generates dissenting perspectives within the narrative. The Oankali biologism initiates a questioning of the nature of humanity, which is made all the more urgent by the spectre of its permanent biological transformation. The reproduction of hybrid human-Oankali children threatens a potential species extinction that creates an anxiety about just what it means to be human. Is the category 'human' a biological, psychological, cultural or historical identity? When does an individual cease to be human and what do they become? These questions invoke an exploration not only of what lies outside the human (the animal, the machine or the alien) but also of how the identity 'human' can be universalized when it is also criss-crossed by differences of race, gender, sex, sexuality, class, age, nationality, ethnicity, culture, language and so on. How can such cultural diversity be encompassed, as the Oankali suggest, by an homogenous human biology?

In opposition to the Oankali biologism, the surviving humans invoke a naturalist, but equally essentialist, conception of their identity. Defining the difference between themselves and the Oankali as an inviolable opposition, they nevertheless work to suppress differences within, between and among humans that might complicate the binary between the self and the alien. In *Dawn* the struggle for a distinct species identity focuses upon the role and nature of sexuality. The humans insist, at times violently, upon heterosexuality (and the relation between sexual pleasure and reproduction) as a defining characteristic of their nature as a two-sexed species. In contrast, the Oankali sexuality involves three or five partners and is focused upon pleasure not reproduction (which is controlled by the Ooloi). Among the humans, deviation from the heterosexual norm is synonymous with the non-human. The spectre of homosexuality haunts the inter-species group matings and is constructed as potentially more threatening to 'human nature' than the aliens themselves. When sexual differences between the humans are stripped of cultural, geographical or historical specificity aboard the alien ship they are re-invested as signifiers of the truly human.[30]

Alien Births

At the end of *Dawn*, Lilith is destined to be the first human mother of a mixed human-Oankali child. But Lilith has not consented to this pregnancy and experiences it as an invasion of her body. The fragile surfaces that exclude the alien and identify Lilith as human have been violated. Her pregnancy is a literal absorption of the 'other' into the self, so that the child she will give birth to will be both flesh of her flesh and an alien corruption of her humanity.

> She stared down at her own body in horror. 'It's inside me and it isn't human!'...'It will be a thing. A monster...That's what matters. You can't understand, but that is what matters.' Its tentacles knotted. 'The child inside you matters'.[31]

Nikanj insists that only Lilith's words reject this pregnancy and that her body welcomes it. But the final scene creates a disturbing conclusion to this first novel. Lilith is ultimately led back to the Oankali, believing that her own humanity is 'lost'.

Butler anticipates this representation of pregnancy as a bodily invasion in an earlier short story in which she also explored the terms of inter-dependency between humans and aliens. 'Bloodchild' won the Nebula award in 1984 for its complex evocation of dependency and revulsion within a cross-species birth.[32] In the story a group of humans, who have fled persecution on Earth, have settled on an alien planet where they are used by the native Tlic as reproductive hosts for their embryos. The young hero, Gan, loves and is loved by his Tlic who feeds his family her sterile eggs, which are both intoxicating and life-enhancing. As the Tlic ambassador, T'Gator also protects the humans from the demands of other Tlic who wish to breed them purely as incubators for their young. Gan is destined to incubate T'Gator's eggs in his body but on the eve of this implantation he witnesses the horror of this alien birth.

> His body convulsed with the first cut...She found the first grub. It was fat and deep red with his blood—both inside and out...Paler worms oozed to visibility in Lomas's flesh. I closed my eyes. It was worse than finding something dead, rotting, and filled with tiny animal grubs. I had been told all my life that this was a good and necessary thing that Tlic and Terran did together—a kind of birth. I had believed it until now. I knew birth was painful and bloody, no matter what. But this was something else, something worse.[33]

The Tlic birth follows the paradigmatic trajectory of genre horror in which there is first invasion and then resolution. The abject other is first incorporated into the body and then expelled from it as the body is physically cleansed and sutured. In 'Blood-child', the Tlic grubs are parasites within the human body, but they are distinct from it and the boundaries between the human and the alien are re-drawn after the birth. In contrast, Lilith's pregnancy at the conclusion of *Dawn* constitutes a permanent erasure of the boundary between humanity and the alien.

Butler has argued that her exploration of power in 'Bloodchild' has been misinterpreted, causing 'some people [to] assume I'm talking about slavery when what I'm really talking about is symbiosis.'[34] That the relationship between the humans and the aliens has been 'misread' in terms that Butler did not intend, however, demonstrates the ambivalences within these definitions of power. The distinctions between slavery and symbiosis are mapped by the structures of control and interdependency which are in turn subject to the demands of compromise and survival. These complexities refuse reification, and the slippages between and within the structures of power disturb this story, as they also disturb the *Xenogenesis* trilogy.

Lilith's response to her pregnancy echoes the ambivalent feelings of those women slaves whose pregnancies were the result of forced matings or rape, and whose children represented an increase in the white man's property. The potentialities of motherhood were undoubtedly overwhelmed in slavery by the imperatives of white economic imperialism. However, Hortense Spillers has argued that the most significant distortion of black woman's maternity was not primarily economic or sexual but ontological.

> Slavery did not transform the black female into an embodiment of carnality at all, as the myth of the black woman would tend to convince us, nor, alone, the primary receptacle of a highly-rewarding generative act. She became instead the principle point of passage between the human and the non-human world. Her issue became the focus of a cunning difference—visually, psychologically, ontologically—as the route by which the dominant male decided the distinction between humanity and 'other'.[35]

In Butler's science fiction this sexually inflected racism, which positions black women on the borders of the human, is literalized as an alien maternity which is fraught with the progressively unnatural possibilities of the 'other'. *Dawn*'s xenogenesis promises a species diversification that will construct humane beings, related to humanity, but no longer fully human. Lilith's body is figured as the symbol of this transformation which represents the interface between the two species, the place in which the designations of human and alien, kin and other will fuse.

For Lilith however this birth constitutes the loss of her bodily integrity, as her womb becomes the abjectified terrain from which an unhuman child will emerge. Butler uses this alien pregnancy to prise open the rhetoric of racism and turn it upon itself. She represents the pain of the historical marginalization of black women, but reconstructs the fear of racial impurity to engender a truly alien birth as the salvation for an over-specialized species. The structures of slavery subtend this birth, but are inadequate to describe the resonances of this new 'miscegenation', which celebrates diversity as the promise and plenitude of life. If, in the *Xenogenesis* trilogy, Lilith's maternity is constructed within the shadow of the slave mother, it is also cast through the iconography of the Madonna.

Xenogenesis and African-American History

In the second novel in the trilogy, *Adulthood Rites*, Lilith's role as the first mother is both despised by the human resisters, who see her maternity as a confirmation of her species' treachery, and also, albeit implicitly, revered. Tino, Lilith's human lover in *Adulthood Rites*, describes the image of Lilith nursing in quasi-religious terms, 'it made her look saintly. A mother. Very much a mother. And something else'.[36] This supplement, the 'something else', defies traditional binary categories of motherhood, which, however elevated or disdained, cannot accommodate this new maternity. When Tino arrives in the construct village, he believes Lilith to be, 'possessed of the devil, that she had first sold herself, then Humanity', that she was, in her words, 'a second Satan or Satan's wife'.[37] Lilith's borderline humanity is characterized by the resister villagers in biblical terms, and, like her predecessor and namesake, Adam's rebellious first wife, Lilith is an unnatural mother whose gender, sexuality and humanity are challenged not confirmed by her children.

The construction of Lilith as a traitor to her species suggests the ways in which her science-fictional reproduction echoes the predicaments of historical and mythical female figures, such as Malintzin Tenepal, who have been used to signify the treachery of female sexuality. Malintzin Tenepal was the mistress and advisor to the Spanish conqueror of Mexico, and is seen as the mother to the mestizo people. Cherríe Moraga writes that Malintzin is 'slandered as La Chingada, meaning the "fucked one"'... Upon her shoulders rests the full blame for the "bastardization" of the indigenous people of Mexico'.[38] However, unlike Malintzin, Lilith is not despised by her children. The final two novels in the trilogy are related from the perspective of the 'constructs' for whom Lilith is not a species traitor but the mother of a new humane humanity.

Stephanie Smith also identifies Lilith with the 'agonizing space of the *mestiza*' but argues that Butler's text does not re-present this colonial history. She further challenges Donna Haraway, who labels the cross-species reproduction in *Xenogenesis* a 'miscegenation'. Smith argues that this charged naming constitutes a 'termino-logical slippage' that 'not only trails a violent political history in the United States but is also dependent on a eugenicist, genocidal concept of illegitimate matings'.[39] The narrative of *Xenogenesis*, however, does trail the violent history of 'miscegenation' in the United States. Haraway's provocative terminology accurately identifies these texts as both a response to the African heritage in America and as a transcendence of that history in the exploration of a progressive hybridity.[40] 'Miscegenation' is a charged category in the history of black oppression in America, evoking various violations of reproductive freedom and integrity, including rape, incest, forced sterilization, forced pregnancies, lynching and murder, human experi-mentation, and child abuse. But the shadow of these abuses haunts the narrative of *Xenogenesis* in which the Oankali forcibly sterilize humans; clone genetic copies of the survivors (so that the humans no longer 'own' their bodies); force non-consenting humans to accept intimate (sexual) contact; and impregnate Lilith with an unwanted child. The narrative representation of this inter-species reproduction is framed by the context of historical miscegenation, but it does not repeat its values.

When Lilith is told about the Oankali 'trade' she misinterprets its nature by attempting to equate it with humanity's own historical narratives.

> 'You are traders?'
> 'Yes.'
> 'What do you trade?'
> 'Ourselves.'
> 'You mean...each other? Slaves?'

'No. We've never done that.'
'What, then?'
'Ourselves.'
'I don't understand.'[41]

Lilith's misunderstanding not only draws attention to several structural features in the text that have an explicit parallel in slavery, but also represents the ambivalence within their repetition. In *Dawn* the humans are the powerless group, but in *Adulthood Rites* it is the non-human 'construct' protagonist who draws upon the conventions of the slave narrative to describe his life among humans as a story of 'abduction, captivity and conversion'.[42] These redeployments of narrative style and historical analogy confuse simplistic identifications of the powerful and the powerless to describe a 'miscegenation' that distorts, as it repeats, history. Through its ambivalent reworkings of the past, the *Xenogenesis* trilogy presents an extraordinary future.

Samuel Delany's representation of his own writing practice within the science fiction and sword and sorcery genres offers a cogent model for an analysis of Butler's use of history in the *Xenogenesis* trilogy. He describes his work as a textual reconfiguration of his experience as a black gay man in contemporary America:

> I'm talking about the experiential specificity of black life. If we—the black writers—are writing directly about the black situation, we use this experience directly. But if we are writing in a figurative form, as I am most of the time with science fiction or sword-and-sorcery, we have to tease out the structure from the situation, then replace the experimental [sic] terms with new, or sometimes opaque, terms that nevertheless keep the structure visible. The new terms change the value of the structure. Often they'll even change its form. I think the figurative approach is more difficult, but it's the best way to say something *new*.[43]

Butler's *Xenogenesis* trilogy draws upon the structures of African-American experience but redefines the values and the possibilities of these structures for the future. The confrontation with the alien challenges the artificially constructed differences between human and alien, self and other. But in its recognition and repetition of the hybridity of history the narrative also challenges and exposes the differences between and within humanity itself. The transformation of humanity within a symbiotic relationship with the 'other', the 'alien', creates a new future through its constructive remembering of the past. When Lilith interprets the Oankali heritage of multiple divisions and diverse matings as a loss of history, arguing that future generations will 'remember this division as mythology if they remember it at all', she is told that 'memory of a division is passed on biologically'.[44] Adele Newson points out the particular resonance of this somatic memory when read against the African heritage in America. She argues that Lilith's concern 'echoes the history or non-history of the African in America, who was forced to mix genes and robbed of a history'.[45] The new 'miscegenation' between humans and Oankali does not repeat the cultural (or physical) violence of that historical miscegenation but guarantees an historical consciousness by inscribing memory within the flesh.

The relationship between the body and the memory or representation of personal and cultural history is a recurrent theme in the work of many African-American women writers. Butler's representation differs from other depictions of this relationship, however, in that this science-fictional body does not bear its history as a sickness or a scar as, for instance, Alice Walker's Meridian or Toni Morrison's Sethe must. The construct children are physically nourished from the time of their birth by the memory of their multiple parentage. The human-Oankali people have their history inscribed within their DNA and their promise to the future is that they will not, cannot, forget their past.

Butler represents this future transformation in a narrative replete with historical echoes, in which the relationship between the Oankali and the humans evokes the power structures of human slavery, colonization and eugenics. She is neither nostalgic about the heroism of the past nor utopian about the possibilities of rewriting history in the future, but identifies a relationship between present, past and future that is fraught with complexity. In her earlier novel, Kindred (1979), she used the motif of time-travel to explore this complexity and to place her heroine, Dana, in direct confrontation with the reality of historical slavery.[46] The use of this motif meant that Kindred, of all Butler's novels, was not given the label 'science fiction'. Butler was forced to publish the book as mainstream fiction and did not receive the publicity she had expected Kindred to generate within the science fiction world.[47] Although not classified as a science fiction device, the narrative strategy which geographically and temporally uprooted Dana to move her from 1970s Los Angeles to nineteenth-century Maryland, paralleled the displacements of slavery itself. Time-travel also features in the Xenogenesis trilogy where the suspended animation pods aboard the alien vessel disrupt the humans' sense of time so that they awaken in a new historical moment.

The sense of temporal distortion in both texts mirrors that of the 'Middle Passage' which transported Africans from their indigenous conceptions of time into Western Christian history. In Dawn the humans are similarly shipped from Earth. Their bodies are chemically marked by individual Oankali Ooloi (who in this way claim the humans as their family) and they are delivered to the 'New World' (which the Oankali have reconstructed from the nuclear wasteland of old Earth, and which they will finally strip to rock when they leave). The humans' journey therefore traces the movement (if not the brutality) of the 'Middle Passage' and reflects the cultural trauma of the transition from 'human' to 'slave'. Hortense Spillers suggests that this historical transition constituted a loss of both spatial and temporal specificity that 'culturally "unmade"' the captives. She argues that:

> those African persons in the 'Middle Passage' were literally suspended in the 'oceanic'…but they were also nowhere at all. Inasmuch as, on any given day, we might imagine, the captive personality did not know where s/he was, we could say that they were the culturally 'unmade', thrown in the midst of a figurative darkness that 'exposed' their destinies to an unknown course.[48]

The cultural 'unmaking' within *Dawn* does not, as slavery did, deny subjectivity to render people as property, but works to transform human identity within the xenogenesis. Butler's narrative retraces the passage of the historical diaspora to describe humanity's deconstruction as a progressive stage in the creation of a hybrid species to whom the brutality and racism that supported historical slavery will be utterly alien.

In *Kindred*, this 'cultural unmaking' draws out the continual fusion of, as well as the distinctions between, the past and the present. Dana is transported through time so that she can save the life of her white, slave-owning ancestor. The genetic and historical relationships between this black woman and this white man, as well as their shared ambivalent expressions of love, power and hatred, demonstrate the complex interconnectedness of gendered and racial experience in the United States. Dana saves Rufus as a child, but kills him as a man when he tries to rape her. Through her time-travel, she experiences a glimpse of an oppositional history of everyday survival which is otherwise submerged beneath the official (mainly white) documentation of slavery. But Dana can never be more than a twentieth-century alien in that past. Missy Dehn Kubitschek identifies the confrontation with history in *Kindred* as paradigmatic of African-American women's writing, which represents a 'tripartite pattern of deciding to excavate history, then accumulating knowledge, and finally reinterpreting it for a forward-looking perspective'.[49]

Butler's *Xenogenesis* trilogy evokes a similar 'tripartite pattern', drawing upon historical narratives and reinterpreting them within a future context. More specifically, the narrative invocations of African-American history present a potentially homeopathic reworking that imbibes the violent structures of the past to create something new.[50] Butler's science fictional translation of contemporary discourses, especially those of genetic and reproductive science and politics, similarly interrogates and teases out the structures of these ideologies, to present them as a modern history which shadows this future 'miscegenation'. However, by situating these terms within the purely organic environment of the Oankali ship, Butler erases the (venture) capitalist orientation of today's decidedly inorganic technology. In this way she might be seen to effect an opposite transformation from the one which Andrew Ross attributes to the cyberpunks of the same period. Rather than making 'the ecosphere becom[e] technosphere' as Ross claims William Gibson does, Butler's trilogy envisages an alternative world in which the technosphere becomes ecosphere.[51]

This is not to suggest that these texts present an environmentalist utopia which denies the hegemony of late capitalism. Butler has disparaged utopias as 'ridiculous', arguing that 'we're not going to have a perfect human society until we get a few perfect humans, and that seems unlikely'.[52] The *Xenogenesis* trilogy biologically constructs 'perfect humans' through a progressive hybridity that values diversity and 'miscegenation' rather than purity and stasis. But the process of this transformation engages in a non-utopian struggle in which the relations of power and powerlessness, consent and coercion, resistance and compromise are all negotiated within the substitute world of the alien ship.

Polymorphous Futures

The final novel in the *Xenogenesis* trilogy, *Imago*, represents a different passage, a metamorphosis from 'construct' to Ooloi that signals the consummation of this new species. *Imago*, unlike the previous novels, is a first person narrative in which Jodahs, the first 'construct' Ooloi, relates its quest for identity and self-knowledge directly to the reader. This textual intimacy invites the reader to identify directly with this new subjectivity, and establishes an empathetic bond with the ultimate 'other'. Like the humans, Jodahs must achieve self-knowledge and self-control to prevent its own destruction. Its polygenetic body has the power to heal or to harm and often injures the things it instinctively desires to touch. Jodahs is a healer who is able to regenerate limbs, change shape, sustain life and give pleasure. This transformative power has been generated by the Oankali manipulation of cancer cells, a human disease which they value as a special gift and a treasured tool.

In *Imago* the progressive alien reconfiguration of the structures of this disease is brought into sharp relief by the human refusal to change. Jodahs's mates, Jesusa and Tomas, are deformed by the growths of malignant cancers that are both disabling and deadly. Their disease is the result of incestuous breeding which marks humanity's desperate desire to conceive 'pure' children, free from the taint of inter-species 'miscegenation'. This destructive over-specialization is contrasted with the multiple mixings of the Oankali heritage. In their celebration of difference and change, the Oankali have found beauty and possibility in the patterns of the tumours. For Lilith cancer is a disease that has killed her foremothers and represents her deadly genetic heritage (a genetic memory within her body). But the Oankali reconstruct this genetic memory, reconfiguring its codes to realise its potential as a source of transformation, empathy and healing.

The Oankali orchestration of the structures of cancer provides a potent metaphor for Butler's writing practice in the *Xenogenesis* trilogy. By drawing from the structures of the American past, in which slavery represents the cancer shadowing the present, Butler transforms the cultural memories of horror and brutality into an exploration of difference and xenophobia. She invokes African-American history, but her representations of these experiences are curative, a homeopathic response to a painful past.

However, Butler's reworking of the past does not constitute a utopian recycling of history that suppresses the dangers or the horrors of the structures it draws from. The short story, 'The Evening and the Morning and the Night' (1987), which is contemporaneous to the *Xenogenesis* trilogy, describes a reconstruction of cancer that has violently inverse effects.[53] The narrative describes Druyea-Gode disease (a condition that Butler has extrapolated from a number of already existing illnesses) which is the tragic side-effect of a miraculous cure for cancer. 'DGD' causes its victims to transform themselves, not through new abilities, but by pulling out their fingers, toes and eyes, and tearing off their skin. The wonder drug, referred to as 'the magic bullet', attacked the cancer cells within the body but, in this offensive, generated new horrors. This allopathic confrontation between the disease and the cure does not attempt to transform the structures of the illness, but simply to obliterate them. In contrast, the Oankali rewriting of cancer, like Butler's rewriting of slavery and miscegenation, acknowledges the complexities of those structures and aims to redirect them rather than erase them, either from the body or the memory.

Fredric Jameson argues that a distinctive feature of science fiction is that it potentially allows narratives to break through to history in a new way, 'achieving a distinctive historical consciousness by way of the future rather than the past; and becoming conscious of our present as the past of some unexpected future, rather than as the future of a heroic national past'.[54] In the *Xenogenesis* trilogy, as Donna Haraway argues, the narrative foregrounds stories of 'captivity and conquest and non-originality' in order to create a 'New World' which has 'a different set of stories attached to it'.[55] These different stories not only reshape history, which is shown to be a polymorphous narrative, but allow for different configurations of the present and the future.

Jodahs's permanent self-fashioning suggests its transcendence of the gendered and racial terms of human 'otherness'. But its performative morphology also locates this dissident identity within an African cultural heritage. Jodahs's shape-shifting talents are evocative of Anyanwu, the immortal, black heroine of Butler's *Wild Seed*, who is based on the Ibo legend of Atagbusi.[56] In this way, the ultimate incarnation of this new humanity reaches through history and myth to promise a polymorphous future.

Notes

1.   Larry McCaffery, 'An Interview with Octavia E. Butler' in *Across the Wounded Galaxies: Interviews with Contemporary American Science Fiction Writers* (ed. Larry McCaffery; Chicago: University of Illinois Press, 1990), pp. 54-70; here p. 54.

2.   Adele Newson, 'Review of Octavia E. Butler's Dawn and Adulthood Rites', *Black American Literature Forum* 23 (1989), pp. 389-396; here p. 389.

3.   Octavia E. Butler, *Patternmaster* (New York: Avon, 1979 [1976]).

4.   Dorothy Allison, 'The Future of Female: Octavia Butler's Mother Lode' in *Reading Black, Reading Feminist* (ed. Henry Louis Gates, Jr; London: Meridian, 1990), pp. 471-78; here p. 472.

5.   Octavia E. Butler, *Mind of my Mind* (London: VGSF, 1991 [1977]); *Survivor* (New York: Doubleday, 1978); *Wild Seed* (London: VGSF, 1990 [1980]).

6.   Frances Smith Foster, 'Octavia Butler's Black Future Fiction', *Extrapolation* 23 (1982), pp. 37-49; here p. 45.

7.   Foster, 'Future Fiction', p. 45.

8.   Frances Beale, 'Black Women and the Science Fiction Genre', *Black Scholar*, March-April 1986, pp. 14-18; here p. 15.

9.   Sandra Y. Govan, 'Connections, Links, and Extended Networks: Patterns in Octavia Butler's Science Fiction', *Black American Literature Forum* 18 (1984), pp. 82-87; here p. 84.

10.   McCaffery, 'Interview', p. 64.

11.   Octavia E. Butler, *Clay's Ark* (New York: Warner, 1984; repr. London: VGSF, 1991); *Adulthood Rites* (New York: Warner, 1988; repr. London: VGSF, 1989); *Imago* (New York: Warner, 1989; repr. London: VGSF, 1990).

12.   Daniel Koshland, 'Sequences and Consequences of the Human Genome', *Science* 146 (1989), p. 189.

13.   Evelyn Fox Keller, 'Nature, Nurture, and the Human Genome Project', in *The Code of Codes: Scientific and Social Issues in the Human Genome Project* (ed. Daniel J. Kevles and LeRoi Hood; Cambridge, MA: Harvard University Press, 1992), pp. 281-99; here pp. 282, 288.

14.   James Watson asserts that, 'the objective [of the Human Genome Project] is, to say the least, heroic…It's to find out what being human is'. Quoted by Pamela Zurer, 'Panel Plots Strategy for Human Genome Studies', *Chemical and Engineering News*, 9 January 1989, p. 5. However, feminist scientists object to this singular interpretation of the human genome, which does not account for human diversity or acknowledge that 'we seem to share ninety-nine percent of our genes with the chimpanzees'. See Keller, 'Nature', p. 297, and Ruth Hubbard, *The Politics of Women's Biology* (New Brunswick, NJ: Rutgers University Press, 1990), p. 83.

15.   This phrase is from Richard Dawkins, *The Selfish Gene* (Oxford: Oxford University Press, 1976) which draws upon economic and well as genetic concepts to promote and naturalize an inherently reductionist model of society. For a critique of this position see Steven Rose, R.C. Lewontin and Leon J. Kamin, *Not In Our Genes: Biology, Ideology and Human Nature* (New York: Pantheon, 1984; repr. Harmondsworth: Penguin, 1990).

16.   Beak, 'Black Women', p. 17.

17.   McCaffery, 'Interview', p. 69.

18.   McCaffery, 'Interview', p. 54.

19.   Quoted by Govan, 'Connections', p. 87.

20.   Donna Haraway, *Primate Visions* (London: Routledge, Chapman & Hall, 1989; repr. London: Verso, 1992), p. 381.

21.   Stephanie Smith, 'Morphing, Materialism, and the Marketing of Xenogenesis', *Genders* 18 (1993), pp. 67-86; here p. 79.

22.   Beale, 'Black Women', p. 18.

23.   Barbara Johnson argues that black women are 'other to the other' in that they are other to both black men and white women who are themselves other to the privileged white male. Quoted by Michele Wallace, *Invisibility Blues: From Pop to Theory* (London: Verso, 1990), p. 227.

24.   McCaffery, 'Interview', p. 67.

25.   *Dawn*, p. 39.

26.   *Rites*, p. 8.

27.   Hoda Zaki, 'Utopia, Dystopia, and Ideology in the Science Fiction of Octavia Butler', *Science Fiction Studies* 17 (1990), pp. 239-51; here p. 242.

28.   Diana Fuss, *Essentially Speaking* (London: Routledge, 1990), p. xi.

29.   The way in which the body is signified as a genetic text in *Xenogenesis* reflects the contemporary discourses about the sequencing of DNA. Hilary Rose argues that because 'one gene…can be made up of a sequence of ten thousand nucleotides stuttering its AACTGCCTATTG along its length…the new genetics mirrors the postmodernist discourse and reduces the complexity of nature to text'. Hilary Rose, *Love, Power and Knowledge: Towards a Feminist Transformation of the Sciences* (Oxford: Polity, 1994), p. 199.

30.   See Amanda Boulter, *Speculative Feminisms: Feminist Theory and Science Fiction* (forthcoming).

31.   *Dawn*, pp. 262-63.

32.   Octavia E. Butler, 'Bloodchild', *Isaac Asimov's Science Fiction Magazine*, June 1984.

33.   'Bloodchild', pp. 45-46.

34. McCaffery, 'Interview', p. 56.

35. Hortense Spillers, 'Interstices: A Small Drama of Words', in *Pleasure and Danger: Exploring Female Sexuality* (ed. Carole S. Vance; London: Routledge & Kegan Paul, 1984; repr. London: Pandora Press, 1992), pp. 73-100; here p. 76.

36. *Rites*, p. 37.

37. *Rites*, p. 48.

38. Cherrie Moraga, 'From a Long Line of Vendidas: Chicanas and Feminism', in *Feminist Studies/Critical Studies* (ed. by Teresa de Lauretis; Indianapolis: Indiana University Press, 1986; repr. London: MacMillan Press, 1988), pp. 173-90; here p. 174.

39. Smith, 'Morphing', p. 75.

40. Haraway, *Primate Visions*, p. 378.

41. *Dawn*, p. 23.

42. *Rites*, p. 226.

43. Larry McCaffery, 'An Interview with Samuel Delany', in *Across the Wounded Galaxies*, p. 76.

44. *Dawn*, pp. 36-37.

45. Newson, 'Review', p. 393.

46. Octavia E. Butler, *Kindred* (New York: Doubleday, 1979; London: The Women's Press, 1988).

47. Beale, 'Black Women', pp. 14-15.

48. Hortense Spillers, 'Mama's Baby, Papa's Maybe: An American Grammar Book', *Diacritics* (Summer 1987), pp. 65-81; here p. 72.

49. Missy Dehn Kubitschek, *Claiming the Heritage: African American Women Novelists and History* (London: University of Mississippi, 1991), p. 51.

50. I am grateful to Michele Aaron and Peter Middleton for discussions about homeopathy and literature.

51. Andrew Ross, *Strange Weather: Culture, Science and Technology in the Age of Limits* (London: Verso, 1991), p. 155.

52. McCaffery, 'Interview', p. 69.

53. Octavia E. Butler, 'The Evening and the Morning and the Night' (Eugene, OR: Pulphouse, 1991) (first published in *Omni*, May 1987).

54. Anders Stephanson, 'Regarding Postmodernism: A Conversation with Fredric Jameson', in *Universal Abandon? The Politics of Postmodernism* (ed. Andrew Ross; Edinburgh: Edinburgh University Press, 1989), pp. 3-30; here p. 18.

55. Constance Penley and Andrew Ross, 'Cyborgs at Large: Interview with Donna Haraway', in *Technoculture* (Oxford, MN: University of Minnesota Press, 1991), pp. 1-20; here p. 16.

56. Butler describes Atagbusi as an Onitsha Ibo woman who was 'a shape-shifter who had spent her whole life helping her people, and when she died, a market gate was dedicated to her and later became a symbol of protection', McCaffery, 'Interview', p. 67.

John Moore

SINGING THE BODY UNELECTRIC:
MAPPING AND MODELLING IN SAMUEL R. DELANY'S *DHALGREN*

Samuel R. Delany's *Dhalgren* (1974) has been characterized as the most ambitious science fiction text ever written and as presenting unparalleled challenges for science fiction readers. Almost nine hundred pages long, containing passages of experimental writing typified by excess, indeterminacy, erasure, and lack of textual closure, *Dhalgren* is neither an easy nor a comfortable read. Nonetheless, Delany remarks in an interview that more copies of this text have been sold in the United States than of Thomas Pynchon's *Gravity's Rainbow*, and this despite the academic cachet attached to the latter.[1] According to the cover on the 1992 Grafton edition, over one million copies have been sold in the USA. This is a formidable achievement for a popular text of such length and complexity, and clearly requires investigation.

In interviews, Delany accounts for the popularity of *Dhalgren* in terms of reader response. The text, he suggests, elicits extreme responses: readers either love or loathe it, and the correlation between these two groups centres 'mainly on discontinuities in the action and the lack of hard-edged explanation for the basic non-normal situation…along with the type of people I choose to write about'.[2] The latter factor is perhaps the most important, as Delany explains:

> …the vast majority of fan letters the book received—many more, by a factor of ten, than any other of my other books have ever gotten—were almost all in terms of: 'This book is about my friends'; 'This book is about people I know'; 'This book is about people nobody else writes of'. These letters came from SF fans and from non-SF fans. For these readers, the technical difficulties of the book, the eccentricity of structure, and the density of style went all but unmentioned. After all, if the book makes any social statement, it's that when society pulls the traditional supports out from under us, we all effectively become, not the proletariat, but the *lumpen* proletariat. It says that the complexity of 'culture' functioning in a gang of delinquents led by some borderline mental case is no less than that functioning at a middle-class dinner party. Well, there are millions of people in this country who have already experienced precisely this social condition, because for one reason or another their supports were actually struck away. For them, *Dhalgren* confirms something they've experienced. It reminds them that what they saw was real and meaningful; and they like that.[3]

For Delany, positive reader response derives from the fact that the text addresses the experience of social dispossession, an experience that remains commonplace for a sizable sector of American society. For readers from this sector, the text's complexities of style are not difficult or problematic, but 'unmentioned', non-significant. The fragmentation and disorientation of the novel's style is accepted as commensurate to rendering the discontinuities of contemporary urban existence. Hence, for this readership, *Dhalgren* is confirmatory and reassuring: it affirms the authenticity and meaningfulness of their experience of alienation and provides a voice for the *déclassé*.

This explanation for the popularity of *Dhalgren* remains inevitably partial. It provides a crucial emphasis on the social context of reception, but neglects to address an issue specific to this particular text: namely, that *Dhalgren* is not a work of realism, but a science fiction. Fan letters recognizing identification between peers and fictional characters might be more understandable in the case of realist texts, but clearly any process of reader identification must operate differently in the case of a science fiction text, particularly given the way Delany conceptualizes the functioning of the genre.

In his critical writings on science fiction, Delany distinguishes between speculative fiction and mundane fiction, maintaining that speculative (or science) fiction is not merely a subgenre of mundane (or mainstream) fiction, but constitutes a discursive order distinct from literary discourse. He indicates that science fiction emerged as a distinct discourse toward the end of the nineteenth century and is characterized by a new way of reading. Science fiction writers, he suggests, write different kinds of sentences from mundane fiction writers, and embed them in contexts in which those sentences become readable. This process generates a new set of codes or protocols which readers must acquire and apply in order to make sense of the science fiction text. As Delany remarks:

> We must think of literature and science fiction not as two different sets of labeled texts, but as two different sets of values, two different ways of response, two different ways of making texts make sense, two different ways of reading—or what one academic tradition would call two different discourses…The encounter, then, is between two discourses, science fiction and literature.[4]

One of the key distinctions between the two discourses remains that, unlike mundane fiction, the language of science fiction enacts a continual defamiliarization of language, a defamiliarization that acts on the reader by opening up spaces for the generation of meaning through techniques such as the literalization of metaphor, thus expanding the range of hermeneutic possibilities.

Given this conceptualization of science fiction, it becomes clear that Delany's explanation of the popularity of *Dhalgren* tells only half the story. Certainly, fans of the novel might recognize aspects of their social condition in the text, but they are also responding to the generic protocols which for Delany determine how sense is made of science fiction. And ultimately they are responding to a writer who avowedly enjoys working within but also challenging the conventions that structure science fiction discourse.

The role of the writer in generating the popularity of a text is a particularly moot point in the case of Delany for a number of reasons. In his critical writings on science fiction, Delany has assumed an overtly poststructuralist stance and remains acutely aware of debates concerning the death of the author. Nevertheless, the issue of the relationship between writer, text and reader remains one to which he often recurs. In his meta-autobiography *The Motion of Light in Water*, for example, Delany contends that 'no simple, sensory narrative can master what it purports', and proceeds to examine the nature of the writer-text-reader relationship:

> That age old philosophical chestnut, the Problem of Representation (in its twin forms, the Problem of Verification and the Problem of Exhaustiveness) makes mastery as such a non-problem, with no need of *haute théorie*. Theodore Sturgeon's fine insight is perhaps germane here: the best writing does not reproduce—or represent—the writer's experience at all. Rather it creates an experience that is entirely the reader's, forged and fashioned wholly from her or his knowledge, of her or his memories, by her or his ideology and sensibility, and demonstrably different for each—but which (according to the writer's skill) is merely as meaningful (though not necessarily meaningful in the same way) as the writer's, merely as vivid.
>
> In short, writing creates not a representation of the writer's world but a model of the writer's purport.
>
> (It creates a representation, in a different form, of the *reader's* world.)
>
> But to model is not to master.
>
> Finally, though, isn't it a question of models that all narrative more or less leads to?[5]

As in Barthes's version of the writerly text, Delany postulates that good writing—characterized as anti-authoritarian because it problematizes referentiality and remains unconcerned with mastery—sets the reader free. Encounters between the reader and the text, encounters in which the reader brings to bear her or his entire sensibility on the text, set the reader free to create a hermeneutic experience that is in key respects her or his alone. But Delany differs from Barthes in insisting on the active role of the writer. Novels are not merely *romans à clef*. Writing does not, indeed cannot, reproduce the writer's experience, but it does model the writer's purport. The writer's experience of the text (or input into it) is as meaningful as a the reader's experience (or output derived from it), but no more so. These experiences may be meaningful in different ways, but there is a parity between them.

Delany's emphasis on reader-writer relations as structured around the issue of a modelling of the writer's purport can be seen as an important factor in accounting for the popularity of *Dhalgren*. In the interview quoted earlier, Delany focusses on reader response to the novel. The other side of this equation can now be recognized as the act of writerly modelling. It is the contention of this paper that reader response to the text is so intense precisely because Delany's writerly modelling is so intense. Delany addresses this issue when explaining his compositional methods and in particular the process of character construction:

> What I try to go through, especially with my major characters, is
> something like this. On the one hand, I want my characters to do things
> that I've done myself; that's so I'll know what it *feels* like to be in their
> situation. On the other hand, I want to have seen at least one other
> person do the same things; I also want to know what it looks like. But
> to try to associate my major characters with me—or with anyone I
> know—is a thankless task.[6]

Rejecting any facile notions regarding the transcription of personal experience into
writing, Delany nonetheless emphasizes the interior and exterior sensory modelling
that informs his textuality. The key term here is sensory: Delany prioritizes the body
and physical participation, and so as a result it is the body and its desires and pleasures
that is inscribed in his texts. This privileging is not unusual in contemporary writing.
What is unusual is that this degree of sensory modelling takes place in the often cere-
bral form of science fiction. Moreover, the fact that Delany engages in this degree of
experiential modelling inevitably determines the kind of science fiction that he
writes and therefore how he defines what he means by science fiction. *Dhalgren* is a
key text in this respect as much of the initial controversy generated by the novel
centred on whether it could or should be classified as science fiction.

The writerly modelling in *Dhalgren* is particularly intense. *The Motion of Light in
Water* provides evidence to support this contention. The autobiography models
episodes from Delany's life-experience which were earlier modelled in *Dhalgren*. A
number of episodes modelled in *The Motion of Light in Water* as coded versions of
Delany's life-experience appear in *Dhalgren* as episodes in the lives of the novel's
major characters. In particular, the meta-autobiography's modelling of the three-way
relationship between Delany, his wife Marilyn Hacker, and their lover, Bob, can be
related to the novel's modelling of a comparable relationship between the Kid, his
girlfriend Lanya, and their lover, Denny.

In light of *The Motion of Light in Water*, then, complex intertextual relations can
be traced between Delany's life-experience in the early 1960s, his 1974 novel, and
his 1988 autobiography. But as Delany maintains in a different context in *The Motion
of Light in Water*, if these accounts are read side by side they will 'obscure, distort, and
contradict one another, producing the aporias that force into conceptual existence
that mental economy which, while it is as much a fiction as any other, alone might
contain them all and which can only be called history'.[7]

The aporia that generates the fiction called history is the subject of *Dhalgren*. In
an essay entitled 'The Column at the Market's Edge', Delany remarks:

> If the experience of the concentration camp—the Jews in Germany, the
> dissidents in Russia, the Japanese Americans in the United States—is the
> experience of the first half of the twentieth century, surely major media
> lies and distortion…is the experience of the second half.[8]

The experience Delany identifies as emblematic of the late twentieth century provides
the context of *Dhalgren*. In the novel, the American city of Bellona—a name

denoting the Hobbesian war of all against all in the capitalist urban space—has undergone an unspecified cataclysm. Social order has collapsed. Buildings randomly burn but are not consumed. A thick haze seals the sky. But perhaps most importantly, media broadcasts cannot leave or enter the city, and as a result the rest of the country agrees to the consensual hallucination that Bellona does not exist. As the Kid remarks:

> Very few suspect the existence of this city. It is as if not only the media but the laws of perspective themselves have redesigned knowledge and perception to pass it by. Rumor says there is practically no power here. Neither television cameras nor on-the-spot broadcasts function: that such a catastrophe as this should be opaque, and therefore dull to the electric nation! It is a city of inner discordances and natural distortions.[9]

The United States is characterized as 'the electric nation', the society of the spectacle. In *Terminal Identity: The Virtual Subject in Postmodern Science Fiction*, Scott Bukatman refers to cyberpunk as the science fiction of the spectacle. For Bukatman, this strand of Eighties science fiction acknowledges its complicity with the society of the spectacle, and hence recognizes and ambivalently accepts the spectacularization of human life. Instead of resisting spectacularization, it recommends seeking empowerment through appropriation of spectacularizing technologies, and in particular a technologization of the body.

In *Dhalgren*, however, the emphasis is somewhat different. The dominance of the society of the spectacle is taken for granted. But Delany focusses on a space which is opaque, impermeable to media penetration and spectacularization, and as a result the spectacle ignores its existence. Such is the power of the spectacle that if Bellona cannot be electronically mediated, then officially it does not exist. Yet within this space that eludes spectacularization and many other conventional structures of social control, power continues to operate. And as power continues, albeit in non-electronic forms, new forms of resistance arise—forms that resist power and spectacularization not by opposing it, but by asserting their otherness, their difference. In Bellona, resistance inheres not in a thorough technologization of the body (as in cyber-punk), but in redefinitions of intersubjectivity through remapping of the body and its pleasures. And the complex textuality of the novel, Delany's redesigning of the corpus of the science fiction text, figuratively embodies this space for the inscription of pleasure.

The city of Bellona is a primary example of what Delany has identified in his critical writings as a paraspace. According to Delany, many science fiction writers 'posit a normal world—a recognizable future—and then an alternate space, sometimes largely mental, but always materially manifested, that sits beside the real world, and in which language is raised to an extraordinarily lyric level'.[10] This alternate space is the paraspace, a rhetorically heightened 'other realm' where language offers an experience of explicit 'otherness'. This space is what Hakim Bey has termed a temporary autonomous zone, a zone for experimentation and the expression of desire that remains relatively free of control structures. But this is a heterotopian space rather than a utopian space, with all the conflicts and contradictions that implies.

At first glance, Bellona seems to be a functioning anarchy, where self-determination and freedom from coercion abound. Early in the novel, the character Tak Loufer, asked why he lives in the city, articulates one of the text's crucial theses on freedom and identity when he replies: 'I think it has to do with—I got a theory now—freedom. You know here...you're free. No laws: to break, or to follow. Do anything you want. Which does funny things to you. Very quickly, surprisingly quickly, you become...exactly who you are.'[11] But anarchy is not a synonym for disorder as Loufer, in dialogue with the Kid, explains when he says:

> 'Oh, we have a pretty complicated social structure: aristocrats, beggars'
> 'Bourgeoisie', I said.
> '—and Bohemians. But we have no economy. The illusion of an ordered social matrix is complete, but it's spitted through on these cross-cultural attelets. It *is* a vulnerable city. It *is* a saprophytic city—It's about the pleasantest place I've ever lived.'[12]

With the collapse of the socioeconomic order, the economic infrastructure that supports the class system has disappeared, but different social groups remain. The relationship *between* these groups has changed, however, as Delany explains in interview when he says of the novel: 'I suppose the central conceit is that what is traditionally socially marginal is replaced at center stage; there's also an economic distortion at work, and a distortion of the landscape, that allows the marginals to take over. All the "decent" people have left the city, leaving only the marginals, who can then go on leading their lives however they want, without the usual exterior pressure. There's still plenty of interior pressure, though.'[13]

The nature of this interior pressure is gradually revealed as the novel proceeds. Its most obvious manifestations occur in the case of the Richards family, a white, patriarchal, petit-bourgeois family unit that continues to live out its now inappropriate routines in the forlorn hope that 'normality' will soon be restored. It is also apparent in the inability by certain characters to countenance the sexual and communal experimentation undertaken by the marginals. But its most sinister manifestation is the figure of Roger Calkins, an elusive Gatsby-like figure who holds numerous exclusive parties in his mansion overlooking Bellona. It is Calkins, ultimately revealed as aspiring to become head of the city-state of Bellona and of its state-approved religion, who attempts to dominate the marginals through 'interior pressure'.

Lacking the resources required for exteriorized social control, Calkins tries to subjugate the marginals by manipulating their definition of reality. He edits, produces and possibly writes the city's only mass communications medium, the *Bellona Times*, a newspaper which acts as a means for establishing hegemonic interpretations of events and thus as a way of imposing his definition of the real. He controls time by publishing the newspaper under random datelines, thus ensuring that all calendrical apparatuses—days, months, years, and even centuries—are under his determination. He, it is implied, also controls space through initiating a sporadic rearrangement of street nameplates. Certainly he holds parties and runs a bar where drinks are free, merely so that his elite guests can enjoy the thrill and spectacle of exotic marginals at play. Everywhere but nowhere—unseen throughout the narrative, only his voice is heard—Calkins represents the diffusion and omnipresence of power that inheres in control structures, in relations of power rather than in the supposedly powerful individual.

The novel foregrounds what might seem initially to constitute the resistance to Calkins: the Scorpions. This multi-ethnic street gang, which the Kid comes through serendipity to 'lead' in an equivocal fashion, with its violence and its sexual and communal experimentation, might appear to pose an alternative and the greatest threat to Calkins's control project. In particular, the apparently transgressive three-way sexual relationship between the Kid (who may be part American Indian), the middle class white woman Lanya, and the lower class white teenage runaway Denny, might seem to challenge the boundaries of race, sexuality, age, and class. But in fact Delany does not code sexuality as subversive. Much of the Scorpions' sexual experimentation incidentally involves the effacement or questioning of power relations, but this is only a by-product of their search for bodily pleasure without boundaries. As Tak Loufer remarks in fully sexualized language, in Bellona, 'You can have your fantasy and...well, besides eating it too, you can also feel just a bit less like you're depriving anyone else of theirs.'[14]

In this radically decentred novel, the perceived threat to control is situated, however, not in the foreground, but in the background of the narrative. The origin of the cataclysm that has struck Bellona remains unclear. One version of events holds that an unspecified catastrophe sparked a riot in the city's black ghetto, during the course of which a black man raped a blonde, blue-eyed white teenage girl. But a close reading of the text indicates that this causal chain could be reversed. The sexual act may have prompted the riot which in turn sparked the catastrophe. But the interpretation of this sexual act needs careful scrutiny. First, because it is this act which makes its supposed perpetrator, George, into an icon in Bellona: posters of his ithyphallic naked form are in wide demand among blacks and whites alike in the city. And second, because it is this act which forms the locus for the inscription of Delany's controversial politics of pleasure.

Significantly, it is Calkins's newspaper that characterizes the sexual act between George and June, the young white woman, as a rape, even printing a photograph of the act with the street riot going on around it. In short, Calkins tries to spectacularize and negativize the event in order—unsuccessfully as it turns out—to defuse its subversive charge. For, as one of Calkins's close associates tells the Kid, Calkins is 'terrified' of George.[15]

George's reading of the sexual act is rather different, and in fact for him the sexual aspect of the act is less significant than the scenario in which it occurred. George admits to Lanya that his source of pleasure is to have sexual relations with women who like to pretend they are being raped. And he maintains June receives similar pleasure from pretending she is being raped. 'Look', George says, 'what it is, is that women wants it exactly just exactly like men do. Only nobody wants to think about that, you know? At least not in the movies. They pretends it don't exist, or they pretends it's something so horrible, making all sorts of death and destruction and needless tragedy and everybody getting killed, that it might just as well not exist—

which is the same thing, you see.' Lanya's reply is significant: 'Yes…I'd noticed. George, people are scared of women doing anything to get what they want, sex or anything else.'[16]

The forces of spectacular control—whether the movies or Calkins's newspaper—deny or negativize the female pursuit of pleasure (sexual or otherwise). Nevertheless, George—aware that June is circling in on him, seeking to repeat their sexual act—maintains that their next erotic encounter will have an apocalyptic effect on the city. Responding to Lanya's claim that like the movies, this characterization negativizes women's pleasure, George asserts: '*That's* the problem—like I say: You see I *like* it like the movies. But when we get together again, we just gonna be doing our thing. *You* all is the ones who gonna be so frightened the city gonna start to fall down around your head.'[17]

George's prophecy of apocalypse eventually comes true, but only after other signs and wonders—signs and wonders denied in Calkins's newspaper—occur. Two moons appear in the sky and the second one is named after George. Later a vast sun rises and covers half the sky, but remains unnamed. An interpretation of these events as symbolic becomes possible when the Kid comments: 'Despite George, and a city consecrated by twin moons, I know there must be some greater, female deity (for whom George is only the consort) a sin yet to name her (as that sun is never named); we have all glimpsed her, sulking in the forest of her knowledge—every tree a tree of that knowledge—and there is nothing but to praise.'[18] Seeking their mutual pleasures, George and (crucially) June become luminous, heavenly bodies. Others code their acts as iconoclastic, as locating a perverse pleasure in the female, as activating deep-seated American myths regarding fears of miscegenation—and for such people the acts of George and June are world-shattering. But the hedonistic couple, the big black man from the ghetto and the petit-bourgeois Aryan teenager, will just be 'doing our thing'. And as the circular structure of the novel indicates, they will keep on doing it. In this affirmation of the body and its pleasures—particularly for women—lies another major source of the text's fascination and popularity.

Notes

1.   Larry McCaffery, *Across the Wounded Galaxies: Interviews with Contemporary American Science Fiction Writers* (Urbana & Chicago: University of Illinois Press, 1990), p. 85.

2.   McCaffery, *Across the Wounded Galaxies*, p. 84.

3.   McCaffery, *Across the Wounded Galaxies*, pp. 84-85.

4.   Samuel R. Delany, *Starboard Wine: More Notes on the Language of Science Fiction* (Pleasantville, NY: Dragon Press, 1984), pp. 87-88.

5.   Samuel R. Delany, *The Motion of Light in Water: East Village Sex and Science Fiction Writing: 1960-1965 with The Column at the Market's Edge* (London: Paladin, 1990), pp. 504-505.

6.   McCaffery, *Across the Wounded Galaxies*, p. 96.

7.   Delany, *The Motion of Light in Water*, pp. 505-506.

8.   Delany, *The Motion of Light in Water*, pp. 559-60.

9.   Samuel R. Delany, *Dhalgren* (London: Grafton, 1992 [1974]), pp. 15-16.

10.   Samuel R. Delany, 'Is Cyberpunk a Good Thing or a Bad Thing?', *Mississippi Review*

47-48 (1988), p. 31.
11.   Delany, *Dhalgren*, p. 23.
12.   Delany, *Dhalgren*, p. 741.
13.   McCaffery, *Across the Wounded Galaxies*, p. 100.
14.   Delany, *Dhalgren*, p. 416.
15.   Delany, *Dhalgren*, p. 538.
16.   Delany, *Dhalgren*, p. 236.
17.   Delany, *Dhalgren*, p. 237. Interestingly, in contrast to George, June insists on the impossibility of her explaining the nature of their sexual conjunction. Her answer to the Kid's question about what happened on that night is: 'You wouldn't understand... if I told you', pp. 218-19.
18.   Delany, *Dhalgren*, p. 767. The quoted sentence contains no full-stop.

Gender

Sue Vice

THE WELL-ROUNDED ANOREXIC TEXT

In this article, I will discuss whether and why textualization and eating disorders, particularly anorexia, should go well together. Is there any link to be made between the various kinds of control (or loss of it) which characterize anorexia, bulimia and compulsive eating, and that which informs the act of writing?[1]

Recently there has been an increase in both representations of eating disorders and theorizations of the link between the body as disordered significatory site, with literary texts. These include work by Mark Anderson, Mary Condé and Maud Ellmann, and join the wider range of cultural and therapeutic studies of eating disorders, by writers such as Susie Orbach, Marilyn Lawrence and Susan Bordo.[2] Even bulimia, which resists representation and is disparaged more than either anorexia or compulsive eating, has featured in Mike Leigh's film *Life is Sweet* (UK 1992) and an episode of the British television series *Inspector Morse*, as well as one of the novels I will discuss. Susan Bordo, in her article 'Reading the Slender Body', convincingly suggests that part of the reason for the increasing awareness of these conditions is that they perfectly replicate, as she puts it, the contemporary 'anxieties of the body politic': the contradictory imperatives to be strictly self-regulating and also to be a large-scale consumer, to partake in excess.[3] Anorexia and obesity are attempted resolutions of the double bind of unrestrained consumption and purging represented by the bulimic, whose 'unstable' position also makes its textual representation unlikely.[4]

The title of this article was inspired by Mark Anderson's article, 'Anorexia and Modernism, or How I Learned to Diet in All Directions', in which he links the sparse, resistant nature of many modernist texts to their depiction of sparse, wasted bodies. More than this, he suggests that the two kinds of minimalism conjure up each other: he says, 'If an ancient trope in Western writing has seen language as a kind of food, or food as a kind of language, modernism confirms their association by negating both'; and that the typical modernist 'textual events' of distance from nineteenth century social reality, the extinction of artistic personality, the perceived disjunction between word and world, are, as he puts it, 'figured' in terms of disgust at food, fasting and wasting away.[5] This is an ingenious way of linking literary history with social reality, and makes the reader wonder if it would be possible, for instance, to redraw the history of women's writing according to the sketch of the changing female body offered by Jean Mitchell, concentrating, perhaps, on the curves of 1950s novels, the emaciation of the 1960s and 1970s, the female Charles Atlas form of the 1980s, and a rarefied cyberpunk textual body, perhaps, in the 1990s.[6]

To return to Anderson's article, there are two issues which seem to fit better the examples of anorexic minimalism which he chooses (these are Kafka, Melville, Beckett, Hofmannsthal, and, in a footnote, Raymond Carver) than the ones I have chosen, which are by contrast all by women and do not conform to the pattern he identifies, of a crisis within language producing a crisis-ridden and dwindling textual body. If anything, in the novels by Mary Gaitskill, Jenefer Shute and Lucy Ellmann which I will discuss, the equation is the other way round: an anorexic or disordered body produces a text which does not reflect an exact image of itself, but one which is either the wrong size or even someone else's. In the case of Shute's novel *Life-size*, an anorexic body casts a large shadow, appropriately reproducing the inability of anorexics to see their own mirror image accurately as thin.[7] Emaciation produces expansiveness. Gaitskill's novel *Two Girls, Fat and Thin* is rather a loose, baggy monster constructed out of sharp, painfully pointed episodes; as the title suggests, this is the textual result of combining the overly large with the small.[8] Ellmann's *Sweet Desserts* is the novel most similar to the ones discussed by Anderson: a short, spare artefact, and one which appears to be representing a compulsively eating and vomiting female body, but ends up actually producing the image of a dead male one instead—or as well.[9]

Anderson does mention this paradox, that the representation of emaciation may actually require expansive verbiage, and describes in one of his chosen texts a language which itself 'remains uncontaminated, offering itself as an artfully prepared and "edible" discourse based on the very images and lush rhetorical periods [the narrator] has supposedly abjured'.[10] However, in Anderson's terms this represents a modernist failure to unite mouth and mind, literal and abstract meaning, while in the novels I am considering, textuality actually represents a way out of the anorexic paradox that 'one is hoist by one's own petard' by it, as a therapist quotes one of her patients saying.[11] The anorexic is entrapped by their own solution to an intolerable problem, which is why the anorexic body is read therapeutically and culturally as presenting two absolutely contradictory meanings: rebellion and failure; egotism and castration. This phenomenon of such a radically ambiguous signifier may be one reason why the textual life surrounding a dwindling or even dying subject is so rich; ambiguity, irony, verbal excess are structural properties of anorexic ambivalence. In anorexic texts, the subject no longer has to to have her cake and not eat it, but can in fact find a way to unite femininity and success, which are otherwise radically divided from each other. By contrast, bulimia as a sign system works rather differently, as the bulimic body does not advertise the presence of a disorder but disguises it; the sufferer's body stays constant, and their social and economic activities may remain unchanged. While anorexia aims for change and movement, bulimia aims for stasis, a clear distinction especially in textual terms: the text may never be written.

Therefore, in opposition to the pattern traced by Anderson, it is not a case of an anorexic text reproducing itself as an anorexic body, but of an anorexic body producing its opposite, a textual shape which is generous, plural and well-rounded.

Further, the body which thus produces its opposite is a female one, another issue briefly raised by Anderson, who notes that all his examples (apart from a passing mention of Marguerite Duras) are of male writers and male bodies, while at least 80 per cent of those actually afflicted with the disorder are female. He says that this 'question of gender' is resolvable because both modernism and anorexia 'involve a crisis of gender that calls into question the very categories of male and female on which such traditional roles are based'.[12] However, concentrating on wasted male bodies in wasted texts is quite a different enterprise from considering the wasted female body in an expansive text. For one thing, the features of the minimalist modernist body mentioned by Anderson—its distance from historical and geographical specificity; its loss of artistic identity—are a special case for men, but more nearly the norm for women. This is the force of anorexia among women, that it merely accentuates what is already the case, as Naomi Wolf puts it in *The Beauty Myth*: anorexia and bulimia 'begin as sane and healthy responses to an insane social reality…The anorexic refuses to let the official cycle master her: by starving, she masters it'.[13] Marilyn Lawrence claims that anorexia is necessarily parodic, as it 'at once exemplifies the feminine stereotype of perfect slimness and repudiates it by making a mockery of it'.[10] Anderson's male examples are limited to a particular literary genre.

The feminine anorexic work reproduces in textual form the attempt at signification made by a subject whose access to self-expression in non-bodily terms may be very limited. Therefore if the text figuring anorexia is also about a female anorexic body, the problem noted by Anderson—'whether the term 'anorexic' is being used figuratively or literally to describe the self-consuming process of the modernist writer'—is resolved. It is (usually) the female body which comes to act as a 'text', uttering its meanings in a material way, well known from instances of hysteria, because other channels do not necessarily exist for it. In the case of the female anorexic, the difficulty of distinguishing between figurative and literal is precisely the point, which is why the textual representation of the disorder is a perfect match of form and content.[15]

Anorexia has been described in psychoanalytic terms by writers such as Michèle Montrelay as a substitute for masculine access to castration, offering a way for women to by-pass the problem of lacking the means to represent lack. There is after all a way of making their bodies the site of signification—by reducing them.[16] The text that follows from this represents the very process that makes it possible; that is, the feminine anorexic text is about its own origins in a way that the masculine one does not seem to be. This is the case in Shute's novel *Life-size*: one among the polyphony of voices which assails the first-person narrator Josie, in hospital for anorexia, commands: 'Next, draw an image of your own body (life-size) on the blank paper provided for you. The therapist will then ask a bystander to draw his or her image of you, next to yours. Finally the therapist will stand you against the wall, arms outspread, while he traces your actual outline with a crayon'.[17] This amounts to a metafictional conceit, but one which is intimately related to the fiction itself: what Josie draws on the blank paper is the text we read, called *Life-size*. She has ironically obeyed the therapeutic instruction, and produced the expected inaccurate outline, inaccurate in being too big and too wordy, just as in the mirror she has seen herself as too big. However, as Mira Dana says, the anorexic mirror-image is perceived correctly, as what it reflects is not the misrecognized, bounded self of the symbolic order, but the anorexic's internal figure.[18] Inaccuracy, indeterminacy, embellishment and self-mythification are all at work in Josie's first-person narrative. They conspire to make it in its fictiveness and multiplicity—incompatible versions of the same event are narrated; hints at cataclysmic occurrences are not clarified—quite different from the minimalist texts discussed by Anderson.

By contrast, Anderson says that in the masculine anorexic text, 'The "fat" of empirical existence is trimmed away to get at the core of an essential writing self'.[19] This is not the case for the feminine anorexic, whose relations to both 'empirical existence' and any 'essential' or 'writing' self are always already put into question. It is as if the writerly male body Anderson discusses moves textually into anorexia; the female one, which already is anorexic, moves out of it by the same means.

In *Life-size*, anorexia becomes the excuse, as it were, or the opportunity, for verbal lavishness and abundance, and indeed for writing at all. This operates on two levels: first, that the novel is an intertextual construction, as the acknowledgements at the back of the book suggest. Shute has drawn together material from works by theorists of eating disorders such as Susie Orbach and Hilde Bruch, and 'genuine' first-person accounts such as Sheila MacLeod's *The Art of Starvation*,[20] as Shute puts it, 'insights from which are woven throughout Josie's story'.[21] The text is rather like Mary Shelley's *Frankenstein*, a fragmentary form containing a fragmentary and monstrous protagonist. Shute's intertextual acknowledgement leads away from the temptation to read autobiographically any first-personal writing by women, particularly a piece of writing like hers which deals with the inner life and the body; in an interview, Shute cited the work's non-autobiographical origins and the fact that precisely because of its particularly confected nature, it appears to be 'authentic': she said, 'I thought the character was so extreme that no one would identify with it, and my sense of humour so perverse that no one would respond.'[22] (The use of pronouns here is revealing.)

The confectedness of *Life-size* also works at a micro-level; it may be about the denial of nourishment, but there is a lively, abundant adjectival presence, fittingly particularly attached to renditions of food or the body. Far from being whittled away in this respect, the text is again expansive. Josie's mother gives her strawberries: 'Stubbornly she passed me the bowl, heaped with fat, dark, and if you looked closely, slightly rotting life-forms: scabrous, papillar.'[23] The description is uncomfortably exact; too accurate, and therefore almost sickening. Later, when Josie is in hospital, an orange slice garnishing a sandwich gets similar treatment: 'This…slice now seems as grotesque, as alien, as a paper parasol in a glass of punch (would you eat that, nurse, gagging on wood pulp, drooling cheap dye?). The more I look at it, with its scaly, reptilian rind and colony of pustular sacs, the more it looks like a section from the dissecting room.'[24] The less there is of Josie's body, the more words there are; and the more cause she has to defamiliarize and describe the medium which assails her, by redescribing her food, again with an excess and not a withdrawal of affect: 'For dinner I eat everything on my plate: corpses, embryos, fluid from mammary glands.'[25]

The effectiveness of the text's verbal vibrancy can be accounted for in terms of abjection, as Julia Kristeva describes it in *Powers of Horror*: 'food loathing is perhaps the most elementary and most archaic form of abjection', Kristeva notes, before describing her own trials with the nauseating skin on hot milk.[26] Abjection is the state the subject is plunged into when the boundaries of its body, clearly established in the symbolic realm at the expense of the pre-œdipal semiotic realm, are threatened by an event such as confrontation with the inedible presented as food. It could be said to operate in Shute's text both formally (for instance in the linking of unexpected nouns and adjectives) and expressively (the food Josie describes is on the brink of turning from an object to a subject, and thereby threatening to send the eating subject into a crisis of abjection). However, the text's adjectival excess is also the exact opposite of the masculzine, minimalist process described by Anderson, whose authors reject 'language as an unclean, tainted food';[27] Josie, on the other hand, rejects the taint of food in order to embrace the burgeoning potential of language. In hospital, the nurse Suzanne offers Josie some toast: 'she holds it out to me, a whole piece, an enormous tilted plate (about 100 calories, counting the—grease; for some reason, even to think the word *butter* seems obscene, lewd and oily on the tongue).'[28] The signifier has become its own signified, in a small instance of what the text as a whole is doing: it is turning the enforced retreat to the body to good advantage, and even turning the retreat *of* that body to advantage.

By contrast, Anderson discusses Hugo von Hofmannstahl's 1904 short story 'Lord Chandos' Letter', in which the protagonist confesses to a sudden inability to speak or write coherently in the following terms: 'abstract words, which the tongue must use in forming a judgment, crumbled in my mouth like mold-encrusted mushrooms'.[29] Clearly, the mushrooms are conjured up by the words, rather than the other way round, as was the case with Josie and the butter.

Like Shute's, the title of Mary Gaitskill's novel *Two Girls, Fat and Thin* is reveal-ing, in its ungainliness, and also in the fact that it is not made clear whether each girl is intermittently fat and then thin, or if it is about two girls, one fat and one thin. In other words, it is unclear if time or space is the novel's dominant mode. In the text, narration alternates between fat, first-personal Dorothy, and thin, third-person-nar-rated Justine, although only Dorothy has a particularly charged relation to food. Her initiation into compulsive eating constitutes the significatory excess of her sections of the novel: 'Summer came and I didn't have to be afraid anymore. I never went out of the house. I stayed down in the basement rec room all day watching *Dialing for Dollars* and eating Sara Lee cheesecake, bags of potato chips, and diet pop. When that was over I'd watch the gladiator movie and then go upstairs to play with my troll dolls or draw pictures of Tarzan and the Lion Queen. Then I'd sit and talk to my mother while she made dinner, and then we'd eat in the anesthetic wind of three fans trained on the table as we watched Walter Cronkite...I gained fifteen pounds that summer'.[30] Unlike the verbal excess associated with Josie in *Life-size*, Dorothy's has a listing, often metonymic quality which reproduces her compulsive eating and her disorderly shape by avoiding any conclusion. Rather like the text itself, both her own narration and her accounts of her eating do not move towards revelation, but simply repetitively defer it: 'In addition [to not brushing my teeth], I began giving in to gross and unhealthy cravings: candy bars, ice cream, cookies, sugar in wet spoonfuls from the bowl, Hershey's syrup drunk in gulps from the can, Reddi Wip shot down my throat, icing in huge fingerfuls from other people's pieces of cake.'[31]

This quality of metonymy and deferral is related to the literary realm from which Dorothy comes, being, as her name suggests, that of the *Wizard of Oz* and fairytale. It collides with Justine's more goal-oriented realm, as her name in turn suggests, that of Sadean pornography, although both genres are transplanted to American suburbia of the 1960s: while Dorothy is sexually abused by her father, Justine abuses other little girls. Justine's distinctive contribution to the text's significatory excess is her perception of other people's bodies, as the rendition of two neighbourhood girls suggests: 'Although their friends described them as "cute", they were not pretty. They were skinny and sharp-boned, with sullen, suspicious eyes, thin, violently teased hair, and faces generic to thousands of suburban little girls. But they were made beautiful by the erotic ferocity that suffused their limbs and eyes and lips.'[32] These descriptions of adolescent female bodies and others, which are old, or male, like Dorothy's lists of food, delay the text's ending, which consists of both women lying on a bed together, their alternating narratives and genres coalesced. This coalescence is rendered by a sudden triangulation of perspective, as Dorothy's genre is described not from within but from the outside, by Justine's: 'for a moment she felt embarrassed to be sitting next to a fat lady wearing hideous chartreuse sweat pants, big red hair and the plastic jewelry of a drag queen with an ironic sense of humor'.[33]

Dorothy and Justine, fairytale and pornography, are narratively brought together by the works of a third possible feminine literary genre, that of pulp fiction, represented in Gaitskill's text by Dorothy's mentor Anna Granite, based on the novelist Ayn Rand. It is almost as if the changing possibilities of writing for women are jokingly likened to female bodily shapes, fairytale voluminous, pornography sharp and slight, as I began by suggesting might be possible. Again, the equation suggested by Anderson only works for masculine disorder; in feminine texts, the body does not figure unease with language, but instead provides the means for circumventing such unease.

Finally, Lucy Ellmann's novel *Sweet Desserts* shares textual and bodily features with both *Life-size* and *Two Girls, Fat and Thin*. Like the latter, it depends on narration shared between two women, using first and third person narration alternately; this time both women are compulsive eaters, and at least one of them is 'pragmatically' bulimic. Like *Life-size*, the body of the text is formed partly out of the disembodied voices of other texts, all of which take a particular rhetorical attitude to the reader; in *Sweet Desserts*, these voices include social security information, recipes, academic articles, letters to the manager of British Telecom, school reports, DIY manuals, phone-in problem programmes, children's diaries. These voices, however, unlike the ones in *Life-size*, are not completely digested or assimilated, and are accounted for within the text itself. It becomes clear that the voices appear at moments of particular pain, so that hearing them becomes a way of avoiding emotion, in this case that of bereavement; after her father's death, Suzy says, 'I knew I was in a bad way when I could no longer read a book…The only things I could now read were personal ads, TV guides, problem pages, recipes, technical handbooks, and junk mail.'[34] In *Life-size*, the act of writing was never accounted for—Josie was clearly not really writing a diary in hospital—but in *Sweet Desserts* both the body of the text and the body of the narrator are formed into their particular shape by the lost paternal body. This is true, again, both formally and expressively.

   In formal terms, the text is an elegy for the father whose death is only narrated
at the end; even on the most pragmatic level, the textual apparatuses draw attention
to the reluctance to end the elegy, or give up the father: the index is a supplementary
narrative in its own right, self-reflexive and quite independent of the narrative it
nominally serves. (In any case, this is a work of fiction—what is an index doing in
it?) In terms of the text's content, the body of the daughter is consistently related to
the father. Suzy states that her fatness is revenge on her art-historian father for his
fascination at his own repugnance at Rubens's women,[35] and when he suggests that
she go on a diet she wants to kill him; when he becomes emaciated through cancer,
Suzy eats even more compulsively, in an attempt to exchange her own sturdy body
for his wasting one. The body of the text acts as a memorial for the body of Suzy's
father, and her own eating habits come to seem like the incorporation and
introjection which characterize mourning and melancholia, according to Freud; the
lost object is encrypted by the mourner when they take it into themselves. It seems
that the story of a male body is told here through and by means of a female one,
which can only tell that story when it is disorderly and too large. It is like an allegory
of the fate of Anderson's article on minimalist anorexia: that tale is best told by a
female voice. Anderson has anorexically limited himself to texts where anorexia
figures diminution and self-cannibalization, whereas, as we see, other kinds of text
can use anorexia and other eating disorders to represent an increased range of
subjects, from pleasure in language to the varied genres of women's writing and
elegiac mourning.

Notes

1.   It is interesting that reading, as well as writing, is also often represented as an
introjective process; Fay Weldon appositely notes, on the cover of the Secker & Warburg
edition of *Life-size*, that she 'devoured it at one sitting', and other readers have spoken of
their 'voracity' (thanks to Chris Walsh for this point; and to Tim Armstrong and Jill LeBihan
for others).
2.   Mark Anderson, 'Anorexia and Modernism, or How I Learned to Diet in All
Directions', *Discourse* 11.1 (Fall-Winter 1988-89); Mary Condé, 'Fat Ladies and Food', in
Beyond the Pleasure Dome: Writing and Addiction from the Romantics (ed. S. Vice *et al.*; Sheffield:
Sheffield Academic Press, 1994); Maud Ellmann, *Hunger Artists* (London: Virago, 1993);
Susie Orbach, *Hunger Strike: The Anorectic's Struggle as a Metaphor for Our Age* (New York:
W.W. Norton 1986); Marilyn Lawrence (ed.), *Fed Up and Hungry: Women, Oppression and
Food* (London: The Women's Press, 1987); Susan Bordo, *Unbearable Weight: Feminism,
Western Culture, and the Body* (Los Angles: California University Press, 1993); Lorraine
Gamman and Merja Makinen, *Female Fetishism: A New Look* (London: Lawrence and
Wishart 1994); Anne Cranny-Francis, *The Body in the Text* (Melbourne: University of
Melbourne Press, 1995); Leslie Haywood, *Dedication to Hunger: The Anorexic Esthetic in
Modern Culture* (Berkeley: University of California Press, 1996).
3.   Susan Bordo, 'Reading the Slender Body', in *Body/Politics: Women and the Discourses
of Science* (ed. Mary Jacobus, *et al.*; London: Routledge, 1989), p. 86 (also reprinted in
Unbearable Weight).

4.   Bordo, 'Reading the Slender Body', pp. 97, 99.

5.   Anderson, 'Anorexia and Modernism', p. 29.

6.   Jean Mitchell, in Lawrence (ed.), *Fed Up and Hungry*.

7.   Jenefer Shute, *Life-size* (London: Secker & Warburg 1991).

8.   Mary Gaitskill, *Two Girls, Fat, and Thin* (New York: Vintage 1991).

9.   Lucy Ellmann, *Sweet Desserts* (Harmondsworth: Penguin 1989).

10.   Anderson, 'Anorexia and Modernism', p. 31.

11.   Wil Pennycook, 'Anorexia and Adolescence', in Lawrence (ed.), *Fed Up and Hungry*, p. 81.

12.   Anderson, 'Anorexia and Modernism', p. 12.

13.   Naomi Wolf, *The Beauty Myth* (London: Chatto & Windus 1991), p. 163.

14.   Lawrence (ed.), *Fed Up and Hungry*, p. 220.

15.   The first, Secker & Warburg, edition of *Life-size* is generously produced, with wide margins and significant spacing between sections. The Mandarin edition, intended for a mass audience, is much smaller, and the textual spaces—arguably as important as the text between the spaces—have been shrunk. In this case the textual body's ability to signify has been literally reduced.

16.   Michèle Montrelay, 'Inquiry into Femininity', *m/f* 1, reprinted in *The Woman in Question* (ed. P. Adams and E. Cowie; Cambridge, MA: MIT–Verso, 1990).

17.   Shute, *Life-size*, p. 218.

18.   Mira Dana, 'Boundaries: One-Way Mirror to the Self', in Lawrence (ed.), *Fed Up and Hungry*, p. 58.

19.   Anderson, 'Anorexia and Modernism', p. 19.

20.   Orbach, *Hunger Strike*; Hilde Bruch, *The Golden Cage: The Enigma of Anorexia Nervosa* (Place: Open Books 1978); Sheila MacLeod, *The Art of Starvation* (London: Virago 1981).

21.   Shute, *Life-size*, p. 232.

22.   Interview in the *Sunday Express*, n.d.

23.   Shute, *Life-size*, p. 105.

24.   Shute, *Life-size*, p. 148.

25.   Shute, *Life-size*, p. 101.

26.   Julia Kristeva, *Powers of Horror* (New York: Columbia University Press 1982), pp. 2-3.

27.   Anderson, 'Anorexia and Modernism', p. 30.

28.   Shute, *Life-size*, p. 82.

29.   Anderson, 'Anorexia and Modernism', p. 30.

30.   Gaitskill, *Two Girls*, p. 86.

31.   Gaitskill, *Two Girls*, p. 58.

32.   Gaitskill, *Two Girls*, p. 88.

33.   Gaitskill, *Two Girls*, p. 274.

34.   Ellmann, *Sweet Desserts*, p. 131.

35.   Ellmann, *Sweet Desserts*, p. 42.

Kasia Boddy

WATCHING THE FIGHT:
WOMEN SPECTATORS IN BOXING FICTION AND FILM

> A boxing match is a story which is constructed before the eyes of the
> spectator; in wrestling, on the contrary, it is each moment that is
> intelligible, not the passage of time.[1]

For Roland Barthes, it is the world of wrestling that represents pure spectacle. In
wrestling there is no logic to the contest, only 'the transient image of certain passions'.
The world of boxing, on the other hand, is concerned with 'the rise and fall of
fortunes', its impetus is distinctly teleological. It is hardly surprising, therefore, that
Barthes, champion of *jouissance* and disparager of naturalism, should prefer wrestling
to boxing. It is not surprising either that the boxing story should constitute an
important subgenre of naturalist fiction.

In his classic exposition of naturalist technique, Zola compared writing a novel
to performing a laboratory experiment; an experiment in which the effects of a
specific heredity and environment on a character or group of characters was to be
observed. One of the most frequently performed naturalist experiments was to test
the thesis that 'living bodies...[can be] brought and reduced to the general mechanism of matter...that man's body is a machine'.[2] For the experiment to be successful,
however, it had to be performed in a carefully controlled environment. The setting
was to be both closely restricted and extreme enough to reveal what were thought
of as the essentials of human nature. Examples of this type of restricted experiment
include 'The Open Boat' (1897) in which Stephen Crane considers the effect of four
shipwrecked men unable to land their boat, and *McTeague* (1899) where Frank Norris
ends his antagonists' struggle for gold in an inescapable Death Valley.

Jack London's experimental settings range from the frozen snows of Alaska to
ships in the violent seas of the Pacific, and to the socially brutal world of the boxing
ring. In such environments, as this fight scene from *Martin Eden* suggests, sophisticated men swiftly revert (or devolve) to what Zola calls 'the animal machine':

> Then they fell upon each other, like young bulls, in all the glory of
> youth, with naked fists, with hatred, with desire to hurt, to maim, to
> destroy. All the painful, thousand years' gains of man in his upward climb
> through creation were lost. Only the electric light remained, a milestone
> on the path of the great human adventure. Martin and Cheese-Face were
> two savages, of the stone age, of the squatting place and the tree refuge.
> They sank lower and lower into the muddy abyss, back to the dregs of

> the raw beginnings of life, striving blindly and chemically, as atoms strive, as the star-dust of the heavens strives, colliding, recoiling and colliding again and eternally again.[3]

In this scene, Barthes's story of the 'rise and fall of fortunes' seems to be straight-forwardly reduced to the colliding of atoms and star-dust, but reading on, the issues are complicated considerably as London introduces Martin's own perspective on the scene. He is described as being 'both onlooker and participant':

> It was to him, with his splendid power of vision, like staring into a kinetoscope…His long months of culture and refinement shuddered at the sight; then the present was blotted out of his consciousness, and the ghosts of the past possessed him…

If the boxing ring is only one of many settings in which the validity of naturalist ideas can be tested and observed, it is the only one in which the act of observation itself is so central.[4] In boxing fiction—where the protagonist performs his rite in front of an audience—there are several levels of spectatorship operating. The fighters survey each other, the crowd watches them, and the writer observes, and interprets, both fighters and crowd. The scientific observation of atoms colliding therefore always exists in tension with the viewing interests—which can be financial, erotic, even æsthetic—of the fictional fighters and spectators. Conflict is not something that is restricted to the activities of the boxers.

Chapter one of Jack London's novella, *The Game* (1905) begins with its protagonists Joe and Genevieve choosing a carpet. They are to be married the next day, but first Joe will fight one last time. Genevieve's response to this is ambiguous. On the one hand, she responds with what London sees as a socially appropriate feminine repulsion. On the other, she reacts in the correct Darwinian manner, 'the masculinity of the fighting male…[making] its inevitable appeal to her, a female, moulded by all heredity to seek out the strong man for mate'.[5] Joe too experiences a conflict of desires:

> He saw only the antagonism between the concrete, flesh-and-blood Genevieve and the great, abstract, living Game. Each resented the other, each claimed him; he was torn with the strife, and yet drifted helpless on the current of their contention.[6]

Before any boxing has taken place then, we see that the central fight of the story is to be between the values of the 'abstract' and 'the concrete'. Contrary to what we might expect, abstraction is allied with 'the Game' while romantic love concerns the physical.

Joe asks Genevieve to watch his last fight—'an' I'll fight as never before with you lookin' at me'.[7] While this might suggest that the fight is to be an initiation test to see if he is ready (man enough) for marriage—an initiation that she must witness—more importantly, as Genevieve notes, it is 'a challenge to the greatness of her love'.[8] The fight is to be a gamble then on several levels. Joe is taking a chance

on his own ability, to prove himself and to win enough money to set up home;
Genevieve is gambling on her ability to win Joe. When she asks why, if he is the
favourite, does anyone bet against him, Joe replies:

> 'That's what makes prize-fighting—difference of opinion,' he laughed.
> 'Besides there's always the chance of a lucky punch, an accident. Lots of
> chance,' he said gravely.[9]

Within the fight then the determinism of animalism is further tested by the operation
of chance, luck and accident. Of course in neither sphere does the individual have
any control.

Chapter two of the novella goes back to consider Joe and Genevieve's courtship,
and to emphasis the importance of what they see of each other in forming their relationship. Genevieve is first described in terms of her 'beauty and aloofness' which has
set her apart from the other neighbourhood girls. The boys are said to watch her in
'a dimly religious way'.[10] When she meets Joe her response is also 'dimly religious':
'whatever it was, he was good to see, and she was irritably aware of a desire to look
at him again and again.' Joe too only knows 'that he wanted to look at her again, to
see her face'.[11] After that their relationship develops to the point where they spend
hours at a time 'merely gazing into each other's eyes'.[12] Described by London as perfect
specimens of masculinity and femininity, as they walk in the park the eyes of passers-
by were 'continually drawn to them', and each observes the glances the other attracts.[13]

The emphasis on seeing and being seen established in this chapter sets the tone
for the fight scene itself. As women are not allowed into the arenas at that time,
Genevieve disguises herself as a boy and watches the fight through a peephole in the
wall. As a boy, indeed wearing Joe's shoes, she is, for the first time in her life, un-
noticed by the men in the hall, 'this haunt of men where women came not'. This,
London suggests, is her first moment of libration from what he calls 'the bounds laid
down by that harshest of tyrants, the Mrs Grundy of the working class'.[14] The next
such moment comes when she sees Joe's 'beautiful nakedness'. She feels guilty 'in
beholding what she knew must be sinful to behold', but, London informs us that,
'the pagan in her, original sin, and all nature urged her on'.[15] The terms in which
Genevieve perceives Joe are, however, far from straightforwardly erotic. Rather her
appreciation curiously shifts between the religious and the æsthetic, and much of it
is feminizing. It is now Joe who is 'godlike', and she feels 'sacrilege' in looking at
him, but his face is also 'like a cameo', a thing of 'Dresden china', and London tells
us that 'her chromo-trained æsthetic sense exceeded its education'.[16] Joe's delicacy,
fragility, smoothness and fairness are also continually emphasized. His opponent, on
the other hand, is the classic 'beast with a streak for a forehead', 'a thing savage,
primordial, ferocious'.[17]

During the central fight scenes, London seems to forget that we are seeing the
fight through Genevieve's perspective, and there are several pages of detailed blow-
by-blow description. Moreover, when Genevieve's perspective does return it seems
confused, as if London was not really sure what do with it. On the one hand, he
describes her attraction to what he calls the pagan values of pain, sex and death: 'She,

too, was out of herself; softness and tenderness had vanished; she exulted in each crushing blow her lover delivered'.[18] Yet, only moments later her responses seem quite distinct from those of the crowd; she feels sick, faint, both 'overwrought with horror at what she had seen and was seeing' and baffled at the whole process[19] As Joe begin to take control of the fight in the ring, the values that Genevieve initially represented—a feminine purity, spirituality—are reasserted.[20] The fight in the ring ends when Joe slips and is caught on the chin with a lucky punch. Chance seems initially to be working for Genevieve, for believing that 'the Game had played him false,' she concludes that 'he was more surely hers'.[21] When she realizes that he is dead, however, it is with the acknowledgment that she had already lost him to 'the awful facts of this Game she did not understand'.[22]

Genevieve's inability to understand the Game is central to the story. Much is made of the lovers' verbal inarticulacy, and their need to communicate with each other through meaningful glances. Men and women look at each other continually, but can they, in naturalistic terms, interpret what they see?

When Genevieve asks Joe what the attraction of the Game is, he first reminds her of its financial rewards (and perhaps we are meant to think of the other connotations of 'the Game'). She expresses dissatisfaction with this answer and he clumsily tries to describe the physical experience. London interprets:

> He lacked speech-expression. He expressed himself with his hands at his work, and with his body and the play of his muscles in the squared ring; but to tell with his own lips the charm of the squared ring was beyond him. Yet he essayed, and haltingly at first, to express what he felt and never analysed when playing the game at the full summit of existence.[23]

Joe conceives boxing as a form of bodily self-expression, and wants her to be present as he expresses himself to her. She responds to the spectacle but not in the way he hoped she would. Her perspective is one of detached æsthetic response. She sees not Joe, but 'the perfection of line and strength and development.'

The Game is finally ambiguous about the status of both the boxer's body (it is a source not simply of violence, but of economic power, and self-expression) and the spectator's interpretation of the body (animalistically, erotically, religiously and æsthetically). It is not only Joe's death that makes the conclusion bleak. He was also gambling on his ability to communicate the meaning of the Game to Genevieve, and that gamble failed as well. The story's conclusion suggests that, had the marriage gone ahead, there would always have been a gulf between the lovers. London's 'finding' then is that women do not understand men, although he of course, understands that female lack of understanding.

The story ends on yet another religious image. Genevieve is reunited by her stepmother, who 'with her fat arms outstretched, ungainly, ludicrous, holy with motherhood', pats her shoulder 'with her ponderous hand'. The mother-daughter relationship is mocking both the male-female relationship and that of the boxers. There is no erotic or æsthetic transcendence possible in such a scene, but it is redemptive.

The Game, along with London's other boxing stories, establishes many of the tropes and themes that subsequent boxing fiction in many cases simply repeats in a more or less sophisticated way.[24] For example, in Leonard Gardner's 1969 novel, *Fat City* (adapted for film by John Houston in 1972) the once successful Tully, now alone in the aptly named Hotel Coma, recalls how he 'had looked to his wife for some indefinable endorsement, some solicitous comprehension of the pain and sacrifice he felt he had endured for her sake, some always withheld recognition of the rites of virility.'[25] Like Paul and Tully, the boxer protagonists of many stories want their 'rites of virility' to be observed by their wives or girlfriends, and the 'female gaze' (sometimes present, sometimes withheld) is a crucial component of the fight itself.

In the 1949 *film noir*, *The Set-Up*, for example, the absence of 'female recognition of the rite of virility' is crucial. Played out in real time, the film presents seventy-two uninterrupted minutes in the life of an aging boxer. Stoker Thompson (played by Robert Ryan) is convinced that if he can win that night's bout he will be back on the road to the top, 'just one punch away' from being able to retire and open a tavern. Meanwhile his seedy manager has accepted $50 from a local hood in return for Stoker throwing the fight. Stoker only learns of the set-up when it is apparent that he is going to win, but rather than taking a fall, he fights on. His integrity, and determination to prove his ability at all costs, leads to a humiliating beating at the hands of the gangsters. The film pays particular attention to the ringside spectators who, like those in *The Game*, are portrayed as an animalistic mass, living vicariously through the boxers. It is notably the women in the crowd who call out most passionately for blood. But they do not represent 'true women', and indeed they are sharply contrasted with Stoker's wife, Julie (played by Audrey Totter). Unable to stop Stoker from fighting she refuses to go and watch him, and her empty seat, in Section C, Row 4, is a constant reminder to him of a world outside the ring.

The film's viewer is thus put into an awkward position. Why, the film seems to ask, are we watching? Are we like the animalistic crowd, baying for blood? And are we not worse than the boxing audience, for they, when the fight is over, simply go home, while we, the viewers, watch as the fight is refought in the streets? Why do we not, like Julie, simply avert our eyes? The moral of the film's ending in which Stoker is forced finally to acknowledge his wife and her values thus seems to be directed as much at the viewer as at Stoker himself.

Such a simple opposition between male and female values is challenged by Joyce Carol Oates in her essay *On Boxing* (1987), and in her two boxing fictions, 'Golden Gloves' (1984) and *You Must Remember This* (1987).[26]

In writing *On Boxing*, Oates is very conscious that she is entering alien territory, and that she must establish her credentials. Her primary strategy is to adopt the impersonal tone of the sweet scientist. Oates distinguishes both male and female perspectives from that of the aficionado. She claims that while women watching a fight identify with the loser, and men with the winner, the true aficionado identifies with the fight itself as 'a Platonic experience abstracted from its particulars'.[27] As an aficionado then, rather than as a woman, she presents herself, and proceeds to dissect the fight game, often pertinently, but often with an unquestioning romanticization of masculinity. The fight becomes 'the body's dialogue with its shadow-self—or Death', 'the very image…of mankind's collective aggression'.[28] She remains loyal to both her natural father, who she evokes throughout the essay, and to literary forefathers such as London in her evocation of boxing as the primary existential experience of masculinity.[29]

The tone of sweet scientist, the coolly observing afficianado, is, however, constantly undercut in the essay by personal confession, and a Genevieve-like attraction or repulsion.

> I feel it as vertigo—breathlessness—a repugnance beyond language: a sheerly physical loathing. That it is also, or even primarily, self-loathing goes without saying.[30]

If self-loathing is what attracts men like Scorcese's version of Jake LaMotta to the ring, it is also (to some extent) what attracts Oates and her characters to boxing. Certainly repulsion is as strong as attraction in bringing together fifteen year old Enid and her half-uncle Felix in *You Must Remember This* (1987).

Uncle Felix is the kind of man familiar from *The Game* or *Raging Bull*, a man whose most intense physical moments have come in the ring rather than in bed. His relationship with Enid is, for the first time, one commensurate with the experience of the ring. This is particularly true after she tries and fails to commit suicide.

> He didn't love her but there was this connection between them now, this bond. A blood bond as if between two men who'd fought each other to a draw. Or say one of them beat the other decisively but the losing fighter fought a courageous fight and pushed himself beyond his limit—the winner was forever in his debt. Yes, she'd had her way.[31]

> a kind of trance was upon them both, a langorous bloodheavy extinction of their minds. She saw he was angry with her, he was sick with desire for her, the rest of the world was distant, obliterated. Enid felt a shuddering sensation of the kind she felt sinking into sleep, into Death.[32]

Oates takes the conventional analogy between sexual conflict and boxing further, however, not only by presenting it from a female point of view, but also by connecting the male experience of boxing (which she takes as representing the essence of masculinity) with what she sees as the essentially female experience of childbirth. In *On Boxing* Oates suggests that:

> Men fighting men to determine worth (i.e. masculinity) excludes women as completely as the female experience of childbirth excludes men.[33]

Although she does not develop this idea further in the essay, both of her fictions which deal with boxing—*You Must Remember This* and 'Golden Gloves'—explore this analogy. The 'blood bond' between Enid and Felix is broken when she forms another 'blood bond' by getting pregnant and then having an abortion. Enid compares the experience to a blow she had not seen coming:

Calmly speculating on the effect an abortion—so extreme a physical trauma, as the medical book said—must have upon the female body with its arsenal of hormones in gear, in dumb preparation for the fetus to grow, to transform itself into an infant, now suddenly the fetus is gone— 'removed'—what does the body think, what does it do...she'd carried Felix's presence with her, he was always with her, inside her, he was her, now she'd be entirely alone, that was the knowledge her body would have to absorb. Jarring, jolting, the head snapped back with the terrible force of the blow. Felix frequently said the dangerous blows were the ones you hadn't seen coming and maybe they hadn't seen this one coming but maybe they had.[34]

Now that Enid has endured a pain and trauma equivalent to that of a boxer she no longer needs to suffer vicariously through Felix. (Previously the only experience she could compare with his was the distinctly unimpressive pain of having her ears pierced.)[35] But there is another dimension to the comparison for Oates not only likens boxing to childbirth, however; she also draws the more familiar analogy with writing. Writers are attracted to boxing, she says, because of 'the sport's cultivation of pain in the interests of a project, a life goal':

> the willed transposing of the sensation we know as pain (physical, psychological, emotional) into its polar opposite...It is an act of consummate self-determination—the constant reestablishment of the parameters of one's being.[36]

Ironically then, Enid's abortion (her equivalent of the unexpected punch) is a form of self-expression for, in Oates's terms, it enables her to reestablish 'the parameters of [her] being'.

In the short story, 'Golden Gloves', Oates explores the analogy between boxing, childbirth and creativity further, and from the boxer's point of view. After an operation to cure his deformed feet, a young boy reinvents himself as a boxer. The story explores the autoeroticism and homoeroticism of the gym as well as providing a potted history of great fights. The boy shows 'promise' but a few weeks before his eighteenth birthday his teeth are broken by a lucky shot from his opponent, and he retires. The story then moves on sixteen years. He is married and his wife, after one miscarriage, is expecting their first child imminently. He identifies his wife's 'rosy bloom' with 'the joy of the body as he had known it long ago', and recognizes the 'plunge into darkness she is to take'. While she sleeps he tells her, 'You'll be going to a place I can't reach'.[37]

Ironically then Oates attempts a male view of pregnancy, as London presents a female perspective on boxing, to demonstrate that men and women are very separate. In London's story, however, this is because (despite gestures towards a female animalism) he finally makes a moral contrast between male and female values. Oates's position is therefore more straightforwardly biological than London's.[38] Men and women are both engaged in 'the Darwinian struggle for existence', yet this fails to provide a connection between them.[39]

Where Oates does depart from London's view of the naturalist boxing story is in her sense of its ending. While in *On Boxing* she argues that the impulse of the fight is tragically teleological, her novel denies this. Although Enid thinks that she and Felix should have had a tragic ending, the novel ends rather anticlimactically (as does *The Set-Up* where Stoker Thompson finally leaves the ring to go and run a pub).[40] Enid leaves to study music and Felix gets married. The naturalist experiment is thus given an alternative outcome; one in which not only the sweet scientist but the protagonists themselves (no mere colliding atoms) can learn something.

Notes

1.   Roland Barthes, 'The World of Wrestling' (1952), in *A Barthes Reader* (ed. Susan Sontag; London: Jonathan Cape, 1982), pp. 18-30; here p.19.
2.   Emile Zola, 'The Experimental Novel', in *Documents of Modern Literary Realism* (ed. and trans. George J. Becker; Princeton: Princeton University Press, 1963), pp. 162-96; here p. 171.
3.   Jack London, *Martin Eden* (1909) (Harmondsworth: Penguin, 1967), p. 118.
4.   Zola distinguishes the simple observational method of realism from naturalism's interpretation of observation. 'The Experimental Novel', pp. 164-65.
5.   Jack London, *The Call of the Wild and The Game* (London: New English Library, 1972), pp. 99-143 (p. 101).
6.   *The Game*, p. 102.
7.   *The Game*, p. 119.
8.   *The Game*, p. 105.
9.   *The Game*, p. 118.
10.   *The Game*, p. 107.
11.   *The Game*, p. 109.
12.   *The Game*, p. 111.
13.   *The Game*, p. 116.
14.   *The Game*, p. 120.
15.   *The Game*, p. 123.
16.   *The Game*, pp. 123-24.
17.   *The Game*, p. 125.
18.   *The Game*, p. 131.
19.   *The Game*, p. 133.
20.   This confusion as to the position of women in relation to the values of physical culture is also apparent in *A Daughter of the Snows* (New York: Grosset & Dunlap, 1902) where in the first chapter, the heroine, Frona Welse boasts of her athletic pursuits—she even boxes herself. As the novel goes on, however, she becomes less interested in her own physical activities and come to represent an alternative moral position. See Clarice Stasz, 'Androgyny in the Novels of Jack London', in *Jack London: Essays in Criticism* (ed. Ray Wilson Ownbey; Santa Barbara: Peregrine Smith, 1978), pp. 54-65.
21.   *The Game*, p. 140.
22.   *The Game*, p. 142.
23.   *The Game*, p. 100.
24.   London's other boxing stories are 'A Piece of Steak' (1909); 'The Mexican' (1910) and *The Abysmal Brute* (1913).

25.   Leonard Gardner, *Fat City* (London: Sphere, 1991 [1969]), pp. 10-11.

26.   Joyce Carol Oates, 'Golden Gloves', in *Raven's Wing* (London: Jonathan Cape, 1987); *You Must Remember This* (New York: Harper & Row, 1987).

27.   Joyce Carol Oates, *On Boxing* (London: Pan Books, 1988 [1987]), p. 73.

28.   Oates, *On Boxing*, pp. 18, 21.

29.   Harry Crews's *The Knockout Artist* (New York: Harper & Row, 1988) reads in places almost like a parody of Oates's essay. It tells the story of a young hopeful who discovers not only that he can be knocked out easily but that he can knock himself out. Eugene (aka K.O.) lives with Charity, whose PhD research he gradually discovers is based on him. 'I'm a scientist,' she tells him, 'I don't invent the world, I only try to discover and describe it' (p. 78). But reading her notes on the metaphysical and religious symbolism of boxing, Eugene discovers that he doesn't really want to be understood.

30.   Oates, 'Golden Gloves', p. 102.

31.   Oates, *You Must Remember This*, p. 168.

32.   Oates, *You Must Remember This*, p. 181.

33.   Oates, *You Must Remember This*, pp. 72-73.

34.   Oates, *You Must Remember This*, p. 386.

35.   Oates, *You Must Remember This*, pp. 43-45.

36.   Oates, *On Boxing*, p. 26.

37.   Oates, 'Golden Gloves', pp. 50-69.

38.   For discussions of Oates in relation to a naturalist tradition, see Steven Bazra, 'Joyce Carol Oates: Naturalism and the Aberrant Response', *Studies in American Fiction* 7 (1979), pp. 141-51 and Sanford Pinsker, 'Joyce Carol Oates and the New Naturalism', *Southern Review* 15.1 (Winter 1979), pp. 52-63.

39.   Oates, *On Boxing*, p. 109.

40.   When MGM initially tried King Vidor's *The Champ* (1931) on audiences, they objected both to an ending in which the protagonist won, and to won in which he lost. The only ending that satisfied them was one in which the Champ (played by Wallace Beery) died.